THE CREATIVE ICE AGE BRAIN

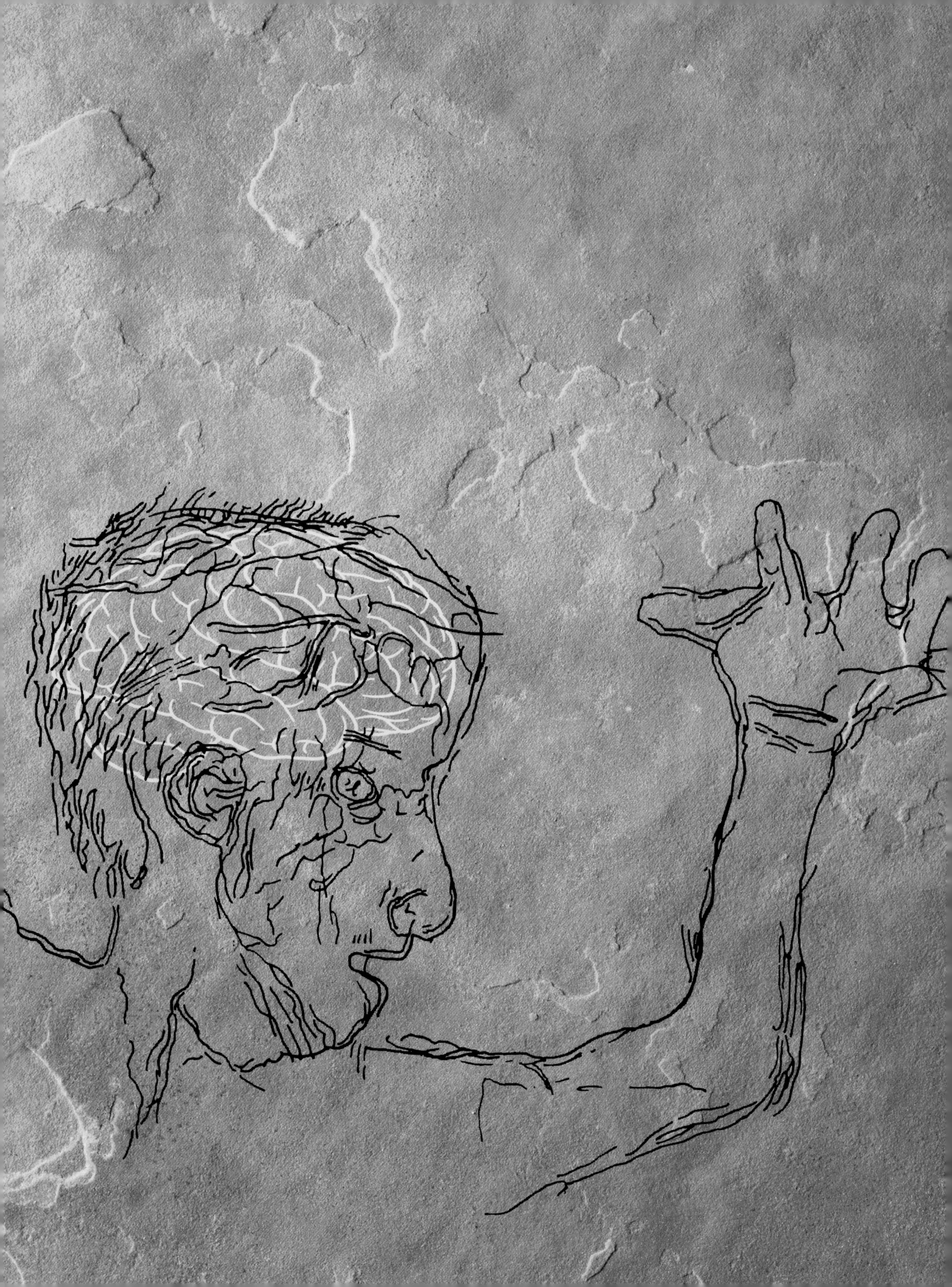

THE CREATIVE ICE AGE BRAIN

Cave Art in the Light of Neuroscience

BARBARA OLINS ALPERT

FOUNDATION 20 21

ISBN: 978-1-934171-10-3

Publisher: Foundation 20 21
Editor: Jane Kepp
Production Direction and Design: Skolkin + Chickey, Santa Fe, NM
Printing: C & C Offset Printing Co., Ltd.
Set in Sabon and Helvetica Neue

FOUNDATION 20 21

www.2021.org

Frontis and page 248. Part of drawing on a stone plaquette from La Marche, discovered by H. Breuil. (After L. Pales)

CONTENTS

FOREWORD

As I read, and reread, Barbara Alpert's wonderful book I came, with growing fascination, to appreciate the ideas that link her world of work with mine. Two guiding themes throw a bridge between Barbara's vividly illustrated account of Ice Age art and the study of the structure and functioning of our brains: first, the thought that these very earliest surviving products of Homo sapiens tell us something profound about our human nature; second, the idea that through their work the earliest artists were, in a sense, beginning to explore and analyse the workings of vision itself.

What makes us human? At the level of biological mechanism the answer must clearly include the brain. We humans lie at the tip of a twig of mammalian evolution notable for its ever-increasing degree of 'encephalisation', the growth of the brain in relation to body size. The brains that result, containing perhaps one hundred thousand million nerve cells or neurons, and around 1000 times as many interconnections, have a reasonable claim to be the most intricately organised systems that we know of in the universe. These extraordinarily powerful organs evolved in tandem with emerging human culture: the use of increasingly sophisticated tools, the division of labour in ever more complex social groups and the beginnings of language were at once the results and the drivers of the brain's increasing size. Our very biology is therefore intrinsically social and cultural.

These developments gradually shaped and transformed the individual human mind. There are several— closely interrelated—candidates for the critical feature that distinguishes our minds from those of our primate cousins: the capacity for language, or for symbol use more generally; the consciousness of self and other, including the awareness of our own and others' minds; going hand in hand with these, the poignant knowledge of our own fragility and transience; the capacity to engage in 'mental time travel', comprising the abilities to recollect the past and envisage possible futures; our propensity, sometimes a blessing and sometimes a curse, to detach ourselves from the here and now, and to imagine things otherwise than they are; our tendency to step back from our immediate needs and actions to contemplate, investigate and document our world, adopting what could be called an 'aesthetic' — or just as well a 'scientific' — attitude.

Barbara Alpert's first guiding theme is that in Ice Age art we see precisely these unique capacities at work, for the first time, in a vivid display of human consciousness. These artists were manifestly symbol-users; their awareness of self and other, and of the finitude of living things, is unmistakable in their depiction of human and animal forms and fates. Working in cramped conditions, in the most dimly-lit of natural studios, the Ice Age artists used visual memory and imagination to summon up the images they captured on the rock. They felt the need that many of us feel today, as we take a photo, make a sketch, jot down some lines of poetry or scribble in our diaries, to rescue memorable moments from the flux of their experience—to capture them, to contemplate and share them. These artists, working as long as 30,000 years ago were, well—uncannily like you and me.

We will never know the finer details of the social context in which these caves were filled with paintings. Barbara's second guiding theme is that whatever ritual and religious purposes the work of the ice age artists may have served, it shares a great many aesthetic qualities with the artworks that we create and appreciate today. Her argument to this effect is in the tradition of the great art historian Ernst Gombrich. His *Art and Illusion* proposed that artists discover and work with keys that turn the locks of perception, exploiting, for example, the power of a few carefully chosen lines to capture character and expression in cartoons (Figure 4.24 depicts a series of astonishing Ice Age caricatures, which could come straight from the studio of Walt Disney). As they hunt for these keys, artists explore the process of vision itself as well as the properties of the visual world. Their exploration is, it is true, in the service of evocation rather than science—but nevertheless, as neurobiologists led by Semir Zeki have pointed out, artists are seasoned experts on sight, and their work has much to teach us about the workings of vision and the visual brain. Barbara's illustrations reveal how successful the Ice Age artists were, in their exploration both of vision and of visual experience. They anticipated their descendants in the classical world, the Renaissance and the 20th century with works that embrace forms of realism, surrealism, cubism. The noble 'horse at Commarque', Figure 3.3, breathes on the wall that reveals him; the 'bird-headed men' of Figures 6.2–6.4 are echoed in contemporary works like those of the colourful Scots painter John Bellany; Picasso's cubist portraits continue the prehistoric experiments with perspective Barbara describes in Chapter 6.

Barbara develops these grand themes with the help of numerous examples, many of them illustrated in these pages. But the book is such a pleasure partly because her range extends beyond her immediate topic, the Ice Age artefacts. She is sensitive to all the arts, and her close attention to the visual qualities of the cave paintings is complemented by analogies with musical form, and seasoned with enjoyable bon mots from artists, critics, writers and scientists. This is a passionate book, suffused by sympathy for its subject, and by a sense of common feeling with our nameless ancestors whose eyes and brains shared so much of what matters with ours.

DR. ADAM ZEMAN,
Cognitive and Behavioural Neurology Research Group,
Peninsula Medical School, Devon, England

PREFACE

When the cave at Lascaux was discovered in the somber, drama filled autumn of 1940, the pictures discovered there filled the imagination with their beauty. Suddenly, it was as if time did not exist and the atrocities of the present were eclipsed by a collective memory of art—inaugurated with Lascaux and kept alive by artists over the ages. Lascaux, product of the Magdalenian period, was not then known to be 17,000 years old, a date later established by carbon 14 dating.

Barbara Alpert, a superb artist, is fascinated by art, by its birth, its fabrication and its diffusion and is in her element in the caves and shelters decorated by the artist hunters of paleolithic Western Europe. An intimacy animates her encounter with the prehistoric artists that she introduces to us with elegance as she gives an expert analysis of their work. She knows the art directly since she has experienced it by visiting those sites still accessible to the public and she has been granted permission to visit sites in France and Spain that are open only to specialists. She has enriched her knowledge of the art by research in preparation for lectures and for articles in archeological publications with the result that her contributions to the material is eminently trustworthy and up-to-date. To her competence, her own work as an artist and her artistic judgement we must add a remarkable knowledge of prehistory as well as of the general history of art, a rare and unusual combination of disciplines which imparts a penetrating originality and genuine critical edge in her approach to the creativity of the Ice Age.

Other cave art, dating from late prehistoric periods to recent historical times, has given Alpert invaluable models for comparison especially when it entails an appreciation of the continuity of structures and the means of elaboration. She finds a universality underlying the radical diversity of iconography seen in art that is spread over the five continents. One of her preferred sources of inspiration is the rock art of the Southwest of the United States. It has ties to an indigenous still living culture linked to historic times so that this rock art is accessible by means of language and can be explained through existing stories and myths. Thus, these images are not mute like those of prehistory but rather reveal their connection to the societies from which they sprang and which they still reflect

Comparisons with contemporary art or classical art, especially that of Europe and America, embellish Alpert's text in a fascinating way. With these artists she is able to engage in an empathic sense of participation and to attain an understanding free of preconceived ideology. She connects these later artists with those of prehistory believing that they shared the same aesthetic impulses. Reading her work, how can one fail to be thrilled by the parallels she makes, for example, between the dot-making found so often on the walls of prehistoric caves and the Pointillism of George Seurat. She is very convincing when she unites, within the phenomenon of 'found art' the prehistoric figures made with formations of rock or bone with the 'ready mades' of Marcel Duchamp.

In the decorated Ice Age caves some animals so naturalistically represented by prehistoric artists (the imitation of nature advocated by Aristotle) may also be depicted in unrealistic positions, for example "inverted", in the section the author calls "paradox". Alpert points out examples of graphic double meaning in the iconographies of other prehistoric people, as well as in modern works of art.

Hominids, marked by bipedalism, evolved during almost 3 million years . The subsequent evolution of the genus *Homo* was marked by encephalisation. In brief, it is possible to say that the principal anatomical difference between early man and anatomically modern man or *sapiens*, is the skull. As accepted by anthropologists, the line of *Homo sapiens* began to emerge in Africa and Eurasia 250,000 to 200,000 years ago. *Sapiens* is characterized by a verticalization of the facial features. The cranial cavity is sharply higher in the frontal section of the head. Evolution in the structure of the skull involved the brain and the development of the frontal lobe. This opened up new cerebral abilities (or amplified in a special way those already acquired in the course of evolution). The cultural evolution of sapiens derives a new complexity in technical achievements, for example in social and economic activities evidenced by new practices in the acquisition of goods and the use of new primary materials.

The socio-cultural innovations of sapiens were clearly more pronounced in the second period of their evolution, revealed in the symbolic behavior first seen in burials The dead were interred with funerary rites a little more than 90,000 years ago in the Middle Eastern shelters of Mt. Carmel. Symbolic practices were later sublimated into art beginning 40,000 to 30,000 years ago. This art belongs to the paleolithic ensemble of the European Ice Age, the great worldwide extension of images, painted or engraved, on rocky walls that occurred over tens of thousands of years. The universality of prehistoric art, expressed with thematic diversity, depending on the region and period, reveals the complete homogeneity of its maker, *sapiens*, the sole master of the globe (now as then).

Art is assuredly born with the evolution of the brain. This is in our mind when we look at the subtitle of Barbara Alpert's book: "Cave art in the light of neuroscience" and the objective which she set for herself. "My concern in this book is the process of art making in all the contexts in which Ice Age art has been found". The expression of the various types of representation which are translated into visual forms would have been impossible except for the brain of Homo sapiens, a brain anatomically like our own. A specific innovation of the brain of sapiens was that it was capable of making representations. As is the case with language art is made and is changed when communicated in a dynamic relationship essential to any society.

The approach to prehistoric art presented by Barbara Alpert is continually enriched and given direction by reflection and analysis that she derives, with knowledge and subtlety, from a study of the cognitive sciences and and from her own practice as an art-maker. With the aid of her artist's eye one sees and actually experiences how a specific form is constructed and how it continues to evolve into the unfathomable creative diversity which artists have been able to generate in an unbroken chain from prehistory to our own day. What a compelling invitation Barbara Alpert offers so superbly to her readers—an invitation, at once delightful and profound -to voyage into both the immensity of prehistoric art and into our own minds.

Professeur Denis Vialou, *l'Institut de Paléontologie Humaine, Muséum National d'Histoire Naturelle, Paris*

For Burt Alpert, my companion in all the adventures that led up to this book, without whose help and encouragement it would never have been completed.

ACKNOWLEDGMENTS

FROM THE FIRST LONG, helpful letter from François Bordes thirty years ago to the present I have had many mentors. Numerous people have given generously of their time and knowledge. I am grateful to them all. This list is far from complete but I want especially to thank the following: Jacques Marsal, Robert Comte de Bégouën, Dr. Jean Gausson, Denis Vialou, Jean Lautier, John Pfeiffer, Campbell Grant, Comte Hubert de Commarque, Alexander Marshack, Kalyan K. Chakravarty, Shankar Tirawi, Edmund Carpenter, Emmanuel Anati, Garcia Guinea, Randall White, Ellen Dissanayake, John Clegg, Kate Sullivan, Lesley Maynard, Neil Lee, Anne Solomon, Gerhard Milstreu, Felipe Puente, José Maria Ceballos, Jesus Altuna, Aurelio Capin, Maria Luisa Quesada Soto, Angel Armendariz, André Alterac, Bernard Gely, Alain Gautier, Brad Draper, Dennis Slifer, Katherine Wells, Polly Schaafsma, Jerry Grimsley, Ekkehart Malotki, Salvatore Mancini, Laurie Whitehill Chong, Robert Patrick and Adam Zeman. Thanks are due as well to the Rhode Island School of Design for a faculty grant to encourage me in the realization of this book. A special acknowledgment goes to Jed Alpert.

THE CREATIVE ICE AGE BRAIN

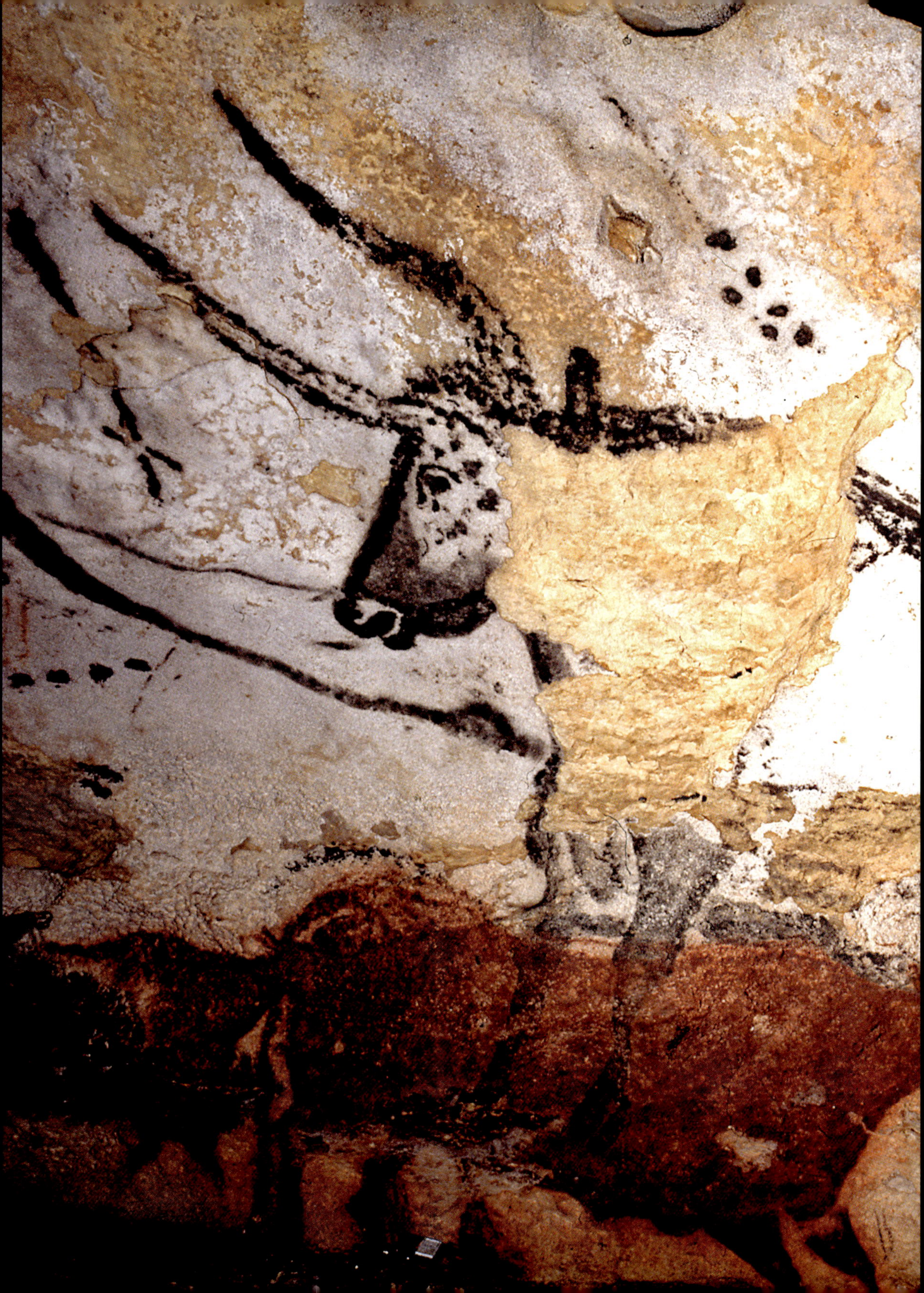

INTRODUCTION

In 1950 the Dutch artist Maurits Escher was in Les Eyzies, in the department of Dordogne in southwestern France, where he spent a two-week holiday visiting prehistoric caves. He wrote to a friend about the painting in the chamber known as the Rotunda at Lascaux (see opposite page):

> It is an image . . . that speaks to us immediately, as if it had been painted yesterday. It touches you deeply. . . . it is a strange phenomenon, that human spirit, that unextinguished spark, that seed that remained alive, the thread we hold in our hands that connects us, across the soundless and pitch-black night, with this member of our species there in the cave of Lascaux, dimly illuminated by a small wick dipped in animal grease and set in a hollow stone.[1]

Twenty-five years later I saw for myself these images of huge animals that seem to emerge suddenly from the dark. For a fleeting moment their overwhelming presence caused me to believe that if I turned I might see the artist standing behind me.

It is difficult to imagine what it feels like to enter the pitch black of an unknown underground space, pass a light over a wall, and see extraordinary images from a distant past. It adds immeasurably to the effect to know that some of the images at Lascaux may have been made as much as 17,000 years ago. Recently, cave explorers in France have found masterful images deep within the cave of Chauvet in the department of Ardèche. If the earliest date for these images of more than 30,000 years ago is correct, then this art is so

Opposite: Head of giant aurochs from the Rotunda at Lascaux. Escher said of this image: "Look! The head of a bull appears on the rock wall, an image so alive that it looks as if it moves. It looks as if the damp nostrils tremble." The entire animal is 5.5 m long. c.15,000 B.P. Photo by J. Vertut. © CNP-MCC

much older than the art of Lascaux that Chauvet is nearly as distant from Lascaux as Lascaux is from us. We know that the people who made the images were, as we are, *Homo sapiens sapiens* and that they possessed brains anatomically like our own. Yet even knowing this, when we step into a cave like Lascaux and stand before the drawings and paintings, we are awestruck.

About 350 European Ice Age cave art sites are known. Important new ones have been discovered in recent years. The art of these caves consists of drawings, engravings, paintings, and occasional bas reliefs and sculptures. Images were sometimes placed on cave floors or on freestanding formations, but because they are primarily on the walls they are called *parietal* art. The relatively few images that can be dated range from roughly 30,000 years ago to 9,000 years ago, which puts them at the end of the last major glaciation. Decorated caves from this period have been discovered in other parts of the world but the greatest number have been found in Europe—from England and Portugal in the west to Sicily in the south and the Czech Republic and Russia in the east. Nowhere is the concentration greater than in France and northern Spain and nowhere has there been as much archeological research.

Another type of Ice Age art, known as portable art, may be found in caves or at sites unrelated to caves. Portable art was made on stone slabs or chunks of minerals, on bone and antler, and even on animal teeth. There are many thousands of examples of portable art, with more coming to light every year.

Other art forms almost surely existed. Animal bones fashioned into flutes, rasps, and percussion instruments indicate that these people made music.[2] Human skulls show that the larynx was by now in a position to allow for speech and song.[3] Solidified footprints in unusual positions suggest dance. But all these remains can only hint at forms of expression that are irretrievably lost, and they can only suggest similarities that might link us to these ancient people.

Despite all that researchers have discovered about Ice Age people, it is only by means of their art that we could ever suspect that humans from such a distant past might have thought and felt as we do. The vast span of time that separates us from the artists and the suggestive silence that surrounds their art pose tantalizing questions. My concern in this book is with the process of art making in all the contexts in which Ice Age art has been found—in the large caves, to be sure, but also in tiny, tunnel-like caves, in cave entrances, on cliff walls, and on portable objects such as pebbles and pieces of stone, bone, horn, and antler. Only by means of the graphic and sculptured artifacts may we hope to understand the sense of kinship we feel with these artists. Researchers have speculated on what the images might have meant. Abbé Henri Breuil (1877–1961), the patient and intrepid recorder of cave art by means of tracing, drawing, and watercolor, was viewed for a long time as having the final word in the interpretation of Ice Age art. The abstract markings were studied and categorized most notably by the archaeologists André Leroi-Gourhan and Annette Laming-Emperaire.[4] Nevertheless, the marks or signs remain enigmatic and will probably continue to puzzle us unless a Rosetta stone is found. The focus of this book is on the figurative art of the Ice Age, because that is the primary thread that connects us to these ancient artists.[5] Figurative art is a remarkable achievement. It is a true leap from the abstract markings that preceded and also accompanied it. One can find antecedents for many of the elements of art making in the behavior of earlier forms of the genus *Homo,* even occasionally of primates, and sometimes of animals even farther from our lineage. But figurative art appears to be something entirely new with *Homo sapiens sapiens.*

The art of *Homo sapiens sapiens* was a result of new possibilities provided by the evolution of the human brain. Scientific techniques now used by neuroscientists and psychologists have resulted in an expanding body of cognitive findings and a whole new field of inquiry called *neuroaesthetics.*[6] Many scientists believe that art making may be the most elusive and fascinating function of the brain. "What is perhaps most extraordinary about conscious human beings," wrote the Nobel-prizewinning biologist Gerald Edelman, "is their art—their ability to convey feelings and emotions symbolically and formally in external objects such as poems, paintings or symphonies."[7]

Examining art making through the lens of cognition is not new.[8] In general, writers who have applied neuroscience to art have done so by examining the best-known examples of the Western canon in the historic period. As an art historian with a special interest in Paleolithic and prehistoric art, I have applied new discoveries in brain function to a different body of work—work that exists outside of history and comes with no written explanations by the artists or their contemporaries. In addition, I am a practicing art maker with experience in a variety of media. This dual viewpoint explains my approach. By applying cognitive findings to Ice Age art, even retroactively, I have gained insights into the intent of Ice Age artists.

Seeing the original of any art is important, but it is especially so with rock art, which is, to use a contemporary term, highly "site specific." The physical context of the art reveals information about the thought processes behind it. In addition, for a full aesthetic experience, the awesome beauty of some of the sites must be taken into account, as the artists themselves undoubtedly did. I have studied at first hand most of the Ice Age art in France, Spain, and Italy that is referred to in this book. The same is true of the Native American, Australian, South African, and Indian rock art that is used as examples.

I have been fortunate to have visited several important caves with their discoverers: Lascaux with Jacques Marsal and Le Gabillou, also in the Dordogne, with Jean Gausson. I was shown the Chumash art of California by Campbell Grant, the "white shaman" panel on the lower Pecos River in Texas by Jim Zintgraff, and the S-Belt of the Betwa source region in India—possibly the longest continuous hill chain of painted rock in the world—by the geologist who discovered it, Shankar Tirawi. In Queensland, Australia, I was taken to the rock art at Laura by one of the sons of Percy Tresize, the first Anglo explorer to find these Aboriginal sites, and I had the opportunity to spend time with Percy Tresize himself. Often the stewardship of prehistoric art remains in a single family. I was shown Trois Frères and Tuc d'Audoubert (Ariège) by the archaeologist le Comte Robert Bégouën, son and nephew of two of the brothers who discovered those caves. Edouard Lepeyre, whose grandfather found La Mouthe (Dordogne), showed me that French cave, and I was taken to immense Niaux (Ariège), in the French Pyrénées, by Dominique Clastres, an archaeologist whose father discovered some of its chambers. I walked the hills of Ardèche with Jean Chauvet and Eliette Brunel, who, along with Christian Hillaire, discovered the cave of Chauvet.

In archeology context is vital. All art is rooted in a specific culture. But art is at the same time an individual expression. The artist and archaeologist Michel Lorblanchet confirms this. Lorblanchet has studied Ice Age art as closely as anyone, devising tools and techniques to reproduce its markings as exactly as possible. He writes: "In the earliest known art in European caves some of the artists appear to have been able to individualize their marks so as to leave a personal stamp on their creations even while adhering to the overall stylistic conventions of their time."[9]

The anthropologist Franz Boas believed that artistic virtuosity resulted from the interplay of tradition and individual creativity.[10] Bill Holm, a Native

American artist and teacher, is the leading authority on the art and customs of Northwest Coast Indians, who work within a very rigid art style. Nevertheless, he recognized the importance of the individual within a style when he wrote that "each object represents the creative activity of a specific human personality who lived and worked at a particular time and place and whose work influenced and was influenced by the work of other artists."[11] Whenever possible, I quote individual art makers from historic periods in their own words to reveal their thoughts as they worked with the same graphic elements and visual perplexities that the Ice Age artists first dealt with. I believe that in order to search for the wellspring of art, it is necessary to view Ice Age art as the creation of individuals who worked within an overarching stylistic tradition and its regional variations. The cultural tradition to which these artists belonged was a remarkably stable and consistent one, lasting for about 20,000 years and extending over a vast territory from the Atlantic to Siberia. It is possible to distinguish different styles from different periods: the Aurignacian from the Magdalenian, for example, and to distinguish art from different geographic areas. It is also possible to distinguish marks of individual artists within specific caves and even on a single panel of images. Although imbedded in a social context, art is made by individuals working alone or in a group. As the art historian E.H. Gombrich wrote, "There is really no such thing as Art. There are only artists."[12]

I believe we will never be able to fully understand the art-making process, neither in the ancient world or in our own time. As with much scientific discovery, the search is analogous to mountain climbing. One peak is successfully scaled only to reveal a whole new range of peaks even higher up. The more we discover, the more tantalizingly mysterious art making appears. By examining it in terms of new knowledge about the brain, my hope is to enlarge our sense of wonder at what humans have achieved. We will follow a trajectory backward from the marks made by the hands to the initiation of the motor response, to the conceptions formulated in the mind, and to the visual or cognitive perception that began the process. In so doing I hope to open the door that permits us to find our way back into the minds of the Ice Age artists. We may gain access to the imagination of humankind at the moment of the creation of the first known art, and we may, as a corollary, be brought closer to understanding the source of the creative spark that is a singularity of our species.

Part One

UNIVERSALS OF ART MAKING

In particular we can ask whether there are such things as artistic universals. . . . The advantage that scientists have today is that unlike philosophers we can now test our conjectures by directly studying the brain empirically.

—V. S. Ramachandran, *A Brief Tour of Human Consciousness*

The neuroscientist V. S. Ramachandran concluded that artistic universals exist and even proposed a list of them. It is encouraging to find that a scientist who studies the brain through research on brain-damaged patients has come to the same conclusions I have reached in my study of the first manifestations of art making in the Ice Age. Coming from entirely different directions and using very different methods, we have reached similar and in some cases almost identical conclusions. The first conclusion is that there are universals in art. Those that I explore in chapter 1 are the graphic elements that first appeared during the Ice Age. Handprints, lines, outlines, dots—sometimes seemingly random, sometimes apparently patterned—are everywhere in Ice Age sites. This art proliferates with marks that humans seem compelled to make. In addition, the earliest known artists organized the marks they made by means of certain basic structures, which I explore in chapter 2.

Artists imposed an order on the cave walls and the stone and bone with which they worked. Sometimes that order was the result of combining the natural features of the cave into well-understood figurative images. Sometimes this imposed order was augmented by the additional structure of symmetry, and at other times, by repetition combined with variation. To use an analogy, we can think of the art elements as a vocabulary for a graphic language, and the structures as a syntax. The elements and structures employed in Ice Age art are seen in the much later art of other prehistoric cultures, such as that of Australian Aborigines, of the San (Bushmen) of Africa, and of American Indians. These elements and structures can be traced all over the world, throughout human history. The recognition and understanding of the language of art provides a link between us and the earliest known artists as they painted, engraved, modeled, or carved often intractable materials to create works that have survived them by tens of thousands of years.

Although the language of art is now much richer than it was at its beginning, I limit my attention to the images, elements, and structures that first appeared in the Ice Age and then give examples to show how they have reappeared throughout the history of art. My long lists of examples may seem excessive, but only by the incremental accretion of examples can I verify my conclusions. Although I offer many examples and illustrations, I could have chosen many more. I hope the lists have the additional advantage of giving readers, as they did me, a tangible sense of the ubiquity of certain forms and concepts.

All visual art is grounded in visual perception, but the first known artists were especially concerned with conveying the look of the world they saw. By means of their art we learn that they made discoveries about how to depict it as realistically as possible. Replication of vision is not a goal to which most of the world's other artists have aspired. Even when the subject was figurative, artists were generally not committed to imitating visual reality with such exactness. The world that the Ice Age artists portrayed was highly selected, and the images they chose were probably meant to carry symbolic meaning. To achieve this meaning they attempted to mimic appearance. Ice Age artists devised drawing and painting techniques now familiar to us. They discovered outline, contour line, cross-contour line, parallel hatching, cross hatching, cameo and intaglio marking, modeling, carving in relief and in the round, champlevé carving, smudging, shading, overlapping, stenciling, foreshortening, use of friezes, and use of plane and void perspective. The purpose of these techniques was to enable them to replicate the way the world looked. Each will be described in this book.

The sophisticated devices used by the cave artists were lost at the end of the Ice Age, perhaps because artists of later societies no longer had the same visual goals. The same techniques were reinvented, however, more than a hundred centuries later in Classical Greece, when artists were again interested in portraying what they saw. They were lost again and then once more rediscovered during the Renaissance. In the period between Classical Greece and the Renaissance, individual artists in some societies attempted to solve problems of perspective, but those attempts seem never to have been fully realized until the Renaissance.

Paleolithic portable art was not recognized until the last quarter of the nineteenth century, and not until the beginning of the twentieth century were the paintings on cave walls accepted as authentic. Lascaux was discovered only in 1940, and Chauvet in 1995. Because of the difficulty of reproducing the images painted in them, it was even more recently that good photographs became possible and that pictures of this art could be made generally available. Many of the Ice Age techniques and concepts had been rediscovered over the intervening centuries, so viewers, when they saw the photographed work, felt an immediate kinship with these most ancient artists.

That lost techniques were invented and reinvented at different places and times in history reinforces the belief that they reveal a universal graphic capacity, first seen in the Ice Age. It is further evidence that artistic universals exist, that they derive from our normal cognitive processes, and that they reveal themselves in the elements and structures of a universal language of art. This language of art gives us access to what we are seeking—an understanding of what was in the minds of these earliest artists, who left the caves of Ice Age Europe imprinted with the work of their hands and even, literally, with the marks of their actual hands.

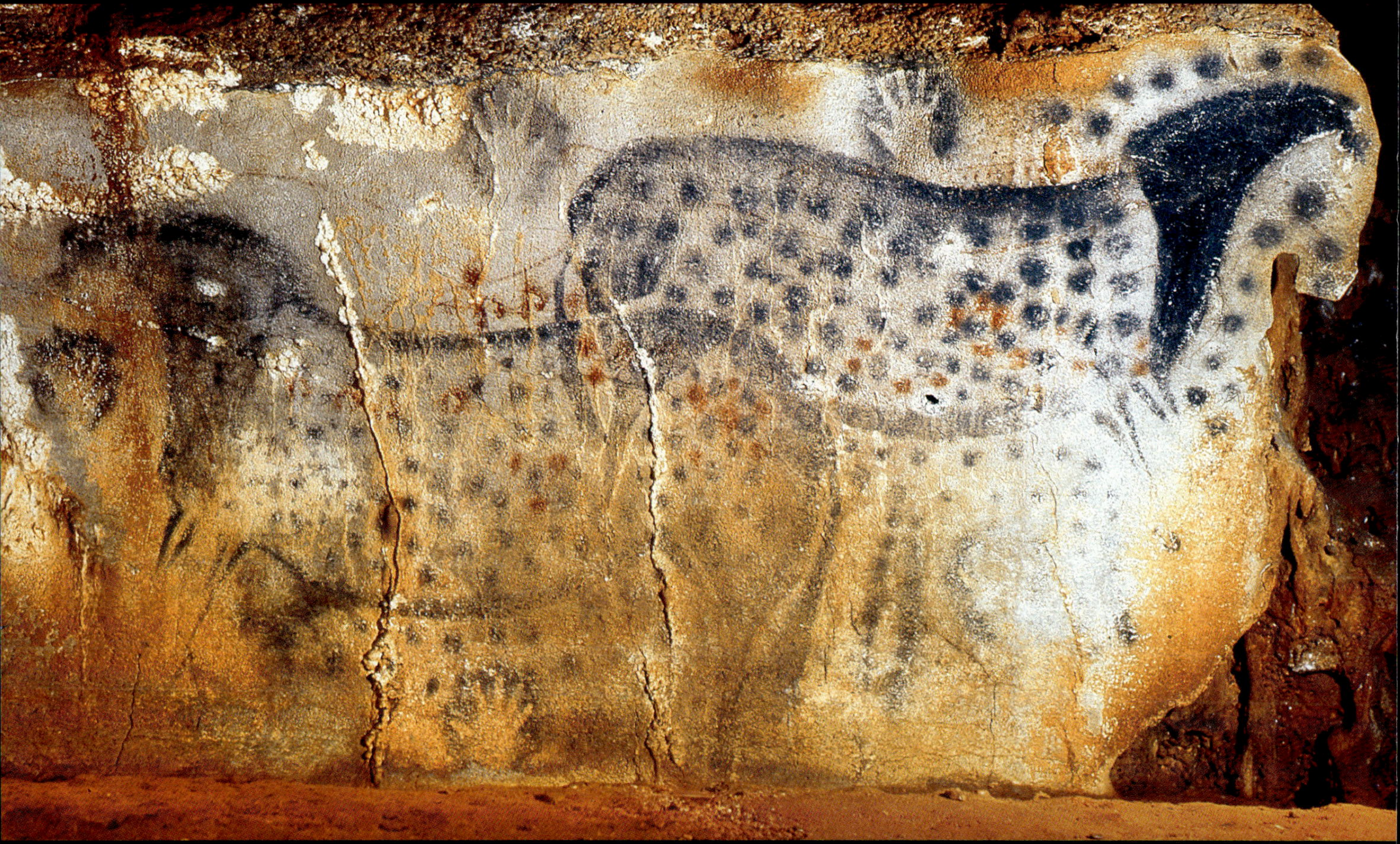

1.

ELEMENTS

The Vocabulary of the Ice Age Artist

The hand is but an extension of sensitivity and intelligence.

—HENRI MATISSE, *Jazz*

IN THE PERPETUALLY DAMP CAVE of Gargas (Hautes Pyrénée), just north of the foothills of the Pyrénées, 150 handprints rise like a procession of suppli- cants on the hardened, clay-coated walls. Gargas is unique among Ice Age caves not only for its enormous number of handprints but also because so many of the prints appear to have missing digits.[1] Handprints, also called dactylograms, are among the earliest images found in caves and are the most ubiquitous of human markings worldwide, found from prehistoric to the present.

In humans the urge to make marks is intense. Perhaps the most primal marks are those made directly by the hand, the hand whose development has played such a large role in making us the creatures we are. Someone drags fingers through the clay coating on a cave wall, creating lines; someone uses a fingertip to daub paint on a stone surface to leave markings of dots. Someone dips a hand in pigment and presses it against a surface, making a print, a duplication of that hand. It is, in a sense, a self-portrait, both figurative and realistic.

POSITIVE AND NEGATIVE HANDPRINTS

Positive handprints are made by imprinting the hand in a soft surface or by dipping the hand in pigment and then pressing it against a surface. At Chauvet, for example, a large panel is composed only of pressed palms. Handprints are seen in many Ice Age caves, as well as in rockshelters and on escarpments representing all periods of human history worldwide. One grouping from American Indian culture in the U.S. Southwest consists of about 50 handprints under a rock overhang. Some of these prints, like those at Gargas, appear to have missing fingers. Also like those at Gargas, they include children's handprints.

Opposite: The right hand "Spotted Horse" in the cave of Pech-Merle (Lot). The panel has handprints, bent finger prints, dots, a circle and a fish in and around the horses. c. 24,500 B.P. Photo by J. Vertut.

Negative prints are made by using the hand as a stencil—pressing it against a wall and blowing a fine mist of paint around it. Negative prints are by far the most common handprints in the Ice Age caves. Australian Aborigines still make handprints this way, taking ocher pigment mixed with water into their mouths and then spraying it out through pursed lips. The prehistorian Michel Lorblanchet demonstrated that it might have been applied in the same manner in Ice Age Europe. He feels that blowing pigment through the mouth is like breathing life onto the cave walls.[2]

Other archaeologists believe the negative prints were made by applying an animal skin impregnated with pigment around and over the hand, again in the manner of a stencil.[3] The Spanish prehistorian Mathilde Múzquiz-Pérez-Seoane found that she obtained results most similiar to prehistoric art by spraying diluted pigment through two reeds bent at right angles.[4] It is also possible that the paint was blown through bent and perforated hollow bone tubes, not unlike the fixative atomizers that artists used before the invention of the spray can. Indeed, bone tubes, often engraved, containing residues of powered pigment have been found in some French caves.

Reggie Miller, an Australian Aborigine who lives at Manyallaluk in the Northern Territories, travels back and forth between his new home and the ancestral part of Arnhem Land, where the majority of his family still lives. He told me that he had made handprints and even footprints at his Arnhem Land home. When asked why, he replied, "To remind. I can go back to our land and I can still see." With this succinct comment he expressed how, for him, a hand sign served as a verification of his earlier presence. Ice Age people who made handprints or who pressed a finger against a surface might have felt, as Miller did, that such marks left a record of their unique presence.

Handprints have signaled human presence in all periods. In 1995 the British artist Marcus Harvey chillingly portrayed the face of a notorious serial child-killer entirely out of children's handprints. In this case the prints indicated not human presence but human absence. Ironically, it has turned out that viewing handprints and fingerprints as surrogates for the person was well understood. Until the advent of DNA analysis they were the best way of identifying specific individuals.

DOTS

Paint-covered fingertips could make points, or dots, another element that may be considered part of a graphic vocabulary. Dots are as ubiquitous as handprints in Ice Age caves. Often the two are associated with each other in the caves, as they are in other parts of the world and at other times. At Lascaux, long lines of dots are ranged along a wall in what is called the Lateral Gallery. Dots are especially prominent at El Castillo (Cantabria), where they are ranged in single or double lines along one wall. In an unusual example at Le Combel (Lot) a ceiling with a natural formation of rounded stalactites was strewn with dots, some made with fingers or pads but others sprayed. The varied application of dots seems to occur worldwide. Sometimes a finger was dipped in paint and pressed on a cave wall. Sometimes it seems that small tampons of fur were dipped in pigment and used as stamps.

Making dots with the fingers (dactylograms) belongs to the same series of physical, creative . . . rhythmic activities as handprinting.

—Mark Verstockt, *The Genesis of Form*

Groups of dots frequently appear next to figures. It is possible that a grouping of six dots may indicate 'the end' in some caves. In the rotunda at Lascaux there is a long frieze of animals. The last and by far the largest animals, an aurochs, has six dots behind its head (see fig. p. xviii). Also at Lascaux, in a pit known as 'the Shaft', six dots punctuate the space behind a retreating rhinoceros.

The celebrated image known as the "Spotted Horses" of Pech-Merle (Lot) includes dots associated with handprints (fig. 1.1). There are at least five nega-

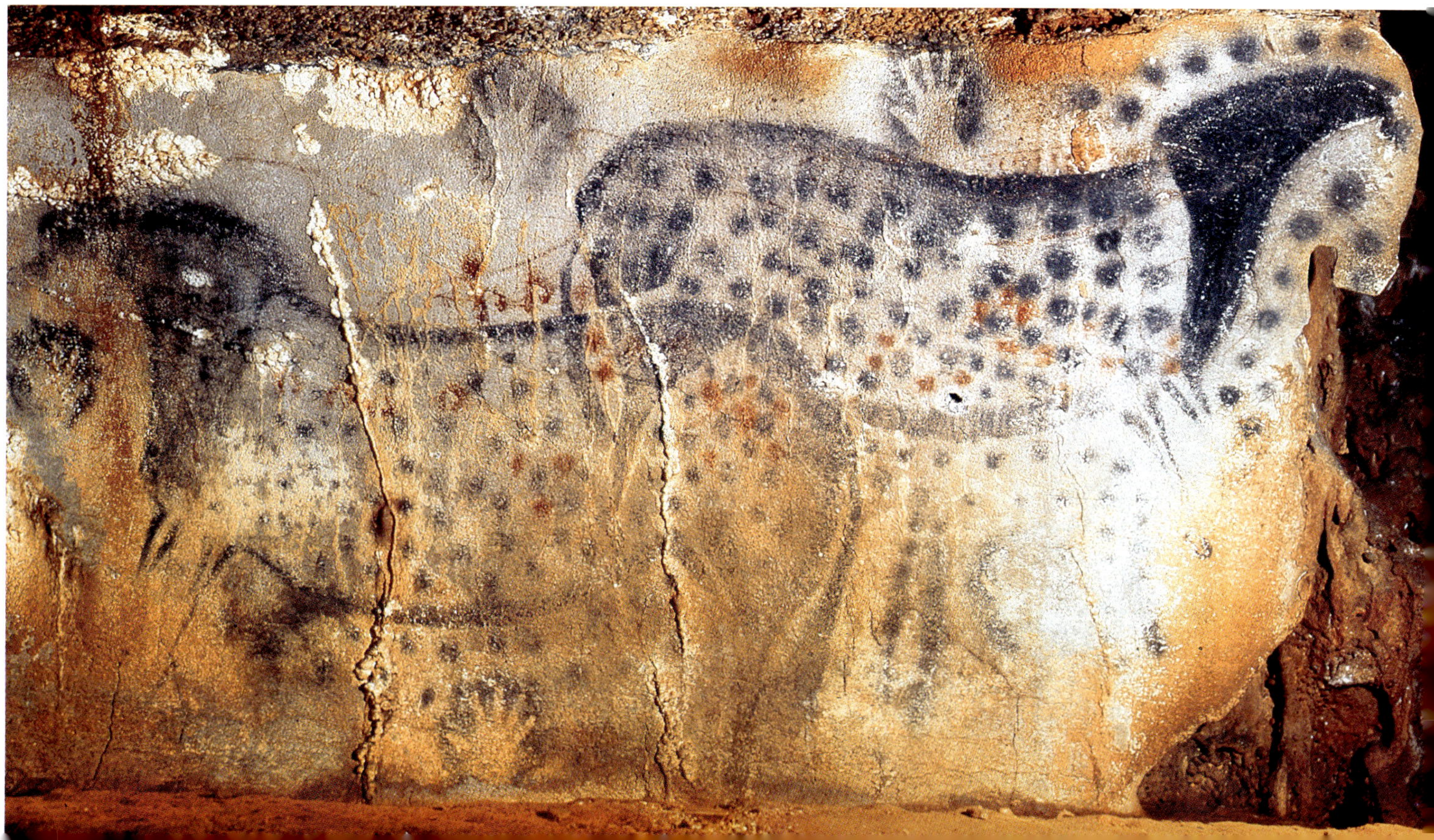

Figure 1.1. The "Spotted Horses" of Pech-Merle. Of five negative handprints, one can be clearly seen over the back of the right-hand horse, and one is under its belly. Another is centered above the left-hand horse, and another is to the left of its neck. There are positive prints of bent fingers in black. On one horse's back is a fish in red, and there is a circle on its chest. Length 1.98 m. Photo by J. Vertut.

tive prints, two of which are symmetrically centered above the animals. There are also positive prints of bent fingers. The spotted horses panel is an important composition to which I return repeatedly as an example of many aspects of cave art. Another association of animals, handprints, and dots is found at El Castillo in Spain; there the animals are not horses but bison. Curiously, a similar example of the association of animal figures, handprints, and dots occurs in a painting made by a San artist at Eland's Bay in South Africa. In this case the image is that of an eland, a species of antelope, an animal that played an enormously important role, both practical and mythological, for the San—a role similar to the apparent role of the horse in Ice Age culture.

The Pech-Merle horses appear in an open space within a vast, labyrinthine cave, its cathedral-like aura enhanced by stalactites suspended from the ceiling. The two horses, facing in opposite directions, are outlined in black paint. They have small, stylized, "duckbill" heads and black-painted manes, and their bodies are filled with and surrounded by black and red dots. These were not meant to describe a variety of spotted horse, as it might appear to our modern eye, because horses of that period had some stripes but no spots. We know this because the horses of that place and time were the ancestors of the historic Przewalski's horse that once roamed the Eurasian steppes and are now native only to Siberia. Some accurate depictions exist in the caves to show the typical striped coat of that horse; one example is seen at Le Portel (Ariège) and another at Lascaux (see illus. p. 144).

Nor does the painting at Pech-Merle seem to show a mythical spotted horse, for among the myriad other horses engraved and painted in Ice Age art, no similar example is known. The dots here seem to follow the dorsal lines of the horses but to ignore the ventral lines, extending below the bellies of the animals and even below their hooves. The horses are surrounded by an array of black and red dots, some of which may have been placed there before the horses were painted. It seems that the mysterious function of these dots was not descriptive.

Multivalent Meanings of Dots

Depictions of other animals in the caves, however, have dots that do appear to be descriptive of the actual markings on an animal's coat. Chauvet has two dotted animals next to each other—the smaller has been called a spotted panther. The larger animal is thought to be a spotted hyena, although it has also been suggested that its spots are not descriptive and that the animal is a bear that for some unknown reason is covered with dots. Dots, perhaps descriptive of the pelt, were also placed on the heads and sometimes the forequarters of several of the monumental extinct Ice Age bulls known as aurochs depicted in the Rotunda at Lascaux. Again at Chauvet, dots were placed on the muzzles of lions. In these cases it is clear that the dots were meant to suggest the animals' whiskers, exactly as they might be used by a contemporary draftsman.

Although my focus is on figurative art, I look at dots in their own right because they constitute such an important part of the art vocabulary. Dots are abundant and often appear to have a specific purpose, but it is difficult to find repeated usages that give clues to their meaning. In Lascaux, it appears that dots were used to mark the ends of some passages. There are dots after the decorated area in the Axial Gallery and the Meander, and two of the most inaccessible paintings, those of the Shaft and the Chamber of the Felines, each conclude the chamber with six dots. Many other dots in Lascaux and other caves seem to have other purposes. Particularly for Ice Age portable art, scholars speculate that dots might have been notational, indicating numbers of animals killed, of days passed, or of full moons.[5] It is also possible that for the cave artist, dots and other signs served as maps of the caves. Some dots seem to function as warning signs for dangerous areas or at least for changes in cave topography.

Dots, like handprints, have been used in every age all over the world. Large clusters of them are found in the pictographic art of the American Indians. Especially impressive groupings are at Mancos Canyon, Colorado, and at Nine Mile Canyon and Black Dragon Canyon, both in Utah. Dots, like handprints, have been used in innumerable other examples. Like handprints, they appear to have multiple meanings. Red dots were found on a mammoth skull from Ice Age Siberia that might have been used as a drum. A buffalo skull from Wind River, Wyoming, used by Arapaho people to temporarily contain the Great Spirit during their Sun Dance ceremony, is decorated with dots made with two different colors of earth pigment. The Indians who used it said the dots had separate meanings—black dots were a prayer for the earth and red dots were a prayer for the tribe.[6] In India, where the patina of the present is translucent, one can look through it into far distant times to glimpse ancient beliefs at work. It is still a custom in small villages to place red dots on the inside walls of houses. The reasons for placing the dots have been variously explained, but all informants agree that they acted as a blessing or charm to ward off evil.

Even within a single traditional society, the meaning of dots may be multivalent. In the Quinkan region of Australia, dots mean sweetness if associated with bees, and eggs if associated with fish. A similar example of multiple meanings for dots is true for masks made by the Yup'ik Eskimos. Artists who still make these masks say painted spots represent the coat of a spotted animal, snowflakes, stars, or eyes, depending on the story the mask is used to illustrate. If it is often impossible to know, without being told, the meanings of such dots in societies for which we have a good deal of information, then how much more imponderable is their meaning in prehistoric art?

One cannot mention the use of dots in art making without referring to the Australian Aboriginal painters centered in the Uluru area in the Western Australian Desert. Geoffrey Bordon, a teacher who was sympathetic to the alienation of the Aboriginal people around him, encouraged them to record traditional images and themes. Their work became the Desert Painters movement. The artists used dots because their traditional sand paintings were composed of dots, and so this method of paint application seemed natural to them. The dot technique may date back to Aboriginal body painting. For ritual body decoration it was the practice to make many pricks in the skin, drawing blood each time, and then, using the blood as a glue, to attach clumps of white plant floss. Australian dot painting was traditionally done on a surface primed with dark paint, a further clue that its origin derived from body painting on dark skin.

Even for a single artist, dots can have many different meanings. For example, the Chinese artist Shitao (also known by his Buddhist name, Yuanji), the greatest of the individualist painters of seventeenth-century China, wrote at length about his varied uses of dots:

> I have dots for rainy, snowy, windy, and clear days and for all seasons. I have negative and positive dots and yin and yang dots complementing each other; dots with water and dots with ink, all mixed together; dots for holding budding flowers, for algae lines, fringes and joining strings; empty, broad, dry, and tasteless dots; dots with ink, without ink, flying white and smokelike; and dots burnt like that I have not been willing to reveal to scholars. There are dots that show no heaven or earth but seem to cut right in front of you; there are also dots that show absolute quietude over a thousand peaks and myriad ravines.[7]

Dots Read as Line

Strings of dots want to be read as lines with a staccato quality, and these dotted lines can be used wherever lines are used. In Spain's Cantabria province, artists working in the small cave of Covalanas used rows of red dots rather than lines to draw deer (fig. 1.2). This technique, favored in that region, was also used at the nearby caves of La Pasiega and La Haza. It is seen in the Basque region of Spain as well, at Etcheberri and Arenaza (Vizcaya). To the north, at Lascaux, we see the use of a dotted line on the neck of one of the "Chinese" horses, so named because they are similar to stylized horses of the Han and Tang dynasties in China. The head of one of the aurochs in the Rotunda at Lascaux is made of sprayed black dots that are seen as solid lines. Dotted lines were used at Combarelles and at Le Portel, where superimposed figures of animals and schematic human figures were outlined entirely by dots.

A line is a dot that went for a walk.

—Paul Klee, *Pedagogical Sketchbook*

But in the Paleolithic art of France and Spain one finds nearly the same animals in comparable settings and in similar positions, whether made by means of lines or by strings of dots. It seems likely that whatever meaning the depiction of these animals had for Ice Age artists was unaffected by the substitution of dots for lines—it was simply an exploratory technical innovation. This connect-the-dots approach to line seems to have been a stylistic preference for rare individual artists. That observation holds for other times and places as well. In seventeenth-century Europe, for example, Pieter Brueghel the Younger—unlike most of his contemporaries—in his pen and ink drawings sometimes deliberately preferred to use a series of dots to indicate a line.

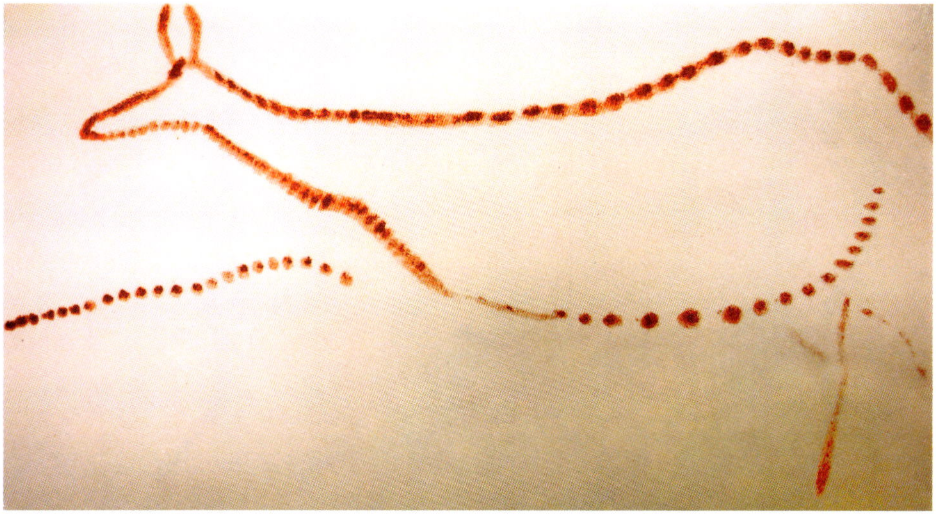

Figure 1.2. Covalanas cave painting of deer with lines indicated by a string of red dots. Length 1,67 m.

The rules of grouping can be treated as applications of one basic principle . . . that the degree to which parts . . . resemble each other . . . will help determine the degree to which they are seen as belonging together.

—Rudolf Arnheim, *Art and Visual Perception*

The Perception of Dots as Mass

Clusters of dots often appear as one mass. It is always unusual to show mass without defining edges, yet in some instances of Ice Age art, animals were made entirely of dots with no containing outline. In the Axial Gallery at Lascaux, some little painted horses are made up entirely of dots. There the dotting results from the granularity of the calcite spike formations of the surface on which they were placed. Drawings done on such a surface have a dotted character because the pigment, in the form of a crayon or pastel, skips along the tops of the bumps, creating an inadvertent dotting. (Of course, had the artist wished to minimize this effect, the pigment could have been blended by rubbing with a damp estompe.) Similarly, in the Rotunda at Lascaux, some heavily carbonate-encrusted walls present rough, cauliflower-like surfaces unsuitable for engraving or fine painting, and paintings on them have a dotted appearance.

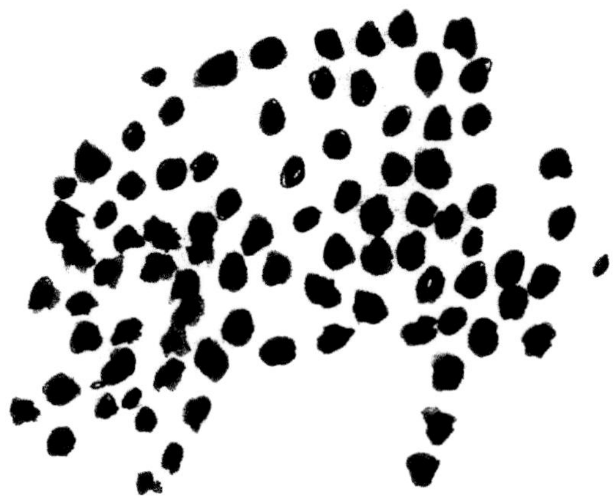

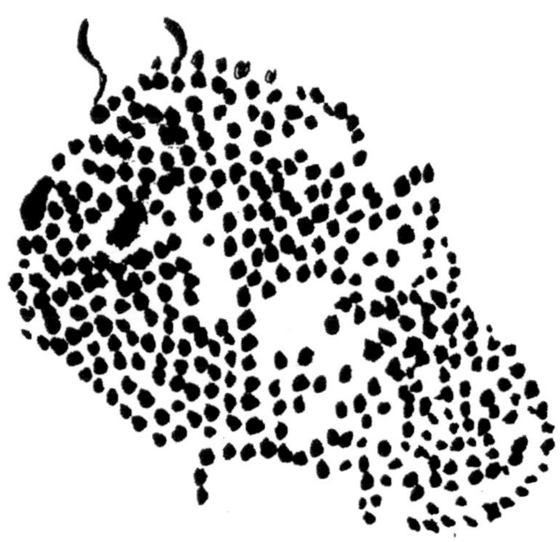

Figure 1.3. Animal at Chauvet made of red dots, possibly a bison facing right.

Figure 1.4. Bison from Marsoulas. 87 cm.

At Chauvet, one group of 92 red dots appears to form an unoutlined animal, seemingly a bison. The dots are believed to have been made by someone pressing a paint-marked palm against the cave wall (fig. 1.3).[8] As much as 15,000 years later, another artist made a bison by means of unoutlined red dots at Marsoulas (Haute-Garonne) (fig. 1.4). These dots are large enough that they do not merge visually but maintain their discrete identity. The dots are each about the size of a large thumb, and we may guess that they are in fact thumbprints. From among the red dots, two black dot eyes peer out. A black mark and an array of dots over the animal may be a horn. This use of the dot technique must have been an independent discovery; it is highly unlikely that the artist at Marsoulas knew of the work of the artist at Chauvet.

The same graphic device was discovered and used in rock art by the San people, also called Bushmen, hunter-gatherers who have lived in southern Africa since about 10,000 years ago. An eland made only with dots was found at Wide Valley, Maclear, in the province of Natal, South Africa. The San parietal art that remains is largely in remote areas such as the Drakensberg Mountains. Like most other rock art, it is difficult to date.

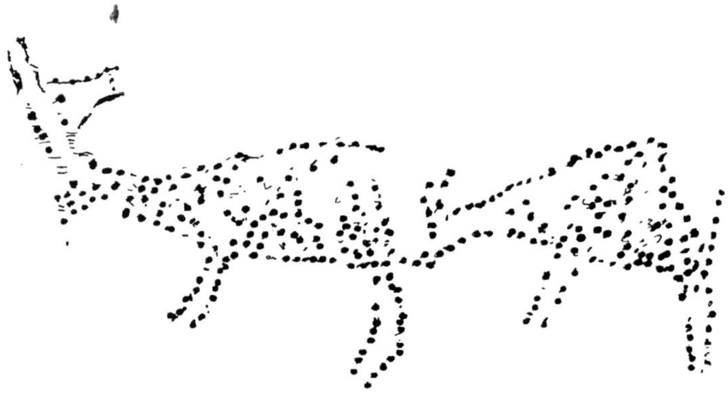

Figure 1.5. Animals from a rock art site along the Pecos River in Texas.

Some of it may be several thousand years old, but because of the fragility of the paint in the exposed rockshelters, it is probably relatively recent.

An uncannily similar discovery was made by yet another artist, this time about 4,000 years ago in a rockshelter at the confluence of the Pecos and Diablo Rivers in what is now southern Texas. There, on a painted rock Art panel, are a number of overlapping figures. One figure is done mostly in dots, which become somewhat elongated into small dashes (fig. 1.5). The use of dots in this way is found worldwide. In Patagonia, at the tip of South America, a feline made entirely of dots and short jagged strokes is dated at 7,000 to 8,000 years ago.

In North America, an ancient artist of the Fremont culture who lived in what is now Dinosaur National Monument, Utah, some 1,300 to 800 years ago left an unusual petroglyph of an anthropomorph. Its face and headdress are depicted entirely by dots, except for the elongated mark of the mouth. The eyes are darker dots, like those in the bison at Marsoulas. American Indian petroglyphs show how technical considerations can lead to a dotted appearance. Unlike the soft limestone walls of France and Spain, the hard basaltic escarpments often used in North America are difficult to engrave. Marking was commonly done with a point and hammerstone. The resulting pecked marks yield a gradual buildup of small depressions. In the interior of a figure they show mass, and when linked together on the exterior of a form they gradually merge to create a line. It was easiest in the obdurate stone to first plan the shape of a figure with dots, the way children in some New England grammar schools were once taught to make letters by pricking dots into a sheet of paper, allowing them to accumulate to form letters. Occasionally one finds what appears to be an incomplete petroglyph for which the outline appears only as dots.

I believe the idea of using dots to show mass without a containing outline was a discovery made independently by a few artists and was always at odds with mainstream stylistic practices. Something about this approach might have appealed to certain restlessly inventive individuals who were interested in exploring the process of perception. In seventeenth-century China, for example, the artist Dong Quichang saw a landscape done by the fourteenth-century artist Wang Meng. He was so struck by what the earlier artist had done that he attempted his own version of it by indicating mass without the structural "bones," as he called outline, of drawing in ink.[9] In this case he used colored washes instead of dots.

We cannot know the motives of these widely separated artists when they looked only at mass and avoided normal contour lines, but we can approach what they might have been after when we observe a parallel technique used by the nineteenth-century painter Georges Seurat. In his drawings Seurat abjured outline and devoted himself entirely to the light-and-dark mass of his subject, which he indicated with irregular dots or strokes. Sometimes he did this by rubbing a charcoal stick gently against a sheet of rough paper so that only the high spots were touched and pigment was left in small jagged marks. Sometimes he used an array of dots on the toothed paper, as in the accompanying picture of his mother sewing (fig. 1.6). The results are murky, and at first one can barely make out the figure. There are no details. The drawing builds up slowly with accretions of small marks—dots, squiggles, rasps—until the surface reaches the proper tone of darkness, giving the form an atmospheric, vaporous insubstantiality. The image gradually emerges to the viewer with the magical inevitability of a developing Polaroid photograph. The result is mysterious and powerful. It lacks the precision and clarity of line but is hauntingly suggestive. Seurat knew well what he was doing; this is Pointillism without its aspect of retinal color theory.

Working with mass alone was one of the exercises used in the Bauhaus in Weimar, Germany, and at Itten College in Berlin in the 1920s and 1930s. Robert Beverly Hale, the venerable anatomy and drawing teacher who lectured for years at the Art Students' League in New York, once wrote: "It is in the realms of mass and tone that students most frequently mishandle details. . . . Remember that details must never be allowed to attract the attention that rightfully belongs to the mass."[10] It is for this reason that a clichéd image of the painter is that of someone squinting before a canvas. Creating purposeful optical blur by squinting makes it easier to lose details, avoiding the sharp clarity achieved by the foveal area of the eye and focusing attention on the more generalized mass of the form.

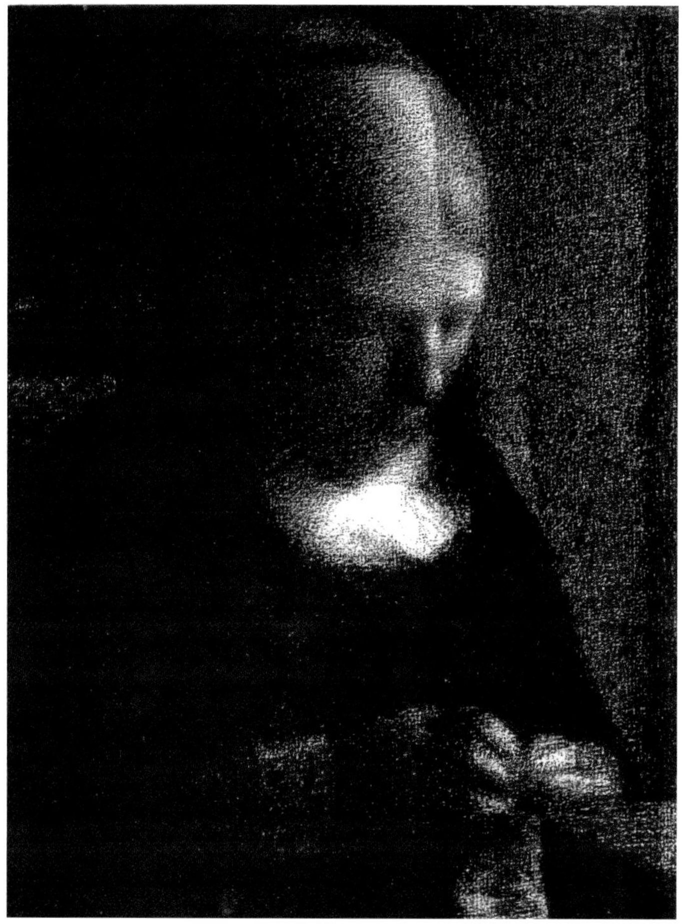

Figure 1.6. George Seurat, (1859–1891)
The Artist's Mother (woman sewing)
conté crayon on paper, 12 ¼ x 9 ½ in
The Metropolitan Museum of Art

Beginning in the Ice Age, artists discovered how to emphasize one type of the brain's visual processing by deliberately filtering out other types. This decision making takes place again and again in the art-making process. A choice is made, consciously or unconsciously, and the artist zooms across the many possible modes of pictorial representation to select one, which becomes the focus of attention. In this case it is mass. Hale continued to emphasize to his art students the importance of getting the mass right: "An accomplished artist is extraordinarily skilled in visualizing forms in terms of very simple mass. . . . When we wish to create the illusion of reality on the surface of a piece of paper or canvas, nothing is more helpful than the ability to visualize in terms of simple mass."[11]

A painting by Salvador Dalí called *Sistine Madonna* reveals this process at work in a striking way, on multiple levels. From a distance of three feet the painting can be read only as dots with slight variations in tone. Backing away to about nine feet, one sees a draped female figure, the Madonna of the title. As the viewer moves still farther away, the Madonna vanishes and a huge ear made of dots unexpectedly comes into focus. Dalí again used dots to create mass in his painting *Portrait of My Dead Brother.* It is the imagined face of the brother who died before he was born. The dots serve the same function but this time, seen close up, are actually cherries and, being red, make one think of drops of blood.

The contemporary artist Chuck Close produced a series of enormous portraits by dividing the faces into grids, in which he stamped subtly varying gradations of inks. Distinctive portraits of photographic accuracy emerged from this seemingly imprecise process. In one group of portraits, Close employed fingerprints made with the use of an inkpad to create the units of lighter and darker shading. He also used dots.[12] Regarding his use of dots to make portraits, Close said, "I discovered about 150 dots is the minimum number of dots to make a recognizable person."[13]

Scintillation and Spirituality

The use of dots often gives an appearance of vibration. Indeed, the avowed goal of many Australian Aboriginal artists is to create a shimmering effect. Traditionally, the Yolngu painters of northeastern Arnhem Land referred to the desired radiance as *bir'gun.*[14] The Aboriginal painters I mentioned earlier, in the Uluru area of Western Australia, wanted their paintings to shimmer as if giving forth light and brilliance. They associated iridescence with the rainbow, with the sacred rainbow serpent, and with life itself.

Contemporary Aboriginal painters still believe that the achievement of scintillation differentiates the exceptional artist from ordinary ones. Such brilliance, for these artists, is a graphic expression of spirituality, not unlike the effect of light pouring through fragments of colored glass in the stained glass windows of Gothic cathedrals or the golden and colored tesserae used in Byzantine mosaics. On the North American continent it is likely that the abundant use of spattering in some paintings on rockshelter walls along the lower Pecos River in Texas, particularly at Cedar Springs, was an attempt to create shimmer. At Horseshoe Canyon in Utah, the intense spirituality of the huge ghostlike figures comes across even to the most casual viewer; parts of at least two of these figures have been colored by spattering paint.

Scintillation continues to be used in modern times. Paul Bonnard collected patterned silver paper wrappers for inspiration in conveying, with little flecks of colored pigment, what he referred to as his "sparkles." Richard Pousette-Dart, in the 1960s, placed little spots of oil and metallic paint on canvas to achieve a similar effect in paintings, especially one called *Radiance.* With all this in mind, we can look back at the unexplained use of dots on the spotted horses at Pech-Merle. It seems to me that their makers might have been using the same device of scintillation linked with spirituality. One has only to visualize the horses without the dots to see how the figures recede into the background and lose the shimmering energy of visual vibration that compels our attention and our awe in the dark, sanctuary-like space.

Some archaeologists believe that the visual vibration of groups of dots is not only a graphic device to evoke a feeling of spirituality but also a literal recording of one of the sensations experienced by the spiritual seeker or shaman. David Lewis-Williams and other proponents of the "shamanic representational" theory believe that groups of dots found in prehistoric art are transcriptions of dots seen during trance states. He refers to them as *entoptic,* meaning that their origin is from within the optic system. Specifically, Lewis-Williams interprets the red lines with white dots found in San art as entoptic phenomena induced by trance-related altered states of conscousness.[15]

Followers of this shamanic theory have applied it to sites such as those on the lower Pecos River, where the large paintings of a vanished prehistoric people are strewn with dots.[16] Another, related explanation is that the dots are meant to portray pods of the peyote plant, a mind-altering drug growing in that region (but not in Europe).[17] Chumash Indians in California painted figures surrounded by white dots. At sacred sites such as Condor Cave, Painted Rock, and Arrowhead Springs, Chumash pictographs are also covered with clusters of red dots. Neuroscientists describe such dots, luminous points, sparks, and flashes of lights as *phosphenes,* "originating from electrical or chemical stimulation of the human primary visual cortex."[18]

Given the ubiquity of dots, it is difficult to believe that all of them, beginning in the earliest art, can be explained by the shamanic representational theory as trance generated. There seems to be no compelling evidence to suggest that dots in Ice Age paintings were trance inspired. It seems probable that dots had different meanings in different contexts but that dot making itself, as an art-related activity, was part of the human repertoire of mark making. In many cases it might have been valued for the kinesthetic sensations that accompanied it.

The Kinesthetic Origin of Dot Making

Many of the elements we associate with art making have antecedents in the higher primates, and sometimes they can be traced even farther back in our evolutionary heritage. They may also be seen in the normal development of the human child. Children begin to make dots when they are about two years old, using pounding movements called *plosive.* The psychologist Howard Gardner described how his young son discovered dot making. He wrote that the boy found the movements and resulting marks to be so pleasurable that he immediately favored them over his earlier linear scribbles.[19] This is understandable for adults as well, because dot making involves a percussive rhythm that affords a kinesthetic pleasure similar to that of drumming. It is important to look at these early manifestations of aesthetic perception in biology and ontology, because they provide the platform of possibilities from which *Homo sapiens sapiens'* leap to art took place.

We know that Ice Age people used percussive instruments. Decorated animal bones suitable for drumming have been found in European sites. Wear marks show that hollow stalactites and stalagmites in caves were struck in order to produce plangent sounds that must have reverberated in the silent caves.[20] It is believed that sound played an important role in some caves.[21] The Black Salon at Niaux, for example, is so formed that one can whisper at one point and hear what is being said on the other side of the amphitheater-like space. Percussion in such a setting might have had a powerful affect. Returning to the painting of the horses at Pech-Merle, one might well imagine that the visual vibration produced by the dots was enhanced by a percussive sound, a musical vibration that augmented the visual vibration of the dotted panel.

How the Brain Perceives Dots

We see the dots in the Marsoulas bison, Dalí's dots, and Close's fingerprints as unified pictures. Gestalt psychologists explained this phenomenon by means of "laws" of grouping. They discovered that the brain perceives individual units such as dots as parts of a larger whole if these units are similar in size, shape, and color—hence their laws of similarity and proximity.[22] For the same reason, we see the very small dots that make up a printed picture and the spots or pixels of light and dark on a television screen as coherent images. In these examples, because the eye cannot resolve the smaller units individually, we are unaware of them and see only the overall image. One could refer to them as being perceptively fused.

Under the right conditions, seeing a series of dots as a line seems to be the working method of our visual system. Each of the many millions of light-sensitive receptors on the retina receives one tiny fragment of the image projected onto it. Artists who work with dots select out one of the steps of the process of seeing and leave it exposed, as though a builder were leaving exposed beams, pipes, and ducts in a finished building to reveal the construction method. Using dots to suggest mass follows the tracks of one aspect of our specialized visual information processing procedure, derailing it at an incomplete state and forcing the viewer to finish consciously the integration of information that would normally be done automatically by our brain.

We transform dots into a visual impression of the real world because the mind is avid for meaning. It struggles to make sense of a barrage of electrochemical data, almost like an instantaneous interpreter who must translate into one language while a stream of speech in another flows on unremittingly. The process seems to have been as true for prehistoric artists as it is today. In the case of the red dots at Marsoulas, the mind interprets triumphantly, "Bison!" In the case of the Seurat drawing, it pronounces, "Mother, sewing." If an artist gets the smudgy suggestivity of the mass drawing exactly right, as Seurat did, then ironically, a more powerful sense of reality may be conveyed than might have been the case with a precisely delineated drawing. This is because viewers must participate in the detective work. Their search for an image they can understand creates a greater intimacy and involvement in the perceptual process. In the same manner, the dotted images made by European Ice Age artists and by members of other prehistoric societies might have resulted from the discovery that it was seemingly more magical if they interrupted viewers' automatic visual processing and coerced them into participating in completing the image.

LINES

Finger markings were often extended to form lines. Rouffignac cave is situated in the Dordogne in France, not far from the caves of Lascaux and Gabillou. More than a mile into the cave, after passing paintings of mammoths and rhinoceroses, one finds a chamber filled with thousands of marks made by people who dragged two, three, or four slightly separated fingers in the red clay of the ceilings and walls. Parallel lines made in this way have been called *meanders, flutings,* or, more picturesquely, *macaroni.*

The first markings of children and our ancestors are tentacles waving in the world to see what the catch will be.
—SYLVIA FEIN, *First Drawings*

Similarly elemental lines appear in many other European Ice Age caves where an unctuous clay surface invited fingers to touch. Examples include Pech-Merle, Gargas, La Baume-Latrone (Gard), and La Croze à Gontron (Dordogne) in France and Hornos de la Peña (Oviedo) and La Pileta (Cantabria) in Spain. Almost identical finger markings are found in the Umtali-area caves in South Africa. More than 20 cave sites have been found in Australia that have the same kinds of serpentine finger markings, among them Orchestra Shell Cave in Western Australia, Snowy River Cave in Victoria, and Koonalda in Southern Australia. Meanders are believed to be among the earliest marks made in some caves. Some in the French caves are believed to be as much as 30,000 years old, and those at Koonalda have been dated to 20,000 years ago.

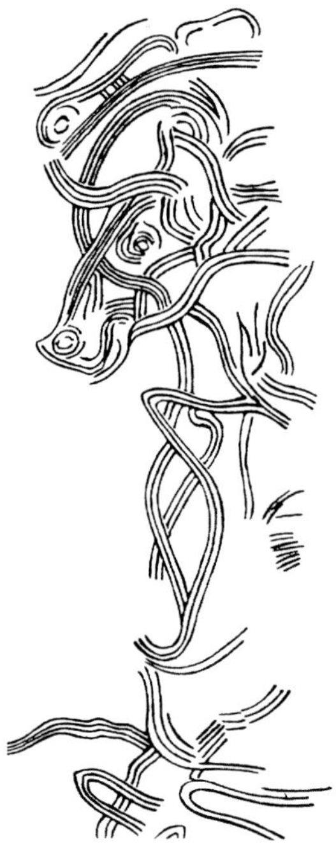

Figure 1.7. Finger-made meanders at Altamira end up to form the head of a bovine animal. Length 5 m overall; head of bovine, 1 m.

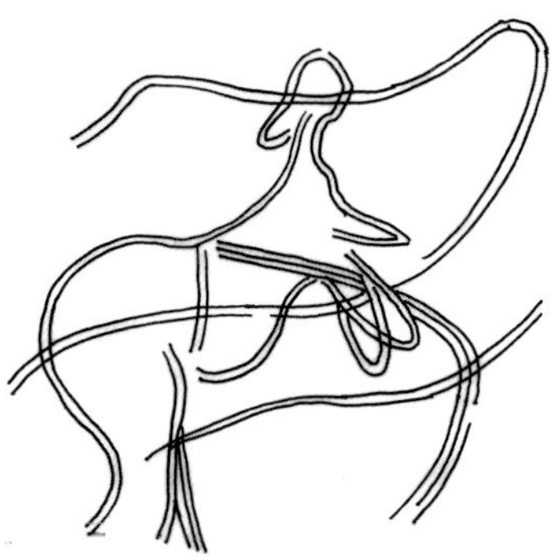

Figure 1.8. Finger-made meanders at Pech-Merle with outlined female figure. Height 55 cm.

As in the case of dots, my major interest is in lines that were used to make figurative art. Lines invite interpretation. Even simple meanders might signify water or snakes, or they might mark sources of water within caves.[23] Sometimes the lines combed against the soft clay of the cave walls suggested figures that, once recognized, were transformed deliberately into figurative images. At La Baume-Latrone fingers dipped in paint seem to start as a meander but are finished as a snake. Abbé Henri Breuil remarked on this transformation: "In the midst of these very primitive drawings, animal figures appear already intensely natural."[24]

One example is from La Pileta (Cantabria) in northern Spain. At Altamira, also in Cantabria, some finger marks began as non-objective scrawls but culminated in the outline of a bovine head (fig. 1.7). At Gargas, from a confused tangle of lines on the cave walls, two eyes and a muzzle emerge to become an animal head. At Ardales (Málaga), red ocher meanders seem almost by happenstance to become deer heads. Someone at La Baume-Latrone drew a mammoth using fingers colored by being dragged on the red clay floor. In some instances, meanders form humans. At Romanelli in Italy, lines become stylized females. At Pech-Merle, in the Hall of the Hieroglyphs, meanders may be seen as forming a mammoth shape. Emerging from these lines is the figure of a female (fig. 1.8).

Meanders are so universal that they seem to have been a kinesthetic imperative to humans everywhere. They are the trajectories of gestures, and when their scale requires it, they encompass movement of the entire body. If this interpretation is correct, then these lines are the touch marks of the fingers extended rhythmically in time and space.

Our early ancestors also used tools to make linear marks. On soft surfaces they replaced fingers with a stiff implement, and when working stone or bone they used a fragment of flint or a stone burin. Alexander Marshack, a noted researcher in prehistory, applied microscopic viewing and sophisticated photographic techniques to an analysis of such tool marks and discovered that a different tool was frequently used for different marks on a single surface. This suggests that some of the marks were made over time and therefore suggested a notational purpose. Others seem to have been purely decorative. Generally we speak of marks made with a hard, sharp tool as *engraving* or *intaglio*. Sometimes, when the underneath layer of stone is lighter than its surface, the engraving produces a *cameo*, so that the drawn line appears to be light rather than dark. This is common in petroglyphs in North America in places where basaltic stone has developed a darker patina.

Deliberate tool markings go farther back in the hominid line than to the modern humans who made the Ice Age cave art. Examples come from Mousterian sites, which appear to have been occupied by *Homo neanderthalensis*, whose exact kinship to *Homo sapiens sapiens* is now in dispute. Some of these sites were occupied at about the same time as the *Homo sapiens* sites. Among the more complicated marks, which would be difficult to confuse with animals' gnawing marks or humans' butchering marks, are a zigzag engraved on a bone fragment from Bacho Kiro in Bulgaria, a double arc on a bone from Riparo, Italy, and a cruciform and a rectangular figure on a mammoth shoulderblade from Molodova-I in Ukraine.

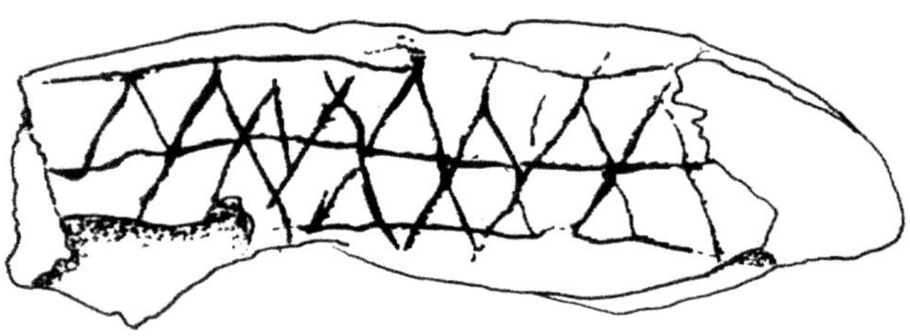

Figure 1.9. One of two intentionally engraved pieces of red ocher from Blombos cave, South Africa, dated to 77,000 years ago. 7.6 cm. The configuration is symmetrical on either side of the central line.

One of the most ancient examples of man-made lines is a flint fragment engraved with concentric half-circles from a Neanderthal site in Quneitra, Israel, dated to 54,000 years ago.[25] Two carefully engraved pieces of red ocher unearthed from Blombos cave in South Africa are convincingly dated to about 77,000 years ago.[26] The engraving tool used on these two pieces was evidently small and required fine motor control. The images suggest considerable deliberation. The larger ocher piece was engraved with three long lines that follow the shape of the stone (fig. 1.9). Crossed lines forming diamond shapes relate to these lines and to one another, and the whole image appears to have been planned so that it would appear both symmetrical and reversible. Such complexity at this early date is difficult to explain. So far the Blombos pieces appear to be isolated examples, but they are nonetheless remarkable in that they hint of a greater sophistication than one would have thought possible at the time. About fifty thousand years later we see the same diamond shape used on figures such as the carved head of a lion from Vogelherd. We have come to accept this as possible, but the Blombos date astounds us.

Origin and Kinesthetics of Line

As was the case with dots, there are antecedents to human line making. Evidence of line making seems to go back to the higher primates and even to other mammals. Most higher primates, having their hands to some extent relieved of the demands of locomotion, are the beneficiaries of a new tactile freedom.

Chimpanzees have been encouraged to draw and paint, and the results have been exhibited in art galleries and museums, where they are often considered "beautiful."

Some nonprimates seem to share this marking urge. Large-brained elephants use their trunks as we use our hands, in a convergent biological development. Despite their awkward look and ponderous size, the trunks achieve a fine prehensile coordination. In zoos, elephants make marks on the ground with their trunks. Bearing this in mind, David Gucwa, an elephant trainer at a zoo in Syracuse, New York, supplied an elephant with brushes and paint so that she could transform her ground gestures into painted marks on paper.[27] Impressed with the results, Gucwa sent her paintings to Jerome Witkin, a prominent abstract expressionist artist, and asked him to judge them without knowing anything about their maker. Witkin pronounced them "lyrical" and "lovely," and he ventured a guess that the mysterious artist was female and in some way connected with the Far East. He was right—she was from Thailand. Now it is relatively common for zoos to augment their funds by selling elephant "art." There is even a center in Thailand where elephants are taught to make specific repetitious markings for tourists, markings that appear to human viewers like flowers or schematic elephants. The results speak of the trainability of these intelligent animals, not of their aesthetic potential.

In humans the urge to mark seems to be intense. There are many instances in which people who have lost the use of their hands have held a marking device between their teeth or toes. An analysis of the art of children may tell us something about the human passion for mark making. Children take up crayons as early as twelve months. After putting them in their mouths, they soon notice that they leave a visible trail. These lines at first seem to record motor activity originating in normal, spontaneous movements of arm and hand. The hand is a restless appendage. At first the kinesthetic pleasure of making marks and the joy of seeing a tangible result might be all that is involved. These first marks are made as accidental by-products of motion, but eventually it is the marks themselves that become the focus of attention.

The Personal Line and Its Psychology

By the time a person has reached adulthood, he or she has developed an individual way of moving, and the lines that result from one's motion are unique. Personal quality of line was true for the Ice Age artists, too, even though they most often made lines with tools that were much less responsive to subtleties of movement than is pencil, pen, or brush. Even engraved lines, made with a stone burin hit by a stone mallet on a stone surface, stone against stone, though relatively crude, allow us to detect differences. Many sites have their own styles, possibly influenced by a master in that region. Sometimes we can discern what appears to be the work of one individual. In the narrow little cave of Gabillou in Dordogne, it appears that the fine line engravings were the work of a single person working alone by the light of a stone lamp. They are as intimate as an artist's sketchbook.

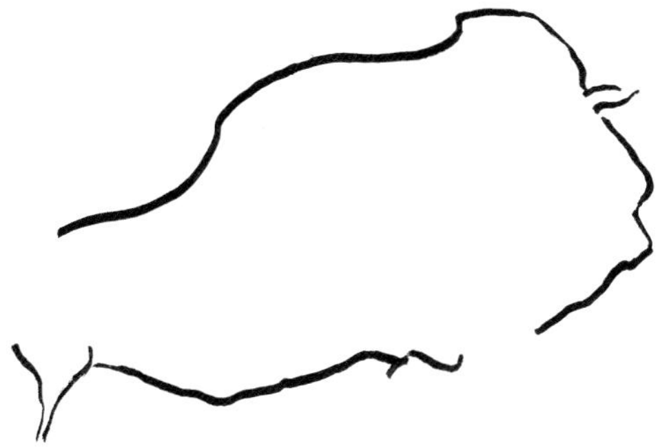

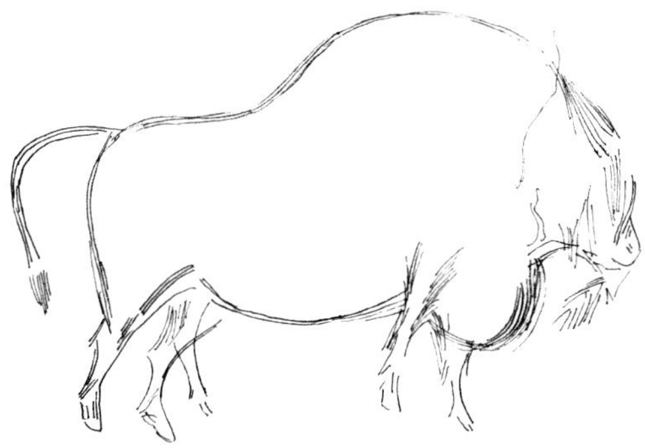

Figure 1.10. Bison at Niaux made with minimal lines in quick gesture. This image is dated to c.13,850 B.P., making it the oldest dated figure in Niaux.

Figure 1.11. Engraving at Peña de Candamo made with hesitant, searching line. 96cm.

The drawn line can be thought of as the seismographic record of electromagnetic surges coursing through our nervous system. Lines are expressive of the personality and even of the mental state of the person who drew them. The most individual and idiosyncratic line is expressed by handwriting. In China, calligraphy has long been considered a higher form of art than drawing. In Islamic countries in which making imagery was forbidden, calligraphy alone had to embody all personal graphic expression. In any art, each individual's lines are as unique as a snowflake, as a fingerprint, revealing temperament and mood even while delineating form or making tangible an idea. In the Ice Age caves, we can see the tour de force of a few quick, confident lines made by the artist at Niaux (fig. 1.10) and the delicate, searching, almost tentative lines of an artist from Peña de Candamo (Asturias). (fig. 1.11).

Such individual differences are evident throughout art history. The cool, taut line of Ingres differs from the impetuous, clotted line of Rembrandt. The cacophonic line of Klimt differs from the hesitant line of Renoir. The exploratory line clusters of Cézanne differ from the whiplash line of Picasso. The analytic line of Mondrian differs from the passionate line of Goya, the pensive line of Klee from the razor-sharp line of Schiele. Then there is the pulsing fluency of Matisse, a result of his wish to follow the line's own "desire." It is as hard to disguise one's line as it is to disguise one's signature.

Cultural Influences on Line

Yet even while artists express themselves as individuals, they can submit to the cultural aura of their time and work within the stylistic rules of a specific period. Broad commonalities within Ice Age art are pronounced enough that some prehistorians have used them as a basis for chronological classification. Stylistic distinctions are much more certain in more recent art history. Art nouveau, for example, with its characteristic self-consciously suave curvilinear line, is notably distinct from German Expressionism. Artists can identify with and adopt the kinesthetic style of an entire culture.

The art of the Pacific Northwest Coast indigenous people uses a particular line called a *form line* (fig. 1.12). The organic elasticity of the line, swelling and narrowing, conveys a specific kind of muscular activity that is also peculiar to their dance movements. Bill Holm, an authority on the Native art of the Northwest Coast, is highly sensitive to the quality of this physical activity: "The constant flow of movement, broken at rhythmic intervals by the rather sudden but not necessarily jerky changes of motion-direction, characterizes both the dance and the art of the North West Coast. I myself have derived a certain satisfaction from the muscle activity involved in producing the characteristic line movement of this art, and there can be little doubt that this was true also for the Indian artist."[28]

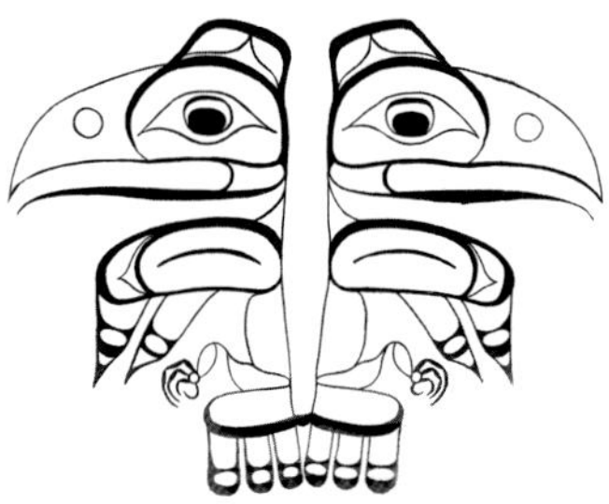

Figure 1.12. Northwest Coast "form lines" can be seen in a Haida split figure of a raven.

Right after the Second World War a group of painters centered in New York began to view marks and lines with a new eye. It may have been partly that some of them had contact during the war with the art of Asia and were made sensitive to Asian calligraphy. Jackson Pollock believed he was influenced by Navajo sand paintings, in the sense that those paintings are made on the ground and the artist often is in the center of the work. If sand painting did influence him, it came about as a misunderstanding of the highly rigorous and disciplined Native American art form. Pollock read into it what he wished to see. For him and others, such as Franz Klein, the critic Harold Rosenberg said, "the canvas began to appear . . . as an arena in which to act."[29] Pollock often painted standing in the middle of the flat canvas or poised on a scaffold over it. From this position he poured and dribbled liquid paint as he moved back and forth like an obsessed dancer. Others worked in a similar fashion, if less dramatically. The movement they initiated was aptly called "action painting."

For almost a generation this approach, later called abstract expressionism, was the dominant art style in the United States and Europe. It was unified by the belief that painting was really about the elements of painting. Because the dots, marks, and lines were, in many cases, the subject of the painting, there was immense concern for their integrity and individuality and for the action by which they were produced. In their emphasis on the motion that produced their lines, these twentieth-century artists, in this regard only, may have been close to the prehistoric artists who made the meanders on cave walls.

Eye, Brain, and Hand

Line is not only a record of the muscular movement of the arm and hand, but in representational art especially, it is also a record of the physical activity of the eyes. The artist can draw with his eyes by following the motion of one area of the eye because it is only in this tiny foveal area that the eye can register an image with fine resolution. Only a minute section of the visual field can be seen with detail at any one instant. From eight feet away, over a whole panorama, we can actually register no more than a four-inch square on the retina with clarity. Because the brain needs more information, the eye and head are in constant motion. Sometimes the lines used by the artist are the direct record of these eye movements. In a certain art school exercise, students are told to draw a figure with their eyes; later, in a variation of the exercise, they might be told literally to draw the figure from memory by reconstructing the remembered movements of the eyes. Some of the intimacy and immediacy of Rembrandt's drawings resulted from his letting the brush or pen follow the motion and pauses of his searching vision. He allowed his hand to linger or burst forward, following the impulse of his moving eye.

In Ice Age art, as well as in other art, a single impulse links eye, mind, hand, and the line which they discharge. Despite the fact that we are modern and these artists were prehistoric, we can experience this because we are highly empathic creatures and because we share with them certain neural structures. If we are open to such experiences we can travel backward from line to hand to eye to experience something of what these ancient artists saw. In those examples of Ice Age art that we deem the greatest, we can feel a connection to the artist. On such occasions we believe we can sense the impulse by which that hand was driven.

FIGURES

A line that returns to its point of origin, enclosing a space, makes us primarily aware of the space it encloses. The space enclosed within a line is called a *figure,* to distinguish it from the space outside the line, which is called the *ground.* The perceptual psychologist Irvin Rock once wrote that "there is a universal and probably unlearned tendency to perceive the region within certain contours as a

Drawing is a series of thoughts with lines around them.

—ROBERT BEVERLY HALE, *Drawing Lessons from the Great Masters*

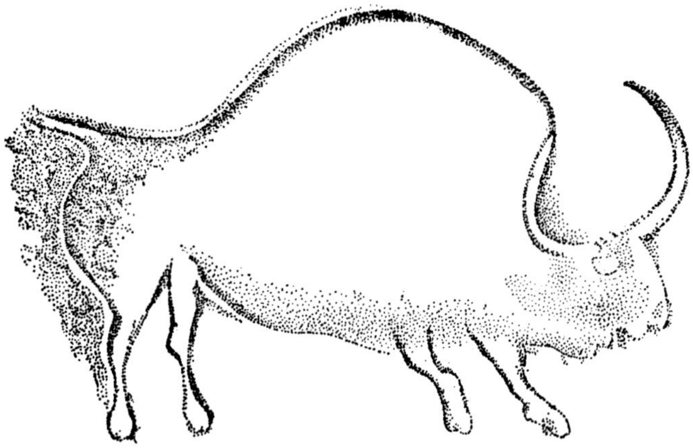

Figure 1.13. The "Bison of the Discovery" at the cave of La Mouthe, first recognized by Gaston Bertoumeyrou in 1895. Length 85 cm.

solid two-dimensional object."[30] This was no less true for Ice Age artists.

About 110 years ago in the French village of Les Eyzies, the farmer Monsieur Lepeyre decided to clean the earth debris from around a small hole in the hillside near his house, probably intending to use the space to store his potatoes. The current farmer, his grandson Edouard Lepeyre, does just that. Not long afterward, four neighborhood boys noticed the newly accessible cave and set about to explore it. Almost 100 yards from the opening, one of the boys, Gaston Bertoumeyrou, noticed clearly incised engravings of animals. A carefully crafted stone lamp lay nearby. One of the engraved animals would later be known as the "Bison of the Discovery" (fig. 1.13), the first rock art to be incontrovertibly dated as Paleolithic, because geologists could date the fine sandy mud that had sealed the opening of the cave to the end of the Ice Age. On the walls of this cave, known as La Mouthe, the boys wrote the date of their discovery: April 8, 1895.

After that discovery, archaeologists were forced to admit that our distant ancestors, once dismissed as brutish cave dwellers, had been capable of the symbolic thinking necessary to create representational drawings. The discovery of an abundance of other Ice Age art followed. A bison almost identical to the one at La Mouthe was found about a decade later in the nearby rockshelter of La Grèze (Dordogne). It has become apparent that some Ice Age artists had such facility that they were able to create figures consisting of a continuous preconceived outline made in one or a few virtuosic gestures, such as the example from Niaux we saw earlier (fig. 1.10).

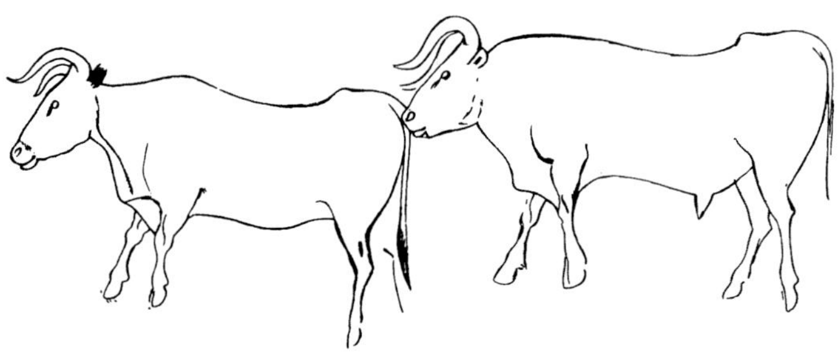

Figure 1.14. Subtle and sophisticated contour drawing can be seen in this engraving of a bull following a cow in the cave of Teyjat. Lengths of animals 55 and 50 cm, respectively.

Contour Line and Cross Contour Line

In outline drawing the artist creates, as at La Mouthe, a primarily two-dimensional figure, visually contrasted against a ground, by using a simple closed outline. A more sophisticated drawing technique, providing real or vicarious tactile information, is called *contour line* drawing. Exploratory touch is important to our visual understanding. Such touch-augmented vision is called *haptic* and is particularly important in representational art.[31] Surprisingly, European Ice Age artists used contour lines in a way that was always assumed to have been devised in ancient Greece and refined during the Italian Renaissance. Yet we now know that Ice Age artists discovered the use of contour line tens of thousands of years earlier. In an engraving of a cow and a bull from Teyjat (Dordogne), for example, the lines follow the subtle, shifting ins and outs of the real and apparent edges of the figure and give the illusion of solid figures (fig. 1.14).

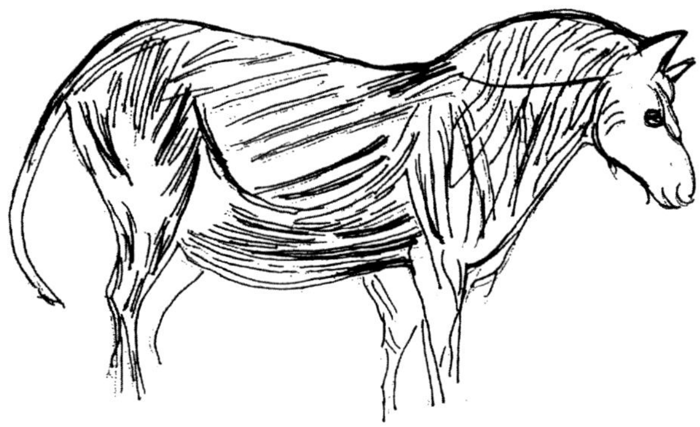

Continuing in this manner, some Ice Age artists discovered how to use *cross contour* lines, which can completely leave the edges of the figure and move over the interior of the implied form to strengthen the illusion of three dimensions. In the tiny cave of El Buxú (Asturias), a horse was engraved using both contour and cross contour line (fig. 1.15). The contour lines describe the head and legs. Interior contour lines describe the belly. Cross contour was used to show the fullness of the flank and, to a lesser extent, the head. Other, purely descriptive lines indicate the mane.

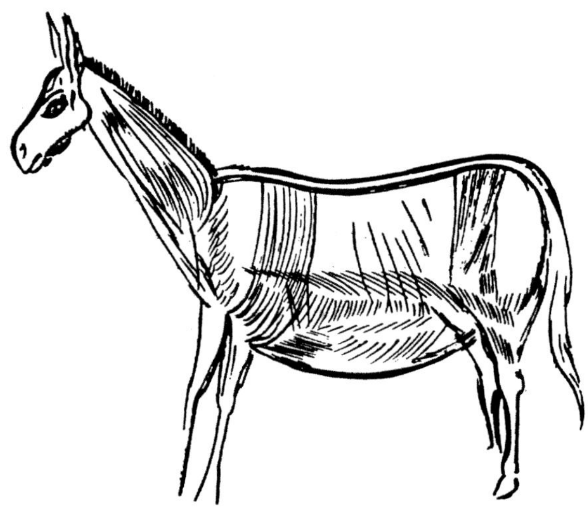

Figure 1.15. A horse at El Buxú displays contour lines on its legs and head and cross contour lines on its flank.

Figure 1.16. Engraving of a wild ass from Trois Frères that shows a sophisticated use of cross contour lines and cross hatching to suggest three-dimensional form. Length 40 cm.

Contour and cross contour lines can suggest the actual presence of three-dimensional forms in space. Indeed, such drawings merge imperceptibly with low-relief sculpture and approach the sculptural panels in which figures partially emerge from their rocky matrix. Cap Blanc (Dordogne) is a prime example. In stone carving, hatching is done by chipping parallel lines with a point or with a comblike tool called a claw. Cross hatching in sculpture occurs when the series of hatch marks overlap one another. In an example from Trois Fréres contour lines are seen on the tail, head, ears, and legs of an engraved wild ass. A variety of cross contour, hatching, and cross hatching lines were used around the body in an attempt to give the swelling belly a cylindrical appearance (fig. 1.16). A surprisingly sophisticated example of contour line is found in the engraving of a lion on a stone plaquette from La Marche (Vienne). Lines move

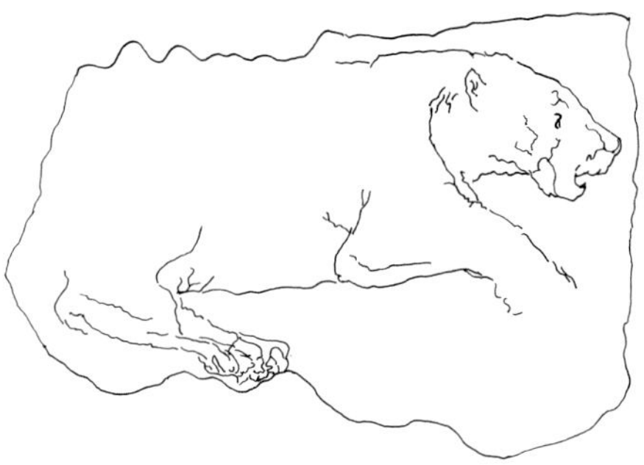

Figure 1.17. Lion engraved on a plaquette from La Marche. The linear image, painstakingly extracted from other extraneous marks, reveals delicate lines. For example, the junction between the foreleg and the body is depicted using contour lines.

from the contour or outer edge of the figure to the inner form, particularly where the legs fold in to join the body (fig. 1.17).

The Search for Visual Realism

Line can be directed toward making schematic forms in a path leading ultimately to hieroglyphics. Alternatively, it can be directed toward exploring and re-creating the visual and tactile sensations of real experience and finding ways to present those sensations in graphic figures. The latter approach has been rare in prehistoric and tribal art throughout the world, and yet the earliest known artists—those of the European Ice Age—chose to re-create such visual reality. Their achievements were lost until the beginning of the twentieth century. Among much later Stone Age artists, perhaps only the San of South Africa were as deeply concerned with the actual appearances of animals. In Europe, after long use of more schematic imagery, the artists of ancient Greece began to search for ways to depict what they saw. Inspired by archaeological finds from Greece, artists of the Italian and northern European Renaissance became obsessed with codifying rules for recording visual reality. Ultimately, the impressionists continued this search in another direction, to the point that Cézanne called Monet "only an eye, but what an eye."[32] Inexplicably, the artists of the Ice Age chose to go in what was to be an unusual direction as they sought to achieve an increasingly greater graphic approximation of optical sensations.

It was with some reason that most prehistorians refused to believe that the paintings in Altamira cave were from the Ice Age when Marcellino Sanz de Sautuola and his little daughter, María, discovered them in 1879. At the time, the most prestigious authorities called the find a fake. Not the least reason for this belief was that Impressionism was the art style of the day. Many prehistorians thought they detected in the Altamira paintings the anachronistic influence of Impressionism. To these scholars the paintings smacked of contemporary forgery, and it did not help that an Impressionist painter friend of Sautuola's had been visiting not long before the ceiling was discovered. The people who were empowered to authenticate the art did not take the trouble to visit Altamira themselves to examine the actual paintings. Almost a quarter of a century later they admitted their error. They were wrong in their arrogant rejection of Altamira, but they were right to see a kindred spirit linking the artists of Altamira and the followers of Turner and Monet.

The Psychology and Neurology of Outlined Figures

Acquiring the capacity to see outlines as containers of meaning is a momentous symbolic step. Very young children discover outlines independently as they play with pencil and crayon. At some point in their experiments with line, the end of a line comes back to its beginning and a closed figure results. The space within this outline takes on a life of its own. The child may see it as an animal or, more likely, a person. Psychologists and art therapists call these figures "cephalopods" because children initially regard the circlelike form as a head from which they cause arms and legs to sprout. This trajectory from outline to cephalopod seems to be a universal phase in the ultimate depiction of the human form.

Howard Gardner, the psychologist, says that outlines "operate as a 'figure' against a background, and create an impression of solidity, substance, thingness."[33] Circles, for example, even those that are not completely closed, may be viewed as sun, moon, bodies, breasts, faces, eyes, or any number of other figures. It is possible that we humans are not the only animals to interpret lines as actual objects. It is much more surprising to learn that the psychologist John M. Kennedy and others have found that even animals such as crows and fish sometimes mistake line pictures for objects.[34] A miraculous coincidence is that lines—whether in ocher on stone or in pencil on paper—produced by human arms and hands have cognates in our perceived world. Almost universally these motor-stimulated lines that enclose space on a flat surface are seen as figures in the three-dimensional world. The spontaneous human interpretation of outlines and contours as figures originates from a serendipitous fallacy. Representational art is, in fact, founded on an illusion that we surely share with our Ice Age ancestors.

The Science of Perception

Perception occurs not in our eyes, as we must keep reminding ourselves, but in the brain. The cognitive process involved in our interpretation of perceived lines was first studied consistently by Gestalt psychologists working in the early part of the twentieth century. They took as their subject the perceptual organization of visual stimuli, and they formulated several "laws" to explain it. For example, the "law of closure" states that when a space is enclosed or nearly enclosed by a contour line, it tends to be interpreted as a figure, distinct from the overall ground on which it appears.

Cognitive scientists have found that line perception is an important step in our visual process.[35] Light signals, in the form of electromagnetic radiation, arrive at the photoreceptor cells on our retinas. The retina, the light-sensitive back surface of the eye, is composed of neural tissue that is an actual outgrowth of the brain. On the retina, the image is elaborately deconstructed, broken down by means of about 120 million rods and 70 million cones, each of which detects only one tiny fragment of the total image. The rods and cones convert light signals into electrochemical impulses, most of which travel from the eye to an area at the back of the brain known as the striate cortex, where visual space is mapped.

Figure 1.18. Four subjective contour lines appear form a square. They show how evenly spaced parallel lines can create a subjective line.

The striate cortex is broken up into segments, each corresponding to a specific tiny section of the retina. Within each segment, columns of cells react to lines. But they can be stimulated only by lines of a specific orientation—horizontal, vertical, or oblique. Certain nerve fibers seem to respond only to sharply defined edges. Other nerve cells in visual areas outside the striate cortex respond to more subtle properties. Some of these cells respond well to incomplete or suggested lines.[36] Indeed, our brains are so strongly predisposed to see lines that we can play tricks on ourselves such that we see what are called *subjective contours* where none actually exists. Beginning in the 1940s, psychologists, especially Gaetano Kanizsa, devised figures to demonstrate these imagined contours (fig. 1.18).

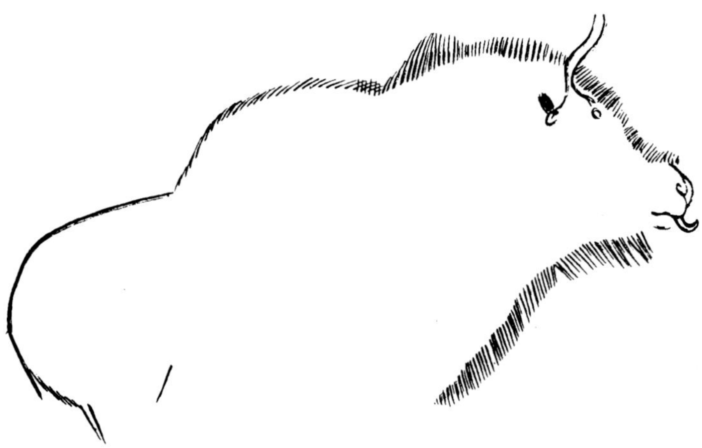

Figure 1.19. Bison at La Pasiega with head and neck indicated by the use of subjective line.

We have evidence that Paleolithic artists understood this phenomenon by at least 13,000 to 14,000 years ago. At Lascaux, for example, the manes and underbellies of horses and bison were almost invariably formed not with simple outlines but by the more indirect use of subjective contours suggested by the direction of the hair of the pelt, approximately a right angle to the imaginary line that our mind sees. At Lascaux, almost all the necks of horses were made with subjective contours created by the parallel lines used to depict the manes. We see the use of subjective contour very clearly in the dorsal and ventral lines of a bison from La Pasiega (fig. 1.19).

Of all the senses, it is the visual system that has most revealed itself to cognitive scientists. Visual signals are processed in more than 30 way stations, or "visual areas," in which the signals are encoded and analyzed in different ways, each area mapping the visual world.[37] All the information that has been painstakingly teased apart must finally be reconstructed in the brain, so that the process of seeing, extravagantly complicated though it is, seems in the end to have been immediate and effortless.

COLOR

A powerful element in the fundamental vocabulary of art is color. If even the chimpanzee Washoe was attracted to red, it is not surprising that this color attracted hominids far back in the human line. Again, the roots of *Homo sapiens sapiens'* aesthetic perception can be traced back at least to the higher primates. It is now known that the primate brain has specialized modules receptive to color. Other primates can respond aesthetically to color even if they cannot use it as we do. Red was one of the pigments most readily available to early humans and to artists in tribal societies around the world, because of the ubiquity of red ocher, an iron ore, in geological formations worldwide. Ocher comes in shades of red, yellow, brown, and purple, and artists have used them all, but red was the most common.

What color do you like best, Tatu?
Black, black!
And you, Washoe, what color?
Red, red!
Why?
Beautiful, beautiful!

—CONVERSATION BETWEEN TATU AND WASHOE, TWO "ART-MAKING" CHIMPS, AND THEIR TRAINER, IN AMERICAN SIGN LANGUAGE, QUOTED IN THIERRY LENAIN, *Monkey Painting*

The use of red ocher for marking purposes has been dated as far back as 900,000 to 800,000 years ago in South Africa.[38] In central Zambia, at Twin Rivers, 342 pieces of ocher in a variety of shades were abraded in a way that suggested they had been used as crayons. At Terra Amata in southern France, 400,000 to 200,000 years ago, members of the hominid species *Homo erectus* left more than 75 pieces of abraded ocher in shades of red, yellow, brown, and purple. Most of these showed wear consistent with a use for marking.

In southern India, at the site of Hungsi, a small red ocher pebble found in a Lower Paleolithic layer also appears to have been used for marking on rock. It is dated at 300,000 to 200,000 years ago. About the same time, a lump of red ocher from Becov Bohe, in the Czech Republic, appears to have been used for the same purpose. An ocher crayon from a site at Nooitgedacht, South Africa, dates from approximately the same period.

Pieces of ocher have been found in a Zimbabwean shelter in association with material more than 125,000 years old. At the burial site of Pech de l'Azé (Dordogne), dated between 300,000 and 120,000 years ago, some fragments of red and yellow ocher were found along with more than 100 fragments of manganese dioxide that were used as black pigment. Many Neanderthal sites include pieces of red ocher and black manganese, rounded and pointed like pencils. Other Mousterian sites more recent than 40,000 years ago with red pigment showing signs of abrasion are Arcy-sur-Cure (Yonne), France, and El Castillo and Cueva Morin, (Cantabria) Spain. Red or black pieces that appear to have been used for marking have been found at about a dozen European Paleolithic sites.

Red ocher has a long history of utilitarian usage. It was employed in tanning leather and may have been used in burials to induce a kind of mummification. It is an insect and parasite repellent in many parts of the world even today, and it has played a role in medicine because of its antiseptic properties and its ability, as a styptic, to stanch blood flow. These practical uses do not preclude other, symbolic uses of red ocher.

The mineral was frequently associated with burial in both Neanderthal and *Homo sapiens sapiens* sites beginning 100,000 years ago. Some uses are intriguing. Red ocher was found on the head of a skeleton at La Chapelle aux Saings in France and on two skeletons at Qafzeh, Israel. In a triple sepulcher at Grimaldi (Liguria), Italy, a thick coating of red ocher was placed over the tops of the heads, as if it were a skullcap. A strange triple burial took place at Dolní Vestonice, a settlement site in the Pavlov Hills near Brno in the Czech Republic. The heads appear to have been sprinkled with red ocher. The single female skeleton had a large patch of red ocher between the thighs, and one of the two males had his hand positioned over her vulva.[39]

At Sungir, near Moscow, at least 25,000 years ago, the bodies of two young boys were laid head to head. When the burial was excavated, their clothing had disintegrated, but the ornamentation that probably had been sewn onto the clothing remained. It consisted of some 3,500 beads of mammoth ivory spread in rows across the entire body, from forehead to ankles. Around this sumptuous burial the earth was stained bright red.

The use of red ocher for burial has also been found in Australia, Southeast Asia, the Middle East, Anatolia, and North America. Around the Great Lakes and northward, two archaic groups that date from about 4,000 years ago, the Glacial Kame people and the Red Paint people, lined burial pits with red ocher. The latter group was named for its prolific use of pigment in this practice.

The most striking use of red ocher, and the one that most concerns us, was in prehistoric art making. Red ocher has been found near paintings in many of the caves in France and Spain, often in the form of crayons, or perhaps more accurately, pastels. Whole blocks of ocher pigment appear to have been dipped in water, possibly to intensify their color. Mortars and pestles for grinding ocher were found at Lascaux. Stones with indentations that were used to hold pigment have been found, and so have shells for the same purpose: a barnacle shell at Tito Bustillo (Asturias), Spain, an oyster shell at Lascaux, two limpet shells at Altamira, and a large sea scallop shell at Mas d'Azil (Ariège), on which one can see the marks of the brush. Palettes may predate *Homo sapiens sapiens* in France; they have been found containing ocher or stained with it at the Neanderthal site of Arcy-sur-Cure

Prehistoric people all over the world have used red ocher in their art. Australia has a number of examples. At the site of Makakanja II, investigators found ocher near a rock painting in which it most likely had been used. At Nauwalabila I on the East Alligator River, specimens of red ocher that show traces of grinding were found with material dated from 60,000 to 30,000 years old. In Queensland, a partly ground block of ocher, a sandstone preparation slab, and ocher crayons were discovered beneath the main panel of Magnificent Gallery near Laura. Kenniff Cave Site yielded 1,248 pieces of ocher. In Africa, a Namibian ocher-stained palette is dated to 29,000 years ago. Beyond the extensive use of red ocher for painting on cave walls, many traces of red have been left on Paleolithic sculpture and artifacts. A 100,000-year-old plaque of mammoth ivory from Tata, Hungary, smoothed and then polished—perhaps by frequent handling as an amulet—had been colored red. The remarkable bas-relief carvings at Laussel (Dordogne) were originally covered with red ocher. A panel of horses at Cap Blanc was also colored red, although now only close inspection reveals traces of the pigment. The archaeologist Paul Bahn states that many bas-reliefs and many examples of portable art, including the generously rotund female figurine known as the Venus of Willendorf, were once painted red. Only fragments of the color can be seen now; most of the pigment has been erased by tens of thousands of years of weathering.

Some people in preindustrial societies managed to mine red ocher in staggering quantities. Between 43,000 and 10,000 years ago in Africa, approximately 1,200 metric tons of iron oxide were removed from a cliff in the area of Lion Cavern in Swaziland. The collecting of ocher could be surrounded by rituals and taboos. Until the first half of the twentieth century, Australian Aborigines still mined two major traditional ocher sources. Because the mines had special sacred significance, women and uninitiated men were not allowed in the vicinity. At one site the red ocher was considered to be the blood of a giant ancestral kangaroo, Wilgie Mia, who had been killed by an evil spirit during the Dreamtime. Seams of yellow ocher were called its liver. Aboriginals leaving the site retreated backward, disguising their tracks so that the evil spirit Mondong could not follow. The journey to the site became a pilgrimage in which supplicants brought gifts for the custodians of the mine. Such pigment mining is a ritual reminiscent of the American Indian salt-gathering ritual in the U.S. Southwest, a pilgrimage people still make from Zuñi to the tribe's sacred salt lake, as well as the Hopi salt-gathering pilgrimage from Oraibi to the Grand Canyon, a distance of about 125 kilometers. There is a parallel, especially if we think of red ocher as a seasoning for the eyes.

The Symbolism of Red

Red is the first color word to have entered the vocabulary of all known languages. In some primitive languages red is the only color named, other than black and white.[40] No matter how it was referred to verbally, the color red almost certainly held symbolic meaning for Ice Age artists. The association of red with blood and hence with life seems to be very ancient. The Hebrew word for blood is *dam,* and for red earth, *adamah.* In the Bible the first human male was named Adam because he was made of this red earth. The Greek word for blood is *haema,* which is the prefix for hematite, or red earth.[41]

The symbolic use of red can be documented in some contemporary tribal societies. The ceremonial pipe of the Sioux—their most sacred possession—is made of a red mineral called pipestone or catlinite. It is found only in southwestern Minnesota and is believed by the tribe to have been formed from the congealed blood of the Sioux ancestors, innumerable dead, caught in an immense ancient flood. The bodies of these ancestors, says the legend, formed a lake of blood that was ultimately compressed into a special stone. Only stone of this blood-red color can be used for the sacred pipes.[42]

The Algonkian people of northern Ontario, Canada, believe that red ocher came from the blood of giant beavers who long ago changed the shape of the land. They also have stories that refer to this pigment as the dried blood of huge sea serpents. Dan Pine, an elder and medicine man from Garden River Indian Reserve, near Sault Sainte Marie, Ontario, said, "Red is a very spiritual color. . . . The spiritual people painted the rock just like the spirits painted the animal's fur. The red paint has a blend of power that overcomes the evil power."[43] Several American Indian tribes continue even now to collect red ocher for healing purposes.

The power of red pigment continues into contemporary times. "Red is my favorite color, definitely," said the French-American sculptor Louise Bourgeois in a statement curiously reminiscent of that of Washoe the chimp. To enlarge on this she added, "It is violent, it is the color of blood."[44]

Other Colors

Color has been used in art making from the earliest examples. At first pigments were to be found only in the naturally occurring iron oxides—red, brown, and yellow—and in manganese dioxide and charcoal for black. By 17,000 years ago a fuller range of colors became available when it was discovered that variations could be created by heating the minerals and by making mixtures of these natural earths with minerals such as calcite and substances such as animal bone.[45] At Niaux, artists devised mixtures of pigment with extenders and binders. At Cougnac they developed a complex method of changing the local yellow ocher into red. Artists were able to get a violet shade by mixing black manganese dioxide with certain reds. One sees this violet at Lascaux and at Tito Bustillo. By mixing the black with yellow ocher, they achieved green. To our eyes, accustomed to a wider range of more brilliant pigments, the subtleties may go largely unnoticed.

Elsewhere in the world artists were also experimenting with pigments. A soft, earthy, yellow ocher called limonite is a natural excrescence on some cave ceilings. It was used in South African rock art for yellow, and it could be heated to produce orange, umber, claret, or black. In addition to the more commonly used carbon and manganese ore, black could be made using burned bone. Pipe clay was used for white in prehistoric Australia and in some areas of North America but not, to my knowledge, in Ice Age Europe. The white found in South African paintings was made from kaolin, gypsum, clay, lime, and even much less permanent termite material and bird guano. A unique blue handprint has been found in a newly discovered cave at Vilhonneur (Charente), France, but at this writing, information about the pigment is unavailable.

The Aesthetics, Affect, and Neuroscience of Color

Most people find a beautiful sunset inspiring, perhaps breathtaking, for a reason we can describe only as aesthetic. It has been suggested that we may share this response with some other primates. A student named Geza Teleki was observing chimpanzees at the Gombe Reserve in Tanzania as the sun set over Lake Tanganyika. He saw two adult male chimpanzees climb separately to the top of the ridge. The animals did not see the student but greeted each other.[46] In a similar example, the Dutch primatologist Adriaan Kortlandt recorded a wild chimpanzee gazing at a spectacular sunset for a full 15 minutes until darkness fell.[47] Humans find pleasure in the grandeur, the evanescence, the array of colors in sunsets and are moved. The Zuñis have a term, *tso'ya,* for the particular aesthetic experience of sunsets; it also includes rainbows and iridescent bird and insect wings.[48]

Color affects our body's responses: "Colors can influence blood pressure, heartbeat, breathing rate, perspiration and even brain wave patterns."[49] Color evokes emotions, a phenomenon that is imbedded in our language. We speak of "seeing red" or being in a "black mood." In our society green suggests envy, and yellow, cowardice. The word *blue* stands for a school of music that conveys a specific mood. Henri Matisse, one of the great colorists, wrote that "simple colors can act upon the inner feelings with all the more force because they are simple. A blue, for instance, accompanied by the shimmer of its complementaries, acts upon the feelings like a sharp blow on a gong. The same with red and yellow and the artist must be able to sound them when he needs to."[50]

Temple Grandin, who is both autistic and a scientist, has written a great deal about her experiences. She says she finds a sunset pretty but nothing more. "I know it's beautiful, but I don't get it." Although she has perfect pitch, she does not relate to music. Nor does music move her. She didn't "get music," she said—didn't "see what it was about."[51] Although she is unusually gifted in spatial concepts and describes herself as a visual thinker, she does not respond emotionally to visual stimuli or to visual art. She has the sense that, for her, some vital connection is missing.

Grandin believes that she and other autistic people have impaired linkages of their visual and auditory sensations to the phylogenetically ancient, emotion-inducing part of the brain. This part of the midbrain, called the limbic system, consists of cell clusters interconnected by long C-shaped fiber tracts. These clusters include the hypothalamus, the hippocampus, the anterior cingulate, and the amygdala, the activation of which is especially important in stimulating emotions.[52] If this is true, then, as the neurologist Oliver Sacks believes, Grandin's mind's impaired connection with the limbic system makes her immune to the emotional content of art. People who for one reason or another have lost this connection often describe everything as appearing monochromatic. A world with diminished emotional response is like a world without color. Drug addicts in withdrawal describe life as gray.

Our emotional response to color is puzzling. After all, the perception of color is merely the result of an operation by the brain on reflected light waves. Receptors in the visual cortex devote their energy to making comparisons between the wavelengths of a selected area and those of its surroundings. This procedure is done separately for the long, middle, and short wavelengths of light. The resulting ratios, computed with remarkable speed, are interpreted by our brains as color.[53]

Although the perception of color is therefore only a comparison the brain makes among ratios of light waves as recorded by the cones in the retina, the results do somehow touch our emotions. This raw feel of sensation, called *qualia,* has presented a problem to philosophers and biologists, who are unable to explain it satisfactorily. Although in a sense unreal, color sensations seem very real and can evoke strong visceral responses. In one example, a 50-year-old man who had been blind from early childhood had surgery that enabled him to regain a great deal of his sight. Oliver Sacks, who followed this patient's reaction to the surgery, wrote that "seeing colors, above all, had been completely unexpected and had a physical and emotional impact almost shocking, explosive." Sacks quoted another patient who had experienced a similar regaining of sight. This patient, too, spoke of the profound experience of once again having color in his world. "I felt the violence of these sensations like a blow on the head," he said.[54]

Painters are often particularly vulnerable to color sensations. Breyten Breytenbach, the South African poet-painter, described how he felt in prison, where he was held in solitary confinement for three years. Under these conditions of sensory deprivation, he wrote that "if even just a thread of material drifted up over the wall you cannot possibly imagine the intensity of the experience. It was as if you'd never seen color before in your life." When released after seven and a half years, he described his return to the act of painting: "There was this richness in just basking in the absolute glory of handling brushes and tubes of paint, simply for their own sake. And then, of course, there was the hunger for color itself: color quite apart from what it means or any of its associations, just color as such—the mad wonderful yowl of it."[55]

The German artist Max Beckmann, a medical corpsman during the First World War, drew many of the horrors he saw. He was limited to drawing in black and white, and in a letter to his wife he expressed a longing to be able to work in color: "Oh I wish I could paint again, color is an instrument which I cannot do without for much longer. If I only think of gray, green, and white, of blackish yellow, sulfuric yellow and violet, a shudder of lust runs down my spine."[56] It seems that the colors he longed for were those that might express the nightmare world in which was then enmired.

Neurologically, we inherit from our primate ancestors, specifically the Old World apes, a color vision system. The primate brain has specialized modules concerned with color, but color perception developed inconsistently in the evolution of primates. The New World monkeys have a simpler kind of color vision that is based on two opsins—visual pigments that are sensitive to particular light wavelengths—and therefore recognizes fewer colors. The Old World monkeys have color vision similar to our own, based on three opsins. Trichromate (three-color) vision began as a mutation about 55 million years ago. Two-color vision had already been in existence for 200 million years at that point.[57] This wider range of color perception gives us access to the three primary colors and thus to a vast spectrum of other colors, enabling us to experience the pleasure of the rainbow. Identification of potential food ranks high among the uses of vision. Arboreal, herbivorous creatures empowered with color vision could much more easily have distinguished ripe fruit from a dense canopy of green leaves. This does not really explain how the perception of color, evolved for utilitarian purposes such as food gathering, became so deeply linked with those parts of the brain concerned with emotion.

When two colors with close wavelengths are juxtaposed—for example, cerulean and cobalt blue, or, on the red end of the spectrum, vermilion and magenta—we experience something like a vibration. It is almost the same effect that comes from the rapid alternation of two close musical notes in a trill. In a sense, it is a color trill. The effect is similar in both color perception and in music. In both instances there results a frisson, a shudder of excitation, as if we had experienced a small electrical charge.

Beginning with the work of Paul MacLean in the 1950s, emotion began to be thought of as consisting of a linked group of structures at the top of the brain stem and at the edge (or "limbus") of the cerebral hemispheres.[58] The limbic system acts as a major switching station, turning external stimuli into emotional responses and emotional responses into action as excitation travels from the hypothalamus to the brain stem. The hypothalamus directs the pituitary gland to secrete hormones, and those messengers aim their chemical excitation toward specific cells in the body. Two limbic structures, the amygdala and the cingulate gyrus, appear to be important in the initial forging of emotional reactions. Three structures, the amygdala, the orbitofrontal cortex, and the cingulate gyrus, are known to control anger, pleasure, and aggressiveness. Researchers in neural science such as Joseph LeDoux now believe that our emotions are not so entirely localized but also involve feedback from other areas of the brain.[59] Light waves are processed in a variety of places, and the resulting color construct somehow stimulates our emotion centers. It acts as a catalyst for increased associative and imaginative powers in our brains as a whole. Color makes us feel more intensely alive.

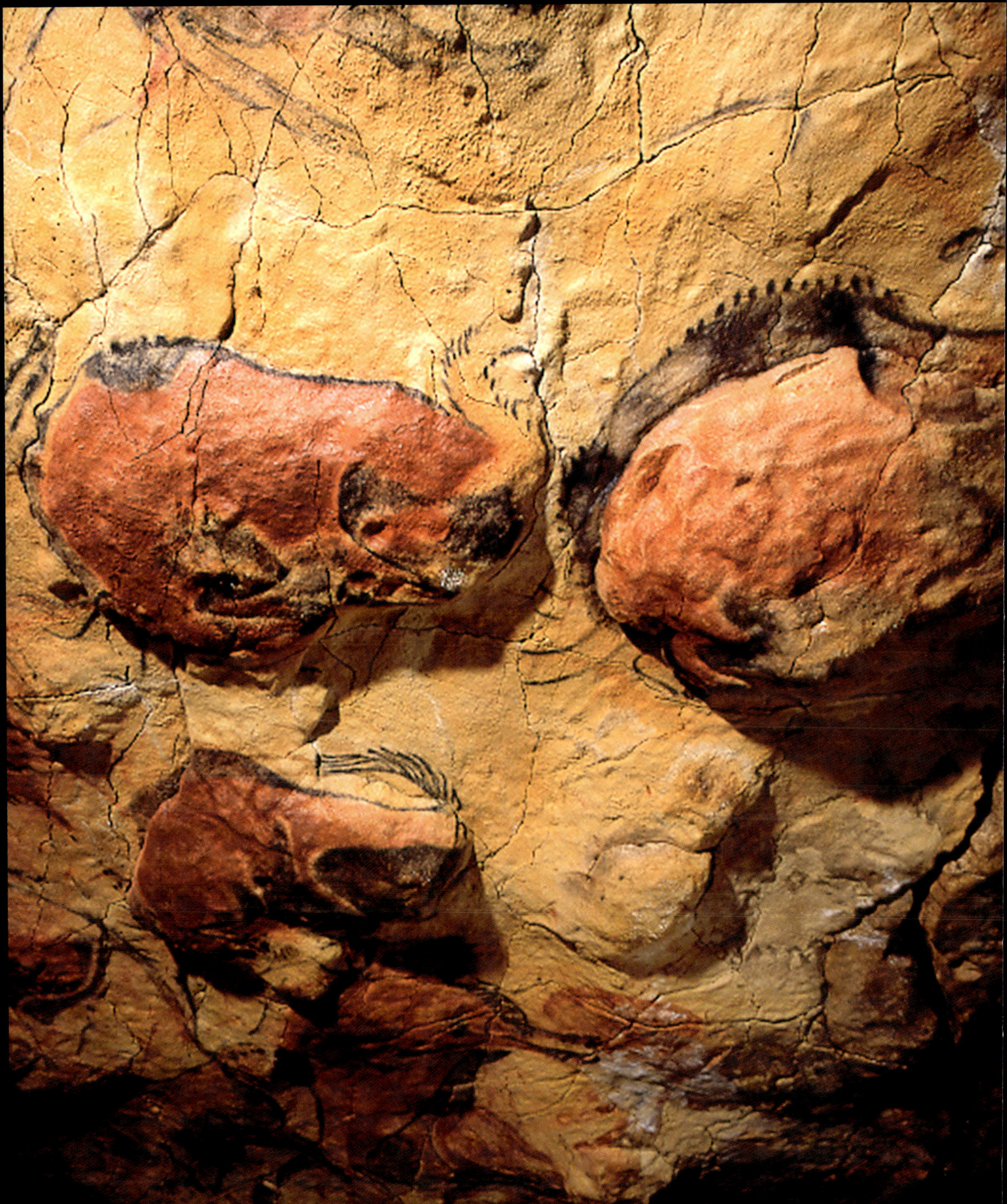

2

BASIC STRUCTURES

The Syntax of the Ice Age Artist

THE FUNDAMENTAL ELEMENTS that Ice Age artists used—marks, dots, lines, figures, and color—can be thought of as a vocabulary on which their image making was based. When such elements are put together in a specific way, we can think of the resulting structures as a kind of syntax. I use the word *syntax* loosely, to parallel its use in language, but it should be understood that calling art a language is metaphorical rather than literal. Syntax, as I use it here, is a way of structuring or composing elements. Two of the most common ways of structuring imagery in the Ice Age and onward have been by using symmetry and by using repetition, often with variation.

Our urge to recognize order . . . in my opinion, this is the basic function of art.

—IRENAUS EIBL-EIBESFELDT, *Beauty and the Brain*

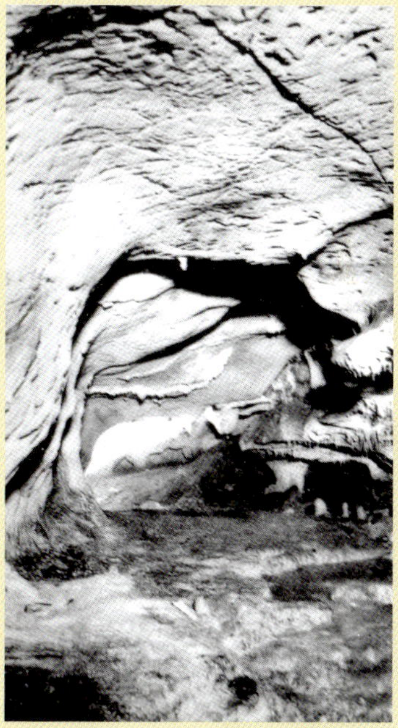

Figure 2.1. A view from the entrance of the cave of El Castillo gives some idea of the tortured surfaces on which Ice Age artists often worked.

Oppsite: Bison on the Polychrome Ceiling at Altamira cave, Spain. C.14,500 B.P. Photo by P.A. Saura Ramos. © Museo de Altamira

Basic to artistic syntax is the fundamental goal of imposing order on the apparent chaos of the perceived natural world.[1] Most caves present chaotic morphological interiors and appear totally unstructured to the human eye. Stone seems to have been twisted and tortured by geological forces (fig. 2.1). Ice Age artists who entered these caves seem to have felt a need, perhaps without being fully aware of it, to bring order out of this chaos. In selected places they took the writhing cave surfaces, full of disordered shapes, and attempted to unify them within an ordered context while also transmitting their more overt messages.

Not far into the small but important cave of Bernifal (Dordogne) is a large pendant of rock brought to life as a bison with the mere addition of two red circles for eyes. Its lowered head and outthrust horns face toward the cave entrance as if to guard against unwelcome intruders. Ice Age artists often imagined rocky formations as animate. The late Magdalenian cave of Font de Gaume (Dordogne), once a rival of Lascaux in majesty, reveals now only a shadow of its former greatness. There, counter to expectation, many incurving surfaces were used to suggest the bulky forms of bison. At both Bernifal (Dordogne) and Font de Gaume, artists gave the irregular surfaces some ordered purpose in a human-directed scheme. At Altamira the ceiling, rough with protruding formations, was tamed by using these forms to create a painted bas-relief of a herd of bison. It is one of the masterpieces of Ice Age art (see illus. p. 40).

Another masterpiece made by imposing order on chaos can be seen at Lascaux. Artists scanned the chaotic surface and the meaningless shapes and then worked them to create comprehensible images. They used leaps of imagination to tie together aleatory natural forms. These forms were subsumed into organized images and given graphic life that radiates power. In one instance, rock outcroppings became the hip and rump of the animal, in this case an aurochs, and nearby depressions indicated the belly. Several adjacent ridges were linked into the line of the backbone. We can almost feel the pleasure the artist took in wresting order from the confusion presented by the cave surfaces.

Often the artists portrayed the great herbivores, remote and powerful like the bison and mammoth or swift and strong like the reindeer and horse. In the Rotunda they painted giant aurochs, one of which is 5.5 m long. The animals race toward the opening of the Axial Gallery and leap onto the walls and ceiling. Animals circle the ceiling or the rounded recesses. A circular composition is important in several Ice Age caves, such as in Niaux's great domed, Pantheon-like Salon Noir and also in Altamira's Polychrome Chamber. At Lascaux, animals are often shown in procession, one following the other. Larger animals are superimposed on earlier, smaller images. They stand proud and immobile in the Nave. These great animals, in all their potency and power, dominate the once inchoate spaces and thus organize and humanize the cave.

With the paintings in place, Lascaux took on awesome but comprehensible dimensions and conveyed meanings to which the Ice Age interlopers could relate. The fearsome underground seemed a little tamer. In this hostile subterranean world, the artist could experience some feeling of control. The dark was illuminated with figures, and meaning was imposed. Few great artworks have comparably achieved the imaging of a belief system: the carved and painted cave temples at Ellora and Ajanta in India, Giotto's Scrovegni Chapel in Padua, and Michelangelo's Sistine Chapel are among those in which artists have undertaken to depict an entire cosmology. We can well imagine that Ice Age artists, in making their art, experienced the exhilaration that all humans feel in imposing human order on an otherwise incomprehensible world.

SYMMETRY

Symmetry is one of the tools of organization in art making, and artists refer to such organization as composition. Initially, Paleolithic wall art may seem devoid of symmetry, but after a first impression of randomness one discovers an underlying order, an attempt to create a balance of figures, often by means of approximate symmetry. The satisfying resonance of approximate symmetry can be likened to that of slant rhymes, or approximate rhymes, in poetry.

Symmetry, the elementary aesthetic form. . .
—FRANZ BOAS, *Primitive Art*

The renowned archaeologist André Leroi-Gourhan was among the first researchers to point out examples of mirror symmetry in Ice Age art.[2] He used this term to indicate a balance between parts on either side of an implied central, vertical axis. A figure on one side of the axis would be a reverse of its counterpart on the other side, in the same way that one's face is reversed in a mirror. Other terms for this are *symmetry of reflection, bilateral symmetry,* and, more technically, *enantiomorphism*. Possibly our bias in favor of such mirror-image spatial organization is that we ourselves are creatures organized, in large part, according to bilateral symmetry.[3]

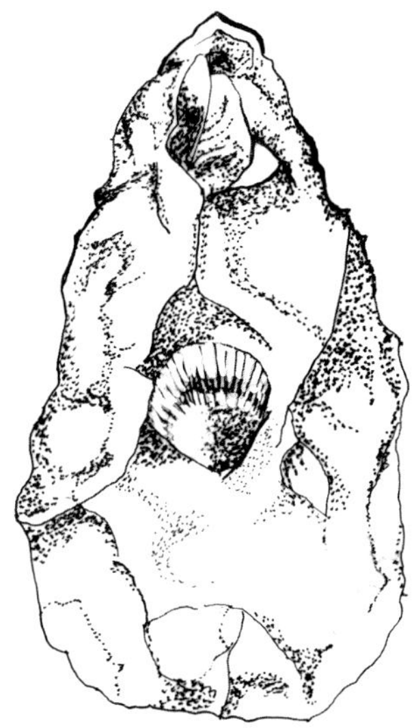

Figure 2.2. Hand ax with fossil bivalve mollusk shell in center, from West Tofts, England, 200,000–250,000 years old. About 13 cm.

We can find examples of symmetry far back in the hominid line. About 250,000 years ago, tool makers living in what is now England fabricated hand axes, universal tools that hominids had already been knapping in much the same way for at least one and a half million years. The tool maker selected a stone, usually flint, that would fracture into sharp fragments when hit and then pounded it symmetrically on both faces and both sides. When finished, the tool was boat shaped so that it could be held conveniently with the blunt edge in the palm of the hand. During its long history the hand ax remained technologically little changed.

Among the English examples, several hand axes have fossils imbedded in the stone—one a seashell, a bivalve mollusk (fig. 2.2), and the other a fossil echinoid with a striking star-shaped pattern. These date from about 250,000 years ago. Each stone ax was worked so that the fossil was left in a central part of the tool. Much later, between 90,000 and 38,000 years ago, a Neanderthal craftsman from the Quercy region of France made a tool, probably a scraper, also with a fossil bivalve imbedded in its center (fig. 2.3). Archaeologists have found other, similar examples. All these tool makers used flaws in their material to make something that was more than useful. It is difficult to believe that they left the fossils in the center of the stone by chance. The craftsman's strategy had to have been carefully premeditated to control the placement of the

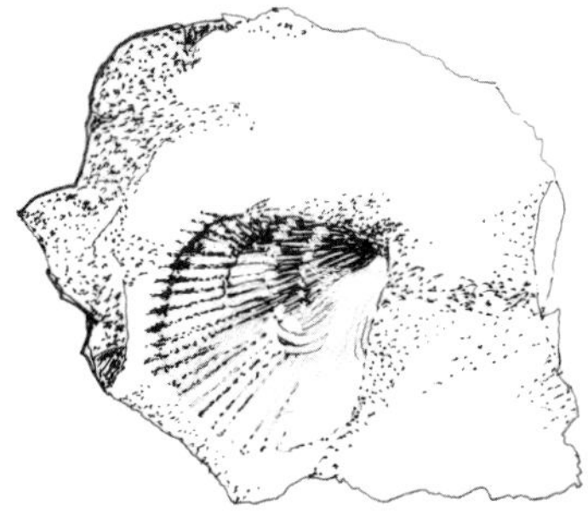

Figure 2.3. A Paleolithic tool, probably a scraper, with a fossil bivalve mollusk shell in the center, from Pech-Merle.

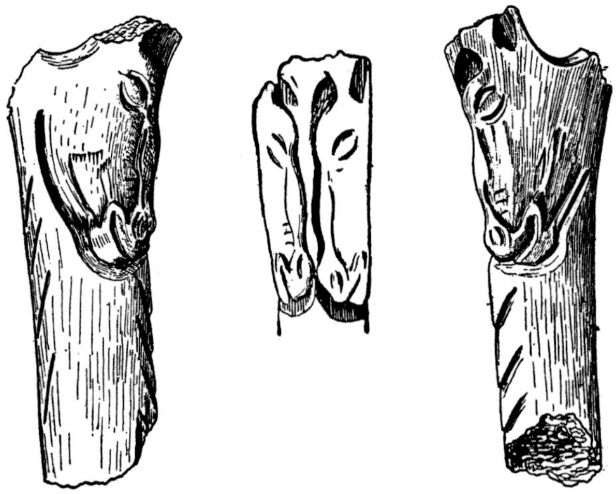

Figure 2.4. Heads of two reindeer sculpted in the round on a perforated reindeer horn from La Madeleine. The antler is positioned to show each reindeer on the sides and can be turned to show the two heads face to face.

fossil. An intent to achieve symmetry must have been constantly in the knapper's mind the entire time the stone was being worked. To have inspired such extra effort, symmetry appears to have been a structure of intrinsic value.

Mirror symmetry exerted a special fascination for Ice Age artists as well as craftsmen. The archaeologist A.-C. Welté found about 100 instances of it, in both portable and parietal art.[4] From La Madeleine (Dordogne), a reindeer horn achieves symmetry by showing reindeer heads facing one another (fig. 2.4). Two mammoths touch heads on a pierced staff from Les Eyzies. A spear thrower carved of antler and found in the deep cave of Trois Frères is surmounted by two reindeer confronting each other as if in embattled embrace. On a plaquette from Gönnersdorf, Germany, two females in profile face each other to create a mirror image (fig. 2.5).

On cave walls there are even more examples of symmetry. At Roc du Sers (Charente), two ibex symmetrically confront each other in a limestone bas relief. Two of the large, painted, naturalistic aurochs in the Rotunda at Lascaux face one another symmetrically. In the Axial Gallery there, two horses stand face to face. Two mammoths mirror each other at Rouffignac (fig. 2.6), and two bison face each other at Le Portel. Two horses are symmetrical to one another at El Castillo (fig. 2.7).

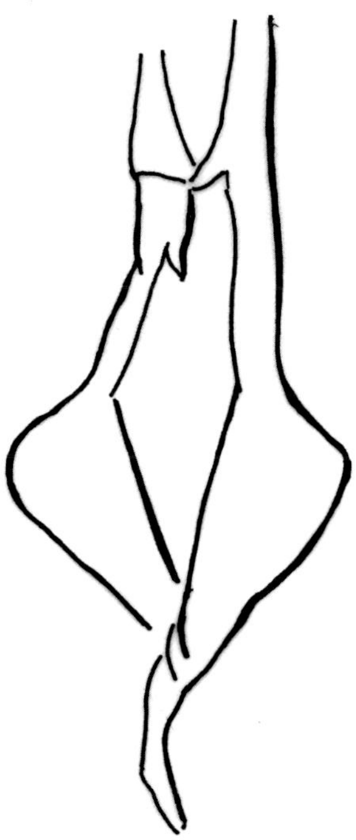

Figure 2.5. On a stone plaquette from Gönnersdorf, Rheinland-Pfalz, Germany, two schematic female figures face each other in a near mirror image that creates an abstract design. Each figure 10.6 cm high.

One of the most surprisingly sophisticated examples of symmetry in Ice Age art occurs at La Magdaleine (Tarn). Two realistic, reclining, nude female figures are sculpted in low relief on either side of the outer wall of the cave with their legs pointing toward the entrance (fig. 2.8). Because of their exposure to weather they are quite eroded, but one can make out the two women leaning on their elbows, legs flexed and slightly parted. It is more difficult to make out the animal figures that accompany the females, a horse on the right wall and a bison on the left.

Symmetry has appealed to many other prehistoric people. Certain American Indian art styles are noted for their use of mirror symmetry, particularly the styles of the Woodland Indians of the Northeast and the Jornada people, a Mogollon group related to the better-known Mimbres culture, in the South-

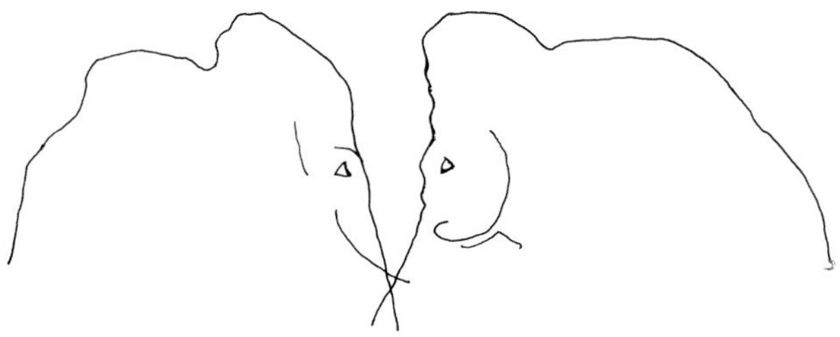

Figure 2.6. Two confronted painted male mammoths at Rouffignac, about 13,000 B.P.

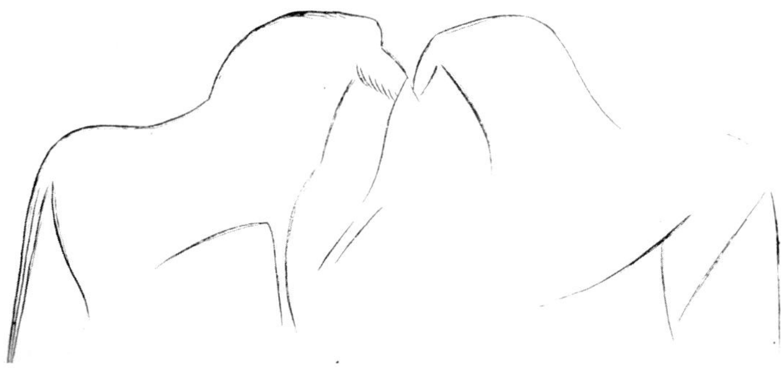

Figure 2.7. Two finely engraved horses face one another symmetrically in El Castillo.

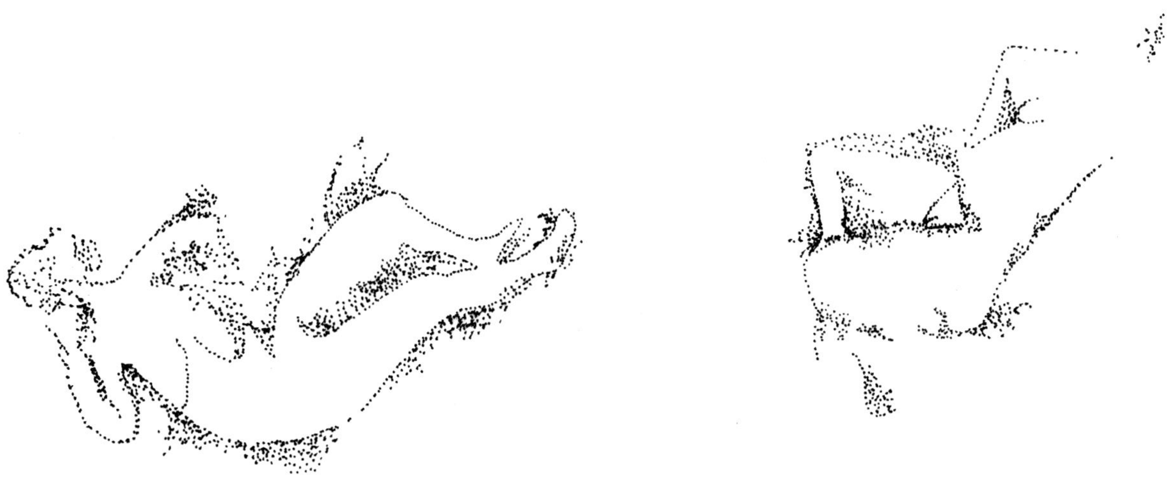

Figure 2.8. Symmetrically placed, reclining nude women at La Magdeleine. These unique images flank the opening to a rock shelter. Lengths 91 and 100 cm; height of each about 70 cm.

west.[5] Much of Northwest Coast graphic art is bilaterally symmetrical, a style achieved by graphically splitting an animal's image and reassembling it as two adjoining, identical halves (see fig. 1.12). Northwest Coast sculpture is balanced in the same way.

Tribal art often aspires to symmetry, but there are exceptions. Near symmetry may be unexpectedly broken, and broken symmetry may be preferred for its innovative excitement. Some tribal people, such as those from Dahomey in Africa, Alor in Malaysia, and Bali in Indonesia, favor asymmetry. As a rule,

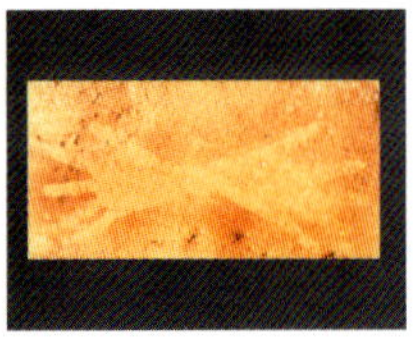

Figure 2.9. Negative double hand image pictograph, Queensland, Australia.

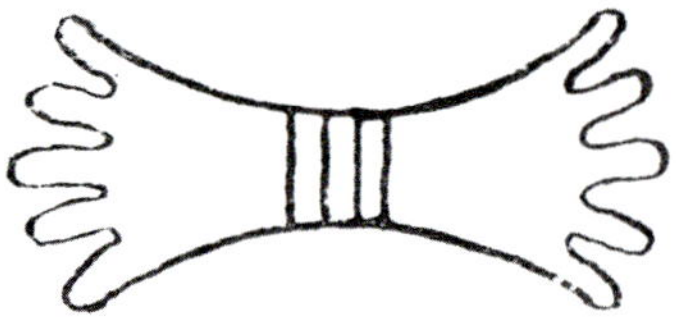

Figure 2.10. Outstretched hands joined at the wrist, from a Hopi petroglyph in Arizona.

however, symmetry is preferred in most tribal societies.[6] A clear example of readily available imagery structured in a symmetrical presentation is a double hand image from a rockshelter in Queensland, Australia (fig. 2.9). Some Pueblo people of North America used a very similar configuration (fig. 2.10).

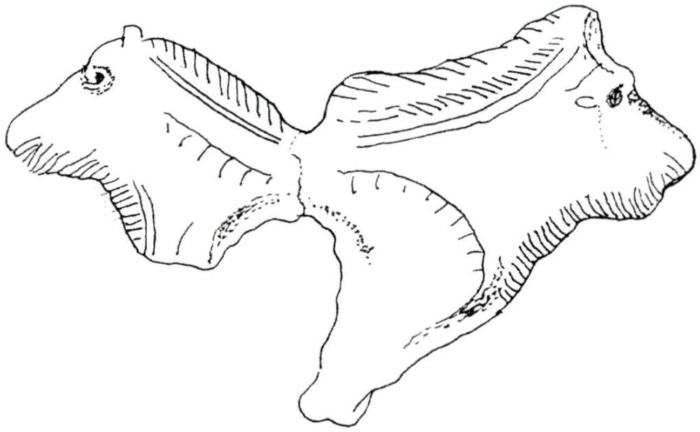

Figure 2.11. Two bison heads, possibly male and female, appear to share one body around a hole in a pierced staff from Laugerie Basse.

Double Heads

The most common expression of bilateral symmetry is the double-headed figure. Symmetrical, two-headed figures are found on all continents.[7] Side-by-side heads are the most common; Janus-style, back-to-back heads are much rarer. It is unusual, but not unknown, to have two heads joined at the top or scalp. The double head theme occurs all over the world, on all continents, and at all periods. It can be found, although infrequently, in the Ice Age caves. An example is a baton from the rockshelter of Laugerie Basse (Dordogne), on which a bison with two heads facing in opposite directions has a single body (fig. 2.11). In the Ice Age caves, double and even triple heads are seen on animals, but they rarely involve symmetrical compositions. In one example at Gabillou, however, two horse heads on a single neck face in opposite directions to create a mirror image (fig. 2.12).

Another example is seen at El Castillo (fig. 2.13).

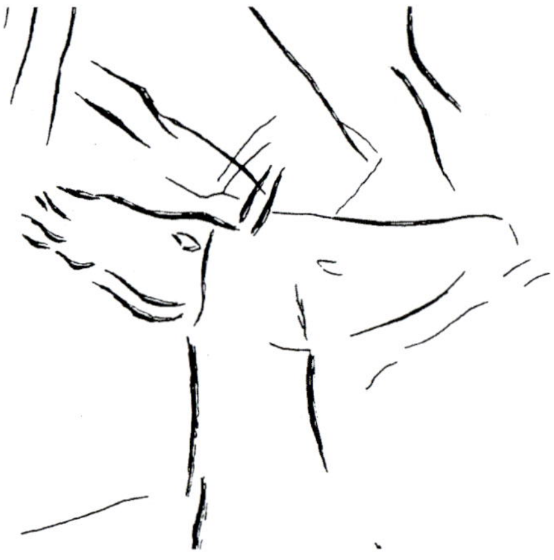

2.12. Horse with two heads in mirror image, from the Red Chamber at Gabillou.

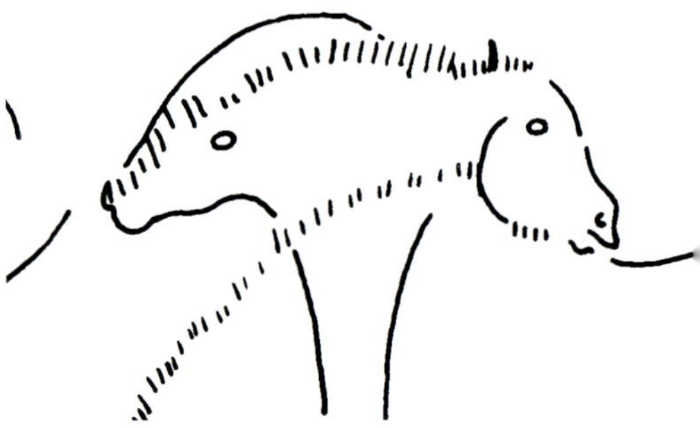

Figure 2.13. Schematic and finely engraved horses in symmetrical position from El Castillo.

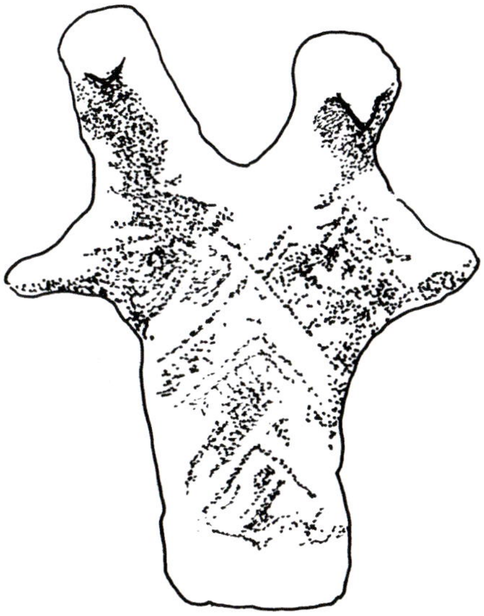

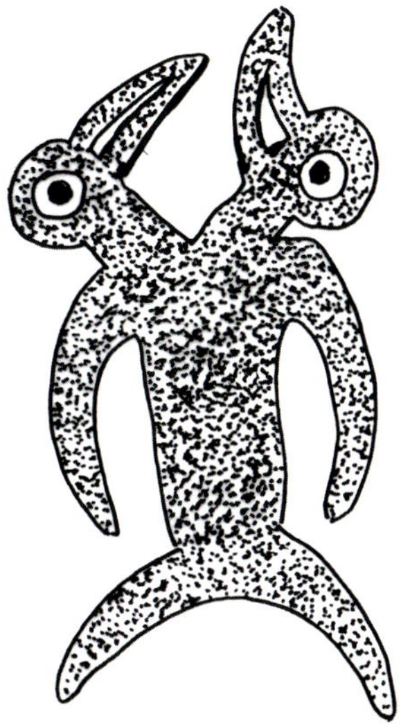

Figure 2.14. Double-headed figure from the Neolithic Vinca culture, which flowered in the Danube River basin about 7.000 B.P.

Figure 2.15. Two-headed bird, Easter Island.

Symmetrical double-headed figures were common during the Neolithic period. The earliest known example, dated to about 8500 B.P., was found at Çatal Hüyük, Turkey. Many have been discovered in the central Balkans (fig. 2.14). Double-headed animal imagery has been abundant throughout the American continents as well, from Eskimo art in the Arctic to indigenous art in Mesoamerica (especially among the Aztecs), South America, and even remote Easter Island (fig. 2. 15). The North American Mimbres pot painters of about 1,000 years ago, who lived in what is now Arizona and New Mexico, made use of inventive double-headed figures. Among numerous examples on their bowls is a fish painted with a single body but with two heads facing in opposite directions (fig. 2.16).

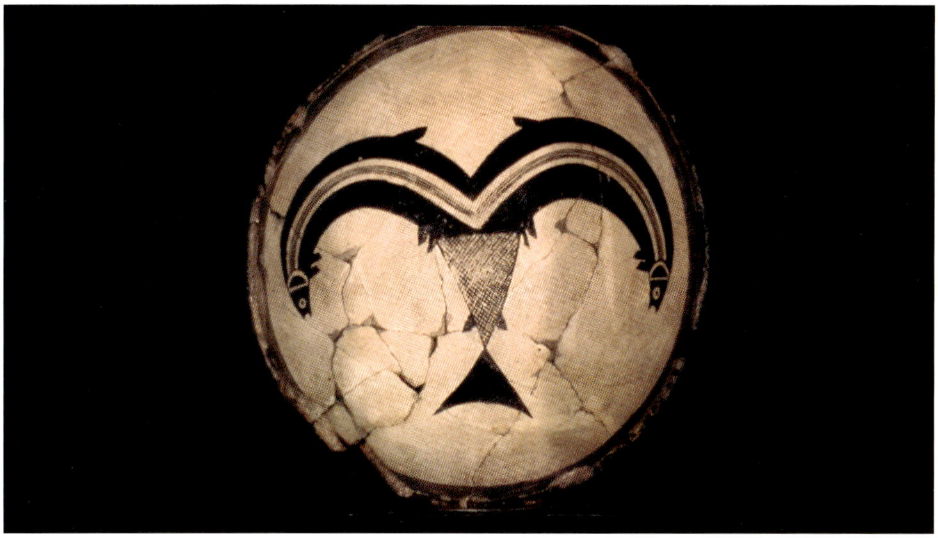

Figure 2.16. Painted Mimbres bowl depicting a two-headed fish. Height 8 cm, diameter 18.2 cm.

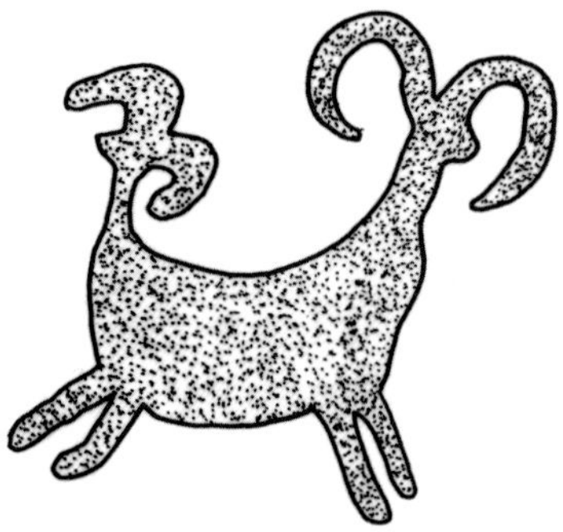

Figure 2.17. Petroglyph of a double-headed bighorn sheep, Renegade Canyon, Coso Range, California.

Symmetrical, two-headed animals are relatively common in American Indian rock art from widely separated areas. Some examples are found in the Great Basin sites of Renegade Canyon and Birchim Spring, California (fig. 2.17). There are petroglyphs depicting such animals from the Fremont culture of 1,500 to 700 years ago, and others from Moab, Utah. At Rochester Creek, Utah, there are two petroglyphs of double-headed bighorn sheep. A two-headed bird was pecked at Zuñi. At Three Rivers, New Mexico, a two-headed quadruped is unusual in that the heads face toward rather than away from each other (fig. 2.18).

The two-headed serpent is a common image in many parts of the world. It may have some basis in reality, enhanced by legend.[8] In the art of the San of southern Africa, the image of the double-headed snake was associated with San legends. A huge example at Birchenough Bridge, Zimbabwe, measures seven and a half feet across, even in its coiled state. In Europe, such a creature appeared as late as the Middle Ages as the monster snake with a head at each end, one of which was always awake.[9] The two-headed serpent is also seen in the Americas. There are petroglyph examples with a head on either end in the Rio Grande area, and a snake with two heads side by side is found in a petroglyph at Coyote Buttes, Arizona (fig. 2.19). Another important example is the Sisiutl of Northwest Coast Kwakiutl and Bella Coola art and legend. This is a double-headed sea serpent–spirit with snake heads at each end and a human head in the center. A

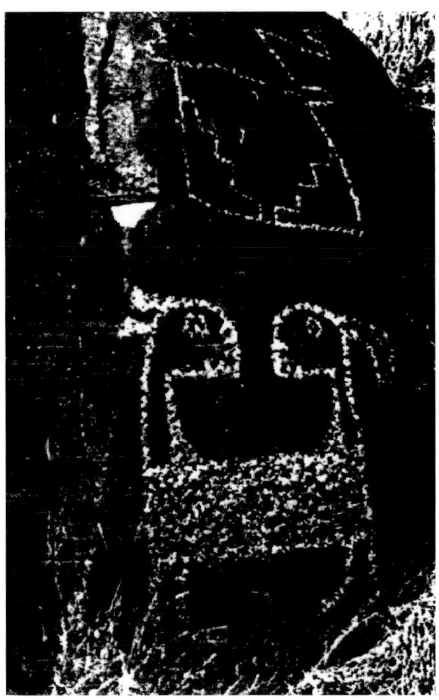

Figure 2.18. Double-headed animal petroglyph, Three Rivers, New Mexico.

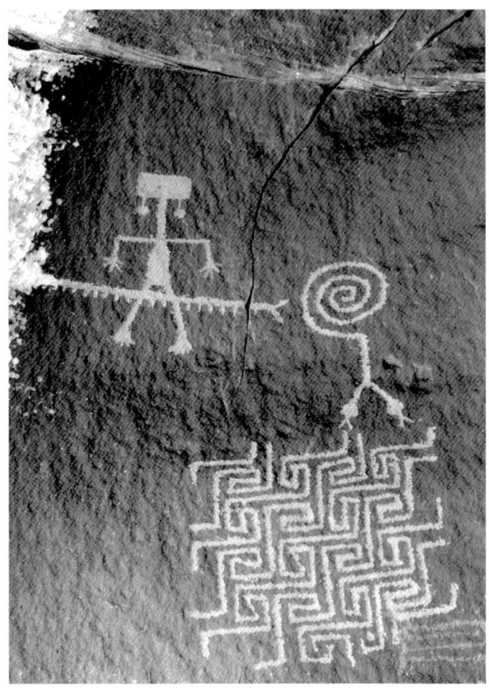

Figure 2.19 Double-headed snake from Coyote Buttes, Arizona. Photo by E. Malotki.

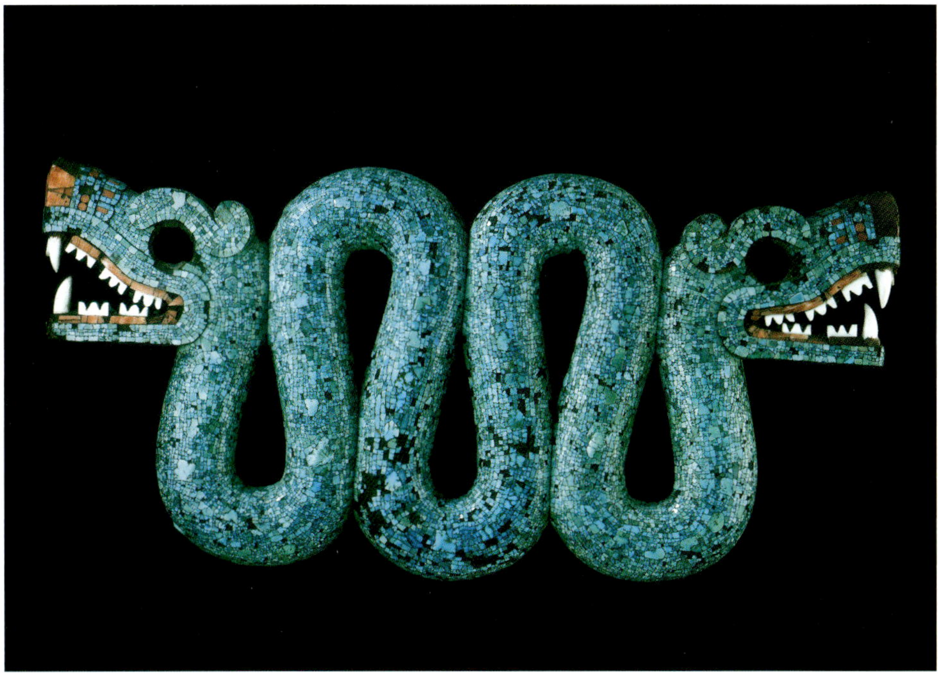

Figure 2.20. Mixtec-Aztec pectoral in the form of a double-headed serpent in mosaic of shell and turquoise over hollow wood. 43.2 cm.

particularly striking example of a double-headed serpent from the Aztec empire in Mexico is one of the symbols of Tlaloc, the Aztec rain god (fig. 2.20).

Most often, two-headed figures are depicted with their heads next to each other, facing in the same direction. Often they are gods—from those of the Aztecs to the gods of India. Sometimes the two heads represent twins. Universally fascinating, twins are prominent in myths. Indeed, there is almost no society that has not developed a complex system of representations and symbols about twins. Twins played a prominent role in early African art. In American Indian mythology, the heroic twin gods represent morning and evening and, at a deeper level, stand for many kinds of duality.[10]

Symmetry in Words and Music

Our pleasure in symmetry is not limited to images. When words are used symmetrically, the result is called a palindrome. Letters, words, and even sentences and paragraphs may be made to appear the same whether read forward or backward. For example, the supposed first words ever spoken were, "Madam I'm Adam." The hearer's reply, also a palindrome, was "Eve." Another example is "A man a plan a canal Panama." A sign proposed for a lawyer's office read, "Sue Zeus." If a mirror is placed vertically on either side of the word "MOM," there will be no change at all, because each of the letters in this word is itself bilaterally symmetrical. The same is true of the entire phrase "TOO HOT

TO HOOT." We find pleasure in the playful manipulation of words and letters leading to the discovery of hidden symmetries.

Composers, too, make use of symmetry. Because music unrolls in time rather than space, the problem is a bit different. What would be called mirror imagery in graphic art is called retrograde motion in musical composition. An early example is by the fourteenth-century composer Guillaume de Machaut, who wrote a palindromic piece called *My End Is My Beginning.* In his organ concerto *The Cuckoo and the Nightingale,* Handel reversed the order of the pitches in the cuckoo's call, a device used much later by Louis Daquin. Bach used retrograde motion in many of his compositions. One notable example is the gigue movement of his *French Suite Number 5 in G Major.*

A canon that can be played backward and forward is called a mirror canon. Bach used mirroring in *The Musical Offering,* his gift to Frederick the Great of Prussia. In one instance a voice goes from beginning to end and another voice, exactly the same, goes from end to beginning in contrary motion, with the musical lines crossing in the middle. In another Bach canon the top line is exactly mirrored in the bottom line. Haydn, frequently playful in his compositions, wrote *Symphony Number 47 in G Major,* called "The Palindromic." Its minuet movement is known as the "Minuet al Reverso." Haydn's *Sonata Number 4* for piano and violin is another example. Mozart, for the third movement of his *Serenade Number 12 K. 388 in C Minor,* wrote a reverse minuet in which the second voice is the mirror image of the first and every theme is repeated either reversed or upside-down. Beethoven used a similar device in the final fugue of his *Hammerclavier Sonata* op. 106.

In more recent times, Bela Bartok used a palindrone structure in his *Second Piano Concerto* and played with similar symmetrical reversals in *Microcosmos.* Alban Berg composed retrograde music in *Chamber Concerto for Piano, Violin, and Winds.* Darius Milhaud did something similar in *Scaramouche.* Messiaen used rhythmic "cells" in a palindromic fashion. Anton Webern wrote some twelve-tone works in which the intervals are the same coming and going. Symmetry is one of the basic elements of the twelve-tone technique. Although its use may not be apparent to the listener, it is important to the composer, for whom reversal is a constructive conceptual element. Alban Berg's *Lulu* contains a musical palindrome. One of the most ambitious uses of symmetry in music is an opera by Paul Hindemith called *Hin und Zurück* (There and Back, or Forward and Backward). It is divided into two halves, the second of which is the reversal of the first. Musically, the order of themes reverses, and so does the action of the story. In all senses the movements mirror one another.

The Origin and Science of Symmetry

When two figures are balanced against each other and one is the reverse of the other, the result somehow delights us. Graphic artists, writers, and musicians all make use of this. And it may be that it is not just humans who are attracted to symmetry. The animal behaviorist Bernhard Rensch found that apes and monkeys tend to prefer symmetrical to asymmetrical visual presentations.[11]

Information theory tells us that the regularity of information presented through symmetry makes for greater predictability and greater intelligibility. It is an important aspect of cognition. With it our brains can more quickly form a hypothesis about the information and more quickly gain understanding.[12] In terms of cognition theory, artificial intelligence devices are notoriously unable to replicate some of the simplest brain functions, but designing computers to recognize symmetry has been relatively easy.

It may be that we feel a satisfaction when information comes to us in a form that fits neatly into our perceptive system. We prefer it because this is what our brains are best suited to understand. Immanuel Kant wrote that "form is judged beautiful if it facilitates the process of perception."[13] Irenaus Eibl-Eibesfeldt, the behavioral biologist, said much the same thing more recently: "What we consider as beautiful may be a type of visual input which corresponds optimally to the processing rules of regularity and symmetry. For this reason it is easier, more economical, and more satisfying on some levels to find regularity. . . . Our perceptive mechanism seeks order, and this quest seems to be a general principle which derives, in part, from the limited capacity of our brains to process information."[14]

The search for symmetry and simplicity inspires many scientists, and they are not reluctant to use the word *beauty* when they discover these qualities. The physicist Anthony Zee wrote, "Following the ancient Greeks, who waxed eloquent on the perfect beauty of the spheres and the music they make, I will continue to equate symmetry with beauty."[15] Einstein wrote that the principles of symmetry or invariance inspired him in his own research. Einstein's son, speaking of his father, said that his "highest praise for a good theory or a good piece of work was not that it was correct or that it was exact but that it was beautiful."[16] Even more apposite for this discussion, Einstein wrote that his appreciation of symmetry in the rarified domain in which he worked was rooted in appreciation of the visual symmetry he experienced in the phenomena of the down-to-earth world around him.[17]

There is a spiritual aspect to symmetry in some societies. In the Pueblo world, two of the most powerful gods are twins. The Iroquois refer to symmetry as one manifestation of their search for balance in all aspects of their lives.[18] The Hopi worldview is based on symmetries of direction.[19] In Navajo sand paintings, exact symmetry is vital.[20] We do not know whether the gods of the Ice Age people required symmetry or even cared about it, but it is apparent that, at least to some extent, the Ice Age artists did.

REPETITION AND VARIATION

Making variations on a theme is really the crux of creativity.

—DOUGLAS HOFSTADTER, *Metamagical Themas*

The art of the Ice Age culture that spread across Europe and Asia featured certain figurative images that were repeated over and over again. In sculpture, women were the dominant theme. There is the sylphlike adolescent figure from Laugerie Haute, but most of the female figures, such as the well-known statuettes of Willendorf (Austria), Laussel (Dordogne), and Lespugue (Hautes-Garonne), are more mature and possibly pregnant. Ripe female figures were apparently made many times over, judging from the numbers that have been found. Vulva images, both engraved and painted, are also found repeatedly. It seems likely that these are examples of metonymy, references to womankind by means of what was considered her most significant part.

Within the caves, repetition was another way of creating order. On the cave walls, where animals predominate, certain ones were repeated with compulsive regularity. Horses and bulls, bison and mammoths, ibex and deer were painted and engraved endlessly at site after site and engraved repeatedly on stone slabs, on antler, and on ivory. Often figures were structured in rows, or friezes: aurochs, horses, and deer at Lascaux, mammoths at Rouffignac, rhinoceroses at Rouffignac and Chauvet. Such processions or friezes of similar animals suggest the animals' abundance as well as their movement in implied space. At times the animals were depicted with detailed accuracy. At other times they were suggested iconographically, with the least information necessary to allow them to be recognized. When they were recognized, it was like a familiar theme being repeated to give structure to the cave walls.

Similarly, in the San art of southern Africa, certain key animals, especially the eland and rows of human figures, often dancing, appear over and over again. In the art of Australian Aborigines one finds repeated depictions of kangaroos and wallabies, broglas (a kind of bird) and emus. All across that continent, in innumerable rockshelters, one sees again and again the image of the mythic rainbow snake associated with the creation of the world.

Besides its importance as a means of graphic organization, repetition may suggest a ritual structure. For example, Pueblo Indian dancers in the American Southwest often repeat every song and gesture to each of the four directions. Then, after an interval of rest, they perform the whole dance again. This process continues throughout the day. The exactness of the repetition is so important that one or more men are assigned the function of arranging any part of a dancer's ceremonial costume—a sash, a garter, an anklet, a headdress—that, because of the dancer's movement, might not be in its precise place. Repetition in the dance seems to lead the participants into a deeply inward state.

The power of repetition is also understood in the major modern religions, most of which use repetition in ceremonies. The Ice Age concern with repetition, particularly in the large "sanctuary caves," may suggest some ritual uses for this art. The constant repetition of the same animals on portable art may suggest that they were associated with myths or stories of significance to that culture. In preliterate cultures, myths and legends such as origin stories tend to have associations that we consider to involve religion. We may wonder whether the repetition of certain images in the caves reflects the important stories, myths, and spiritual beliefs of the Ice Age people. Some of it, I suspect, does, but the answer is more complex. My message throughout this book is that the art must have had many uses and meanings.

Repetition and Perception

Repetition gives us a sense of control. Instead of working with new information, our brains can recognize what they have already categorized and stored in memory. Perception is the act of processing an endless incoming stream of information. Repetition facilitates this process of organization. Things that are the same can be recognized easily and placed, without much effort, with things that are similar. Symmetry can be seen as a form of repetition varied by rotation in space, often to create a mirror image.

In both art and life, however, there can be too much repetition. Although it makes perception easier, repetition also tends to make it less intense. Too much may be anathema to a work of art because it dulls the senses in the same way an odor that we smell for any length of time becomes unnoticeable. The endless engravings of horses in cave after cave would soon dull the viewer's interest if there were no variations in the way they were made and if the differences between caves and walls did not create constant variation of context. We need variation to keep our senses alert. The use of variation within a repetitive pattern enables artists to keep work fresh and stimulating while maintaining the order the brain desires.

Theme and Variation

Delight lies somewhere between boredom and confusion.
—E. H. GOMBRICH, *A Sense of Order*

In Ice Age art, themes are repeated over and over, but always with variation. We see this, for example, with horses. In their book *Palaeolithic Cave Art,* Peter Ucko and Andrée Rosenfeld showed reproductions of 22 horses' heads drawn from Ice Age images.[21] The range of styles used to present different recognizable representations of the same subject is surprising. The same is true for bison, about which the prehistorian Jean Clottes wrote, "In the Cave of Niaux . . . where painted bison are legion, none are identical. The fantasy of the artists, their talent, and their aesthetic pleasure are given free rein and explain the variations on a common theme. The individualizing of the figures, more evident for the bison than for any other animal, translates true artistic intention, a freeness that transcends simple religious or material concerns."[22]

Within the stylistic unity of specific periods and geographic locations there is always variation. In Ice Age Europe, depictions of the same kinds of animals made in the same cave in what we believe to have been the same period show individual diversity. Even paintings made by what appears to be the same artist vary. It is as if the artists were not repeating what they already knew how to do but were continually seeking new solutions. It is interesting to observe the depiction of the hooves of bison, which change from region to region and from cave to cave (fig. 2.21). There is even greater variation in the attempt to capture horses' hooves—as round balls, cloven circles, and many other graphic vari-

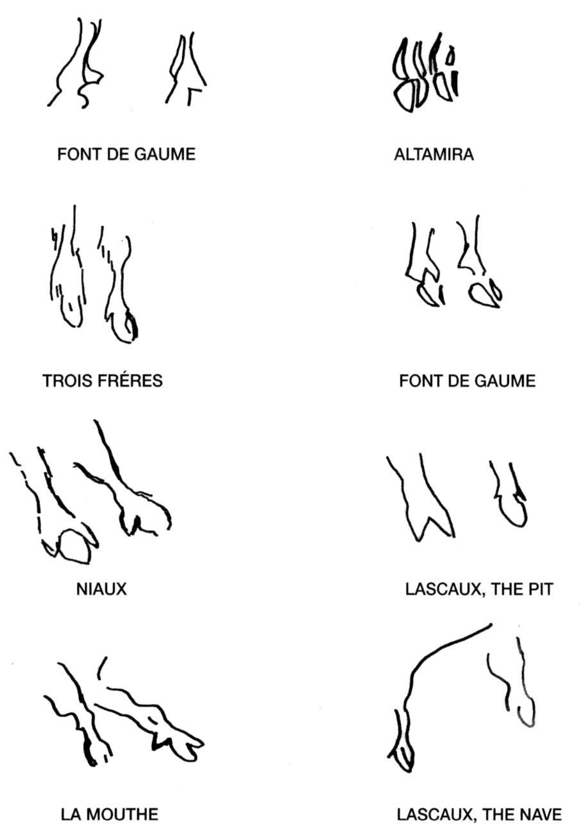

Figure 2.21. Varied solutions for the depiction of bison hooves in Ice Age art.

ations. At Gargas, one artist was particularly experimental, making variations in the feet of a single bison (fig. 2.22).

The same kind of experimentation can be seen in far different times and cultures. At Sanchi in Madya Pradesh, India, stand two Buddhist stupas dating to about 1,400 years ago. Both are covered with stone carvings that are outstanding even for a culture whose artistic genius seems to have been best expressed in sculpture. The carvings on Stupa II are daringly fanciful. On one medallion, a horse in bas-relief has each hoof carved in a different manner. In the rockshelters of South Africa, endlessly repeated Paleolithic dancing figures are similar to one another but not identical. On the American continent, each panel of petroglyphs is unique, even though the rock art of a specific cultural group in a specific time period tends to portray the same themes and images repeatedly. It seems that beginning with the Ice Age, the impetus for the artist has been to repeat a theme and then to invent variations upon it.

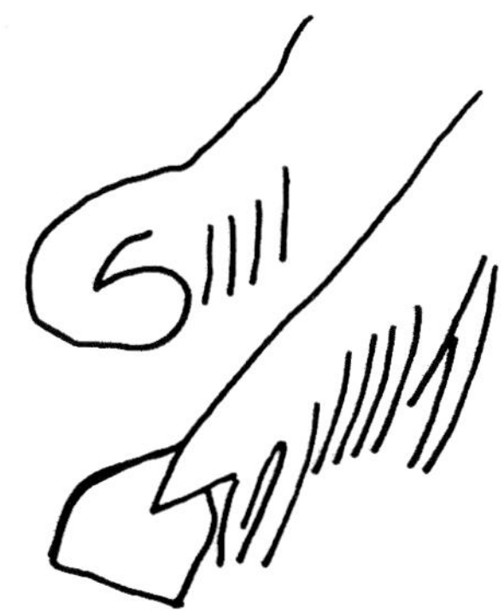

Figure 2.22. Two front legs of a bison at Gargas show variation of graphic treatment.

Artists often work the same material over and over again. One explanation for this was given by Degas: "One must treat the same subject ten times, even a hundred times. . . . One loves and endows with art only what one is accustomed to."[23] Degas himself, however, never exactly repeated the same subject. Rembrandt's self-portraits, Monet's haystacks, Cézanne's apples, Morandi's bottles are all examples of a repeated subject with variations. So, too, is the tendency for artists to work in series of paintings that deal with the same subject but each time in a different way. Part of the appeal of work by the contemporary artist Wayne Thiebaud is the use of variation within repetition. For example, his platters of sliced pies show each one wedge-shaped but slightly different from the next.

Symmetry, as I mentioned, is one example of repetition, but in art, symmetry is rarely exact. The subject is not precisely repeated when rotated or reflected. Instead, we most often find a variation on perfect symmetry in which the image is slightly altered or skewed, making it seem more alive than if it were repeated exactly. Christopher Tyler, a neuroscientist, studied 170 portraits by famous artists in the western European tradition from the last 500 years and found that, despite the impression of being centered, the face was almost never symmetrically placed on the canvas.[24] The artist almost always reserved the center of the painting for one of the portrait's eyes. The faces gave only the illusion of symmetry. It appeared that skilled artists working in this stylistic format felt an intuitive need to create a subtle tension between appearance and actuality.

Repetition and Variation in Music

Art and music have much in common in their use of variation within repetition. Maurits Escher wrote: "General elements such as rhythm and repetition, which play an important part for the auditory sense in music and for the visual sense in plane division, also indicate a certain affinity between the two. . . . the hand executes movements that repeat themselves rhythmically as in a dance."[25]

Music and visual art can be compared in many ways. As with graphic art, it is possible to find suggestions of what we might call music in other animals, and this gives us some clues to the biological component of music. The German ethologist Bernhard Rensch reported that an elephant he had worked with could distinguish 12 musical tones, remember simple melodies, and recognize them over a year later.[26] The neurologist David Sulzer, who is also a composer, working with Richard Lair, found that a group of captive elephants shown how to make sounds on instruments devised distinct melodies without being taught to do so and then repeated and varied those melodies.[27]

In such situations, people have tampered with the natural behaviors of animals. But there is some indication that some aspects of music also occur when animals are in their natural settings. The California bass marsh wren presents music-like themes that are reiterated by a neighboring bird, much the way humans do in call-and-response singing. In Western music such repetition would be called a canon.[28] Some whales make noises that would fit our description of music; humpback whales ornament their calls with what musicians would call trills, arpeggios, and glissandos. Whale songs generally consist of a sound phrase followed by an elaborated variation. This is followed by a return to a slightly modified repetition of the original phrase. One might liken this to a version of the A-B-A form so common in human music—a form of theme and variation.[29]

Repetition is a fundamental principle of musical structure, but overused, it can be deadening. Bach called the work of a fellow composer "pedantic" because he stuck continuously to his principal subject without variations.[30] Bach himself was a master of variation. The chaconne movement in his *Partita in D Minor for Unaccompanied Violin* is a gigantic set of variations on a harmonic pattern derived from four measures continuously repeated. His most famous example is a work for clavier known as the Goldberg Variations. Bach was commissioned by Count Kaiserling, who suffered from insomnia, to compose music to be played for the count during his sleepless nights. He wanted music that would cheer him—not, as legend has it, something that would put him to sleep. The resulting composition consisted of 30 variations on a single theme. One of Bach's pupils, a brilliant clavier player named Johan Theophilus Goldberg, stayed in an adjoining room and played Bach's composition for Kaiserling when he could not sleep.

According to the polymath Douglas Hofstadter, the ability to make variations is the key to the definition of art: "Spinning out variations is what comes naturally to the human mind and it is ever fertile."[31] Perhaps theme and variation are satisfying to us because they enable us to experience a feeling of recognition, of greeting the familiar, while they do not lull our minds but rather stimulate them with novelty. We wait eagerly to recognize an old friend beneath the newest disguise. As we see in their work, Ice Age artists must have experienced such feelings as well.

Part Two

WINDOWS INTO THE MIND

Therefore, O Lord, let me preserve
The sense that does so fitly serve,
Take Tongue and Ear—all else I have—
Let Light attend me to the grave!
—THEODORE ROETHKE, *Prayer*

HUMANS HAVE EVOLVED to be very sight-oriented animals. Visual perception serves as one of our brain's most important functions. We perceive wavelengths of light that range between 375 and 750 nanometers, for which we have an astonishing number of light receptor cells—an estimated 160 million. Each of these cells influences hundreds of thousands, perhaps even millions, of neurons. If we include all the cells involved in vision, some scientists estimate that there are over 1,000,000,000 million neurons in more than 30 interconnected brain centers, each of which helps to map out the visual field.[1] In anatomically modern humans, the cells devoted to visual processing take up between 40 and 50 percent of the total cortex.[2] The brain is often described as having been formed in layers, like an onion; vision is at the core, and verbal ability is one of the last thin layers of the onion.

It is evident that drawing and painting are visually inspired, but it may be surprising to discover that activities directed toward verbal and scientific creativity are also often inspired by vision. Even now, in our highly literate world, complex thought often occurs primarily as images. Problems that seem to involve nonvisual logic are sometimes solved only after one finds the right mental picture. When we have understood something, we say, "I see." The mathematician Jacques Hadamard, in his study of creative thinking, refuted the idea that verbalization is necessary for thought, even in abstract fields such as mathematics and physics, where we might not expect imagery to be important. Speaking of his own work, Hadamard said that images were an absolute necessity. His most dramatic evidence of the importance of the visual image for creative thought came in a letter he received from Albert Einstein, who wrote:

> The psychical entities that seem to serve as elements of thought are certain signs and more or less clear images, which can be "voluntarily" reproduced and combined. . . . The above-mentioned elements are, in my case, of visual and some muscular type. Conventional words or other signs have to be sought for laboriously only in the second stage, when the mentioned associative play is sufficiently established and can be reproduced at will.[3]

There is so much evidence of scientists' relying on visual images for their discoveries that it cannot be dismissed as the idiosyncrasy of a few. Niels Bohr, the physicist, found that complex atomic models came to him intuitively as pictures or images.[4] Donald Glaser, inventor of the bubble chamber used in particle physics, was inspired while sitting in a local bar watching bubbles forming on the side of a beer mug.[5] James Watson, who with Maurice Wilkins and Francis Crick discovered the double helical structure of DNA, said that his moment of insight came while he was drawing the fused rings of adenine on paper. This drawing, he claimed, helped him recognize the profound implications of such a structure, and new possibilities were opened to him.[6] Mitchell Feigenbaum, one of the founders of chaos theory, the revolutionary way of calculating complex nonlinear problems, said that when his inspiration came, it became etched in his mind in the form of a bright, sharp image of two small wavy forms and one big one.[7] Benoit Mandelbrot, founder of fractal geometry, in describing how much his work was influenced by visual images, said, "I do everything by eye."[8] The theoretical cosmologist Stephen Hawking is limited in his research by the severe disability of Lou Gehrig's disease. Out of necessity, he mentally translates mathematical problems into geometrical problems that can appear as images, and these, Hawking says, can be pictured in his mind.[9]

In literary creation, often called a "left-brain" activity, images can nevertheless be all important for some writers. George Orwell wrote: "Probably it is better to put off using words as long as possible and to get one's meaning clear as one can through pictures or sensations."[10] Harold Pinter said that many of his plays began with images. The Canadian writer Robertson Davies wrote that his ideas often appeared first in pictures. The brain appears to have separate verbal and visual storage areas, and the memory capacity for pictures appears to be higher than that for words. J. J. Gibson, a psychologist of visual perception, gave an explanation for the use of imagery in unexpected instances when he wrote, "Visual thinking is freer and less stereotyped than verbal thinking. . . . As every artist knows, there are thoughts that can be visualized without being verbalized."[11]

As our culture becomes increasingly saturated with visual information from film, video, and computer, pictures have become a dominant form of communication. Yet despite our being bombarded with images, they remain potent. We are made newly aware of their iconic power when we see the bulletproof glass and armed guards protecting Picasso's *Guernica* in Spain. In a thirteenth-century painting by Duccio di Buoninsegna, *The Last Temptation of Christ,* the face of the devil still bears deep scratch marks. Recently Rembrandt's *Danae* was slashed and sprayed with acid. There are many examples of the potency of pictures through the ages. They might well have been considered receptacles of power and even magic to the Paleolithic viewer.

Our perceptions can be disturbing when they result in visual deceptions and visual illusions. When we receive competing, opposed clues we may interpret them as simultaneous, contradictory messages leading to alternative possibilities of interpretation. We can see an illusion even while we know it is false; we can experience it and be fooled at the same time. Psychologists such as Alan Leslie have found that the illusions, misinterpretations, and ambiguities that result from the very nature of the visual processing system can present windows into the mind.[12] They offer clues that can help guide us to a clearer understanding of how our brains work and therefore a more complete understanding of ourselves. In Part Two, I look at the ways in which artists have used illusion and the related concepts of ambiguity, paradox, and analogy—searching, by means of these, for windows into the artist's mind.

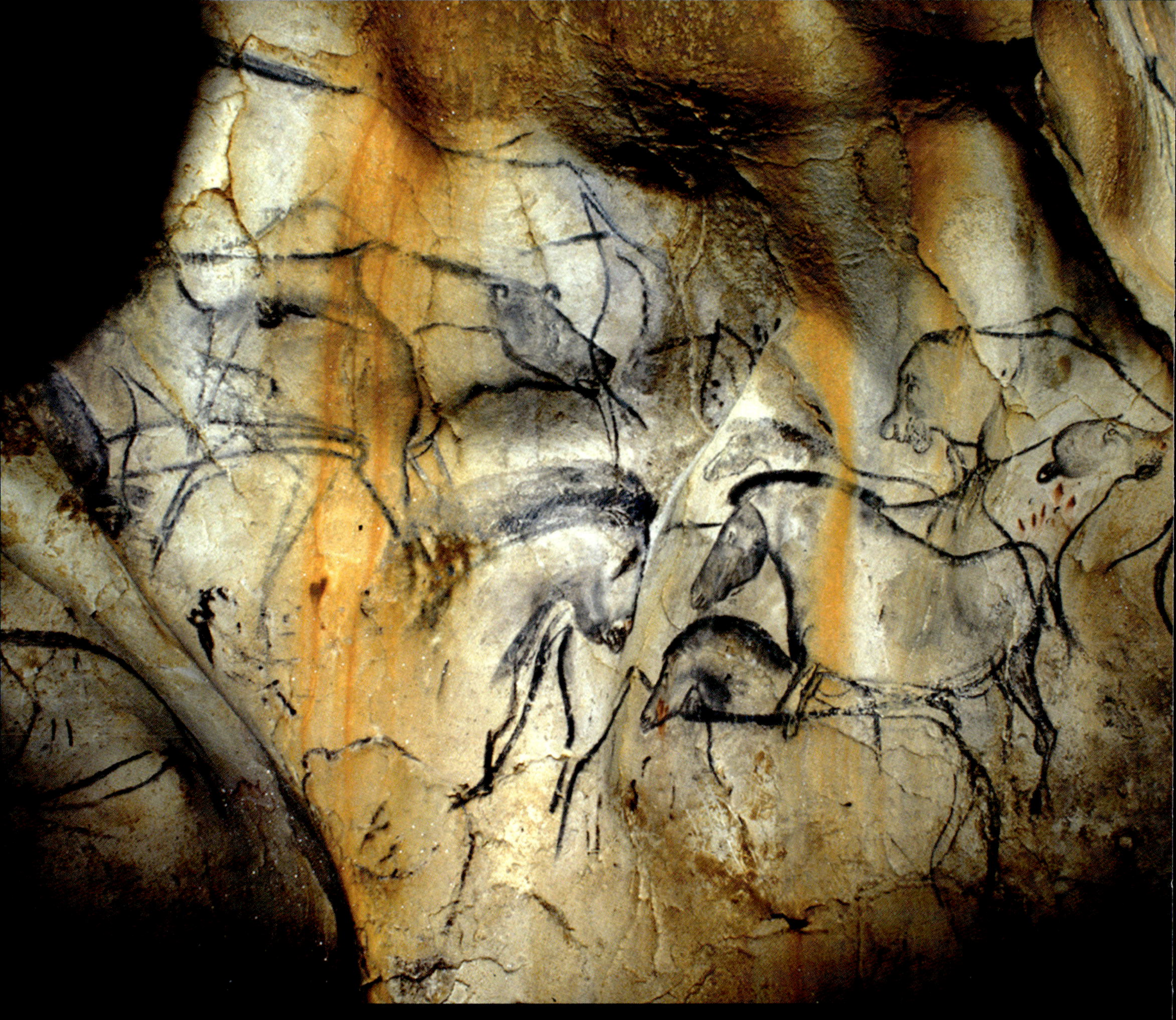

3

ILLUSION

Making the Imagined Seem Real

> *It may be that susceptibility to illusion is necessary for being creative.*
>
> —R. L. GREGORY, *Illusion in Nature and Art*

THE WAY INTO THE DEEPEST CHAMBERS of the cave of Tuc d'Audoubert is long and arduous. Squeezing through increasingly narrow passages, attempting to avoid sharp, hanging rock, one finds it difficult to light the way. Disoriented by the darkness and the silence, the visitor feels both spatially confused and alienated from the normal passage of time. After what seems like endless walking and crawling, one passes evidence of former human presence, along with cave bear skulls half buried in calcite. Eventually one enters a narrow crack, or *chatière,* so tight that there is a real danger of getting stuck.

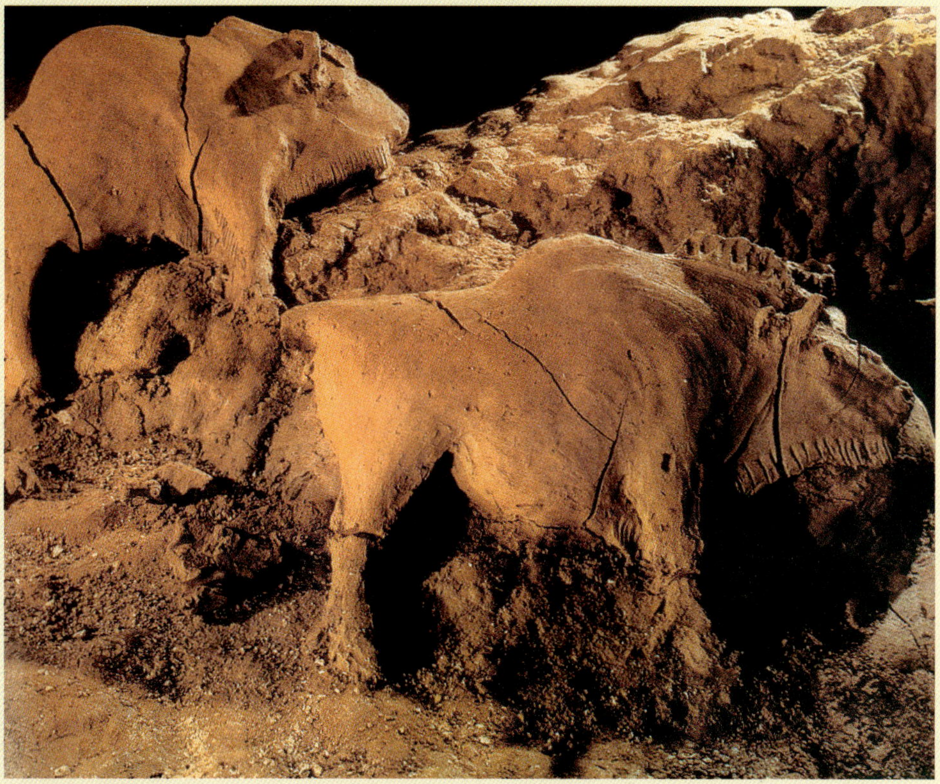

Figure 3.1. Clay bison, Tuc d'Audoubert. The preservation of this work, made of unfired clay, is astonishing. The cow, to the right, measures 61 cm long; the bull is slightly smaller. Photo by J. Vertut. CNP-MCC

Finally, after about three-fifths of a mile—though it seems much longer—one squeezes through the narrowest passage into a circular chamber where, in the distance, in the dim light of the lantern, appear two bison that for the briefest moment seem to be apparitions (fig. 3.1). They are modeled of unfired clay that has miraculously lasted in the damp cave for 150 centuries. In this theatrical setting, after the long journey in the dark and the exaltation of the entry into light, we are ready to be deluded. The sculptor of the bison, like artists of all subsequent times, was an illusionist.

The word *illusion* comes from the Latin verb *ludire,* meaning to play—specifically, in this context, to make believe or pretend. In many cases, to evoke illusion requires the viewer's collaboration and collusion. When we view a painting by Velázquez up close, for example, we see a grouping of brush strokes. As we step back, the strokes suddenly become a hand or a face. We move forward a step, and they dissolve again. We can move back and forth over this imaginary line, losing and finding the image. On one side of the line are brush strokes with some inexplicable order of their own; on the other side those same strokes become recognizable images. That step back and forth over the line is an examination of our brain's ability to perceive masses and to flesh them out as convincing likenesses. We are watching a cognitive process at work. Illusions occur not in the eye but in the brain. In the Velazquez we see ourselves being fooled before our very eyes. That step is the means by which we examine the ability of our brains to arrive at a convincing interpretation of amorphic forms. All the while we are aware of the trick, and all the while we are examining our own perceptive process just as much as we are examining the illusory figure itself.

There seems to be a natural pleasure evoked in both the making and the recognition of realistic images. . . . this is the "miracle" of the upper Paleolithic; not art, as often stated, but representation.

—JOHN HALVERSON, "Art for Art's Sake in the Paleolithic"

The Ice Age artists' apparent desire was to portray the world as they saw it, and especially to replicate the appearances of the animals that were important to them. In order to do so, like all other artists everywhere they had to act as illusionists. They had to devise ways of representing reality that caused viewers to suspend disbelief and allow themselves to accept the art as equivalent to reality. In this chapter I examine three forms of illusion that Ice Age artists employed to achieve their goal. These are replication (mimesis), closure (synecdoche), and projection (the Rorschach effect). The artists did not entirely hide their graphic tricks; unlike later Greek artists, they doubtless could not have done this. So viewers were aware of the means by which their senses were fooled and understood it as an act of transformation meant to confound the real and the imagined.

REPLICATION, OR MIMESIS

In their figurative art, Ice Age artists sought to portray the world as they saw it. This is not a goal to which most of the world's early or tribal artists have aspired. Even when subjects have been figurative, they generally have not been based on visual realism. The world that the Ice Age artists portrayed was highly selected. The images probably were often meant to carry symbolic meaning, but the means used to convey meaning was to replicate appearance as closely as possible.

At the Ice Age site of Trou Magritte in Belgium, the finding of a red deer's canine tooth would not have been unusual except that the tooth was actually carved from limestone (fig. 3.2).[1] The imitation was good enough that it might have fooled both the people who used the perforated tooth as a bead and the archaeologists who much later found it. It attests to the maker's skill as an illusionist in this most direct form of representation, the replication of a natural object in another medium. Animal teeth, particularily stag teeth, were imitated in ivory, stone, bone and antler during the Ice Age.[2] Paleolithic people in Europe also took bits of bone or limestone and rounded and polished them to make imitation cave pearls, rare objects that in nature form when calcium carbonate precipitates from limestone in supersaturated pools of cave water, in the same way nacre is coated around an intrusive body in a mollusk. Cave pearls were probably considered as rare and serendipitous as pearls from oysters seem to us now.

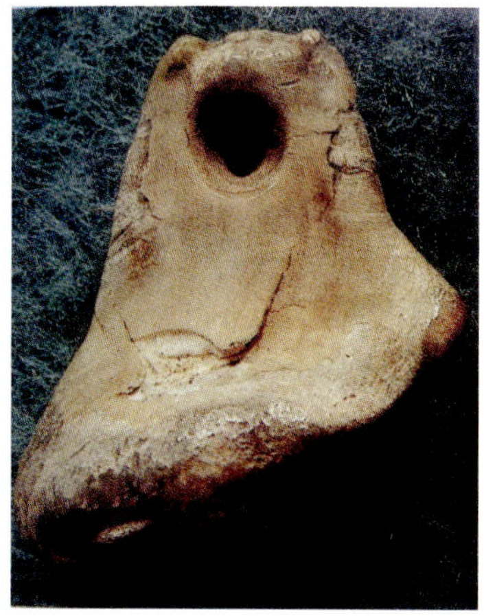

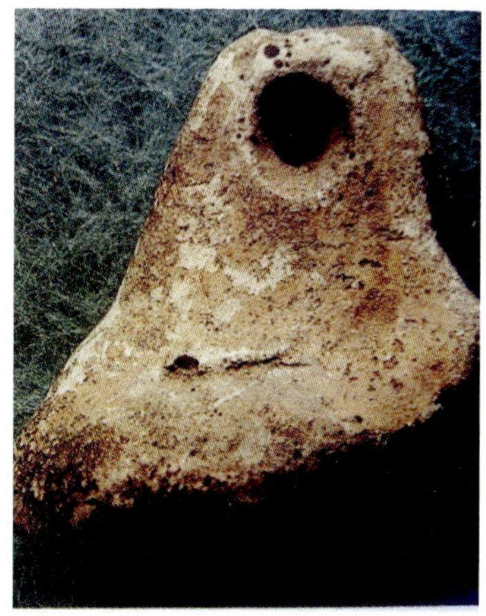

Figure 3.2. Top: Pierced red deer canine. Below: A carved limestone replica of a red deer's canine tooth. Both are from the site of Trou Magritte in Belgium and are about 30,000 years old. Photos by R. White.

From a much later date, a ceramic triton shell was unearthed in Hittite ruins. In the still later Minoan culture, a favorite subject was the nautilus shell, naturalistically represented, often in faience. Similar replication appears on other continents. In North America, for example, a pottery vessel from the Mississippian period imitates a conch shell. From later periods, bears' teeth have been found carved from shell. Carved basalt replicas of conch shells have been found at Tenochtitlan, Mexico. Turtle shells were favored in North America in myth and ritual. One, carved in stone and then incised with the pattern of the shell, was found in the mounds of the Ohio Valley, dating from about the thirteenth century.

In 1993 the Whitney Museum displayed as high art, carefully isolated in a glass case to underline their precious quality, 11 pairs of stones by the Latvian-California artist Vija Celmins. These small stones, about the size to be picked up and held easily in one's palm, varied in size and shape but were unremarkable in any way, typical of what one might find on a casual walk. One of each pair was made of cast bronze and painted with acrylic to duplicate as exactly as possible the real stone with which it was displayed. The curator's description of this show said that it posed "questions about the nature of representation." The work appeared to strike a chord with viewers, who hovered over the glass case with evident pleasure. There was indeed a marvelous quality to the work, which appealed directly to our delight in being fooled. But the ploy works only if we are aware that we are being fooled; otherwise it is pointless, and we would see nothing more than pairs of stones. What the viewers really marveled at was the oscillation between reality and simulacrum, the dual sensation of being deceived by their senses and simultaneously aware of this deception.

Verisimilitude has a special appeal, as we can see in a waxworks museum. It is easier to achieve this kind of illusion with three-dimensional sculpture than with two-dimensional drawing or painting, which requires much greater abstraction. Some prehistorians believe that sculpture preceded painting.[3] Well-dated, realistic small sculptures appear very early in human art. Figures carved in mammoth tusk ivory found at Hohle Fels cave in southwestern Germany have been dated from 30,000 to 33,000 years ago. A carved horse from Vogelherd, Germany, is about 30,000 years old. At Dolní Vestonice, in the Czech Republic, numerous modeled clay figurines, dating from about 26,000 years ago, have been found. They depict humans, primarily females, and animals, primarily carnivores. These figures have been kiln fired. It is remarkable that ceramic technology was discovered about 15,000 years before it had previously been thought to have been discovered. It is even more surprising that this technology was used for artistic purposes before it was used to make utilitarian vessels.[4]

The difference between the cognitive requirements for modeling and those for carving is significant. A modeling material such as clay allows form to be built up slowly and corrections to be made along the way. Carving requires an opposite way of thinking. Rather than being additive, it is subtractive, involving a more convoluted mental process because the completed figure must be visualized and adjusted to the shape and amount of material before the work begins. Corrections are difficult if not impossible. Nevertheless, carvings in stone, bone, and ivory were made very early in human history, and some still survive. The survival of clay, especially unfired clay, over so long a time is rare, another reason the bison from Tuc d'Audoubert are so remarkable.

Representing Reality

The developing child makes the giant leap into representation at approximately three years of age. Children find a natural pleasure in representing objects and people. For those who observe children at this period, the process seems magical. Apes and chimps, given art materials, sometimes produce what looks similar to children's art, and for that matter even some adult art, but no matter how attractive their work, for apes and chimps the breakthrough into representation never comes. Many cultures have portrayed their world realistically to a greater or lesser degree, but it is unusual for a society to base its style on a search for visual verisimilitude. Yet some of the earliest artists we know about, the artists of Ice Age Europe, sought to create just such a duplication of visual sensation.

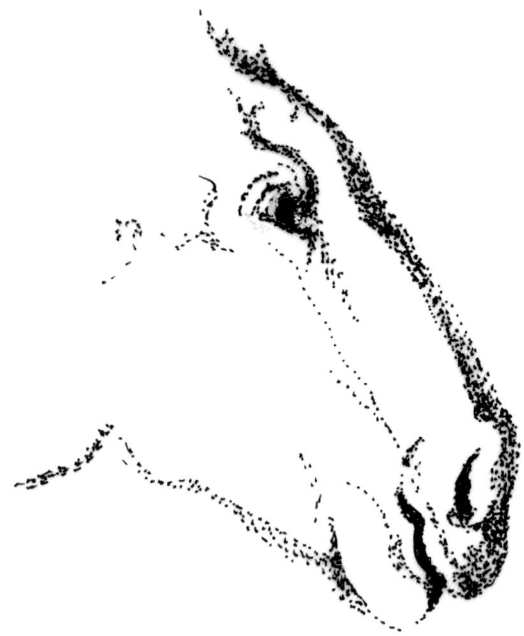

Figure 3.3. The horse at Commarque. The complete animal is carved, but the head is most fully realized and best preserved. Height of head 70 cm.

One of the great works of art of the Ice Age, and indeed of all time, is the horse at Commarque (Dordogne) (fig. 3.3). It is in a small cave under a twelfth-century chateau still in the possession of the family of the Comte de Commarque. The body of the large horse, carved in low relief, is eroded so that it is difficult to see, but the profile of the head, in slightly higher relief, is well preserved. The horse's head is about life size, 68.6 cm long, and is an accurate depiction of the Przewalski's horse. Because of the position of the relief in the narrow corridor, less than 91.4 cm wide, it seems larger than life, even monumental. The carver was able to model the form with parallel hatchings and to achieve extraordinary subtlety. The artist made use of a natural hole for the nostril and, despite the roughness of the stone, was able to suggest the muscles and veins in the head, the tender mouth, even the pupil of the eye. Warmth and moisture seem to emanate from the distended nostril. The eye is wild and focused. The horse has been given the illusion of life but not of freedom. It strains toward the cave entrance, but like Michelangelo's carved *Captives,* who remain clearly imprisoned in their blocks of stone, the Commarque horse is doomed to remain embedded in the cave wall for eternity. This impassioned animal might well be compared to the consummately carved horses of the Parthenon.

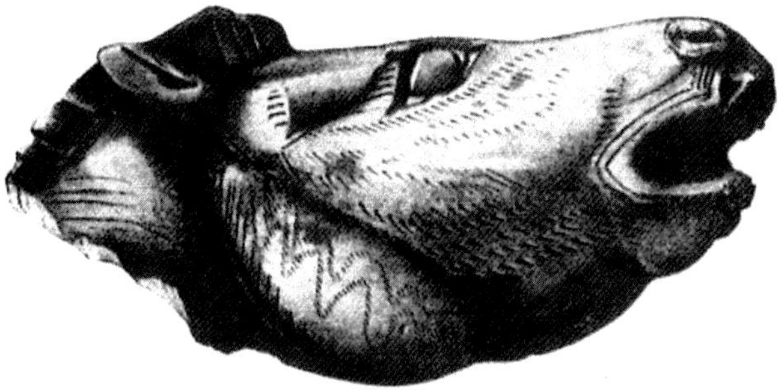

Figure 3.4. Horse's head carved from reindeer horn, Mas d'Azil. 6.5 cm.

Another example of the genius of an Ice Age artist is the depiction of a horse found in the enormous cave complex of Mas d'Azil. Carved from a bit of reindeer horn just over 5 cm long, it manages to show the modeling and the details of the horse's head as well as the passion of the animal (fig. 3.4).

Not until Classical Greek civilization arose about 25 centuries ago did artists systematically focus on creating an illusion of realism comparable to that achieved by the Ice Age artists. Artists of Classical Greece were equally obsessed with mimesis, the realistic mimicry of the natural world. The success of a painting of horses by the Greek painter Apelles of Cos was judged on the way real horses reacted to it. According to Pliny, Apelles' won a contest because the real animals neighed only in front of his painting. Pliny also wrote that the painter Xeuxis won a competition when he pictured grapes so authentic in appearance that sparrows came to peck at them. A rival artist, Parrhasius, invited Xeuxis to his studio to demonstrate that he could do as well. Preparing to appraise his rival's work, Xeuxis asked Parrhasius to pull back the curtain covering the painting, only to discover that it was a painting of a curtain. Xeuxis acknowledged defeat, saying the "whereas he had deceived the birds, Parrhasius had deceived him, an artist."[6]

Greek artists painted stage sets for the theater, which played a vital role in their culture. In 460 BCE, while painting a stage set for a tragedy by Aeschylus, Agatharchus of Samos worked out the underlying principles of linear perspective in an attempt to convey the illusion of depth.[7] An aspiration to *trompe l'oeil* realism in the landscape backgrounds of stage sets likely set a standard for art used in other contexts. It is possible that a similar need arose in the Ice Age. If some of the caves were sites of rituals—for example, the great amphitheater-like spaces in Lascaux, Pech-Merle, and Niaux—then the cave art could have served as backdrops. The actual presence of humans in the caves might explain the lack of need for depiction of humans in the art. If, as in Greece, the cave art was intended to be a backdrop for dramatic ceremonies, then the Ice Age aspiration to give the illusion of visual reality would be easier to comprehend.

Mimetic art, which Michelangelo likened to imitating the work of God, became important once again during the Renaissance and inspired anecdotes similar to those from Greece. A horse painted by Bramantino appeared so real that it was attacked by actual horses. Giotto painted an insect on one of Cimabue's pictures. That celebrated artist, who was Giotto's master at the time, tried to flick it away before realizing his error.[8] The painted insect mistaken for real was a common theme in Asia as well as Europe.

The term *visual realism* refers to art that attempts to imitate the visual sensations we experience when confronted with an object or scene. Sometimes we consider the acme of such an approach to be the photograph and "photographic realism" in painting. The camera, in its early version the camera obscura, served as impetus for the Florentine artist and engineer Filipo Brunelleschi in his formulation of scientific perspective, known also as Renaissance perspective. The camera is now enormously more sophisticated and produces far subtler images. Yet there is a deception in calling the camera image more realistic than other ways of depicting reality. The photographic process remains very different from the process of vision, if only because it is monocular and static, whereas we humans see with two constantly moving eyes.

Interpreting three-dimensional reality in sculpture is relatively straightforward in comparison with the requirements of translating it onto a two-dimensional surface. In that case, reality must be abstracted in such a way that it conveys information to our senses similar to that which we receive when viewing an actual object. Much of the history of representational art is about the ways in which tricks have been devised to facilitate the artist in this ruse. Much of it involves manipulating the mechanism of our visual perception so that when we look at a two-dimensional image, our brain may override signals of stereopsis that would normally tell us the picture is actually flat. The possibilities of experiencing and abstracting reality from our vision are richer and more varied than the limits of the camera image would have us believe.

Mimesis in Music

Mimesis and music have coexisted from very early in music making. It is possible that much of the earliest music was meant to imitate birdsong. Both the recorder and the American Plains Indian flute were originally used that way, and for the latter the avowed purpose was courting.[9] At the Pueblo of Acoma in New Mexico, the notes of the swallow have been set to Native words. Western European composers wrote music that mimicked bird calls at least as far back as the thirteenth century. The oldest known piece, believed to date to the mid-1200s, may be *Summer is icumen in,* with the call of the cuckoo. Many subsequent composers liked to mimic that distinctive two-note, falling call. In the 14th century Jehan Vaillant wrote a virelai using bird call imitations of the cuckoo. In the same song, *Par maintes foy*, he played that call against those of the dove, the lark, the thrush and the nightingale.

The beautiful and varied nightingale call was also imitated. The blind Dutch composer Jacob van Eyck incorporated variations on nightingale calls in some of his recorder music. The melancholy song of the turtledove appealed to composers as well. An anonymous piece portrayed the murmurs and coos of a dove. Jacobo da Bologne wrote such a piece in the fourteenth century, and Jacques Gallot composed a lute piece called *The Dove.* In the sixteenth century Pierre Passereau wrote a piece imitating hens. In the eighteenth century Jean-Philippe Rameau wrote a harpsichord piece called *The Hen,* using clucking sounds. Michael Praetorius imitated the crowing of roosters in a piece about a century later. The Italian composer Ottorino Respighi incorporated many of these bird pieces in an orchestral work called *Gli Uccelli* (The Birds) about two centuries after that.

In his *Pastorale Symphony,* Beethoven imitated both the three-note call of the European quail and the two-note call of the cuckoo. Olivier Messiaen was passionately fond of birdsong, spending much of his time transcribing it and then using the sounds in his music. Antonin Dvorák wrote a symphonic poem, *To the Wood Dove.* Mozart used a starling's song in the closing variations of the piano composition *Concerto in G,* also known as "The Musical Joke," which is strangely unlike Mozart's other work. Musicologists have determined that its peculiarities can be explained by the work's having been based on the normal off-key calls of starlings, and as if in confirmation, they discovered that the piece was written six days after Mozart's pet starling died. Starlings appear to have an unusual ability to recognize, remember, and imitate song patterns.[10] Maybe Mozart recognized that he shared some musical capacity with his starling.

Leos Janácek wrote a *sinfonietta* imitating the sounds of the forest. Insect sounds have also been used—the cricket in the madrigal *El Grillo* and the mosquito in Bela Bartok's *Mosquito Dance.* In a wealth of examples, musical instruments imitate other sounds. Ferde Grofé put the clomp of donkey hooves in his *Grand Canyon Suite.* Saint-Saëns used the noise of frogs heard from the Nile in his concerto *The Egyptian.* Heitor Villa-Lobos used the sound of a train as did Arthur Honegger in *Pacific 231.* One of the ultimate uses of mimesis in music is heard at the beginning of Richard Strauss's *Death and Transfiguration*, for which Strauss composed music that imitated the labored breathing of a person who was terminally ill.[11]

Kinds of Pictorial Mimesis

In graphic art there are degrees and kinds of mimesis. Sometimes replication is made down to the smallest possible detail. The ancient Greek approach was probably of this kind. In another, subtler form of mimesis, enough information is given to enable the mind to fill in what is only suggested. Because of our involvement in creating the image, this approach is even more potent than complete mimesis. Impressionism is the most deliberate vehicle of such deception. In this case, what one sees depends on one's viewing distance from the painting. But as we saw in the earlier example of a Velazquez painting, this device was not new with the Impressionists, and it did not end with them.

The Postimpressionist painter Paul Bonnard studied subtleties of visual perception in a unique way. He turned his attention from the camera-like clarity of central foveal vision to the softer and more ambiguous vision with which we scan most subject matter using peripheral vision. Contrary to usual painterly practice, Bonnard placed objects that were more vaguely depicted in the middle of his canvas and objects shown with more detailed clarity on the edges. He thereby coerced the viewer to explore the painting surface using peripheral vision and as a result delayed recognition.[12] Reality viewed in this way not only causes a more gradual and more dramatic discovery of images but also makes our brains work harder and yields a stronger illusion of volume and space.[13]

Many artists remain more strictly mimetic. The seventeenth-century Dutch artist Cornelis N. Gysbrechts and the nineteenth-century American artist William Michael Harnett both specialized in portraying assemblies of low-relief objects in a manner so convincing that viewers might feel the objects could actually be picked up. A contemporary sculptor, Ray Charles, has used visual confusion in a number of his works. *Ink Box* (1986) is a shiny black cube, three feet on a side, filled to the brim with shiny black printer's ink. The ink looks so like its metal container that its surface seems to be the top of the container and cannot be distinguished as ink unless the viewer reaches out to touch it. When the piece was exhibited, many viewers did exactly that, with disconcerting results. The sculptor Duane Hanson has made such consummate contemporary use of mimesis in his figures that he walks a razor's edge between waxworks mannequins and "art."

The experience of such exact replication underlines the fact that mimesis, even when painstakingly achieved and amazingly accurate, cannot by itself be considered art. "Exactitude," said Matisse, "is not Truth."[14] One might add that exactitude by itself does not make art. Some Ice Age artists who left us masterpieces may have aimed for mimesis. The realism they achieved may have succeeded by their standards, but in our time, acclimated as we are to photography, it seems less than real. Yet the greatest artists of the Ice Age, if they aspired to visual realism, went beyond that goal to imprint their work with something more. Looking back at the horse of Commarque, we see the difference between slavish imitation and what we call art.[15]

CLOSURE, OR SYNECDOCHE

. . . humans are wired up to respond to archetypes, to "partial representations." . . . The part stands for the whole.

—JUDITH HOOPER AND DICK TERESI, *The Three-Pound Universe*

The vast cave of Pech-Merle, which contains the famous spotted horses, also has a panel of wall art known as the Black Frieze (fig. 3.5). There, 11 mammoths are painted in a tightly compacted mass, ranging from one that is fully delineated in all its hairiness to others in varying degrees of succinct silhouette. The animals become increasingly abbreviated as they proceed from bottom to top of the frieze, until, at the very top, two ponderous animals face each other, trunks overlapped. It is amazing that we can see them as fully realized mammoths, for in truth they consist of nothing but two brief gestures made rapidly with a brush dipped in black paint.

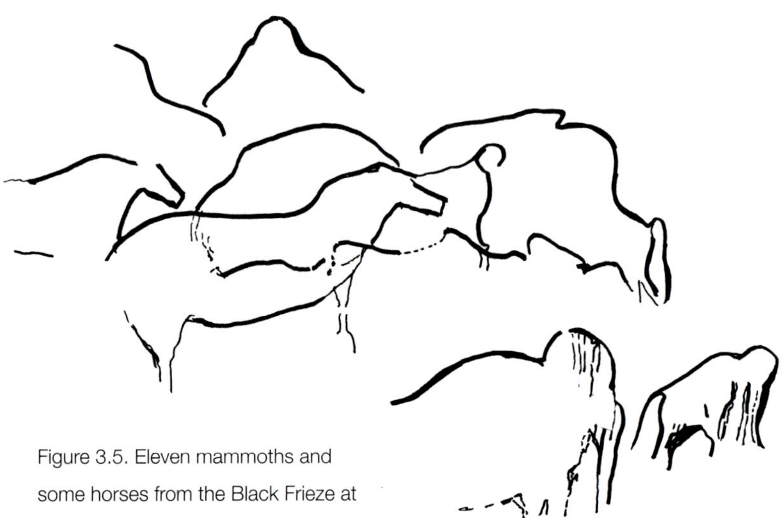

Figure 3.5. Eleven mammoths and some horses from the Black Frieze at Pech-Merle. The entire panel measures 7 by 2.5 m.

Closure is a term used by Gestalt psychologists, whose "law of closure" describes how our brains "close" incomplete lines to form a recognizable figure. *Synecdoche,* a literary term, refers to a figure of speech in which a part can stand for the whole. In a process similar to visual closure, one is presented with a partial description, and the mind fills in the missing verbal information to arrive at the complete concept. The example usually given is that the word *crown* denotes the monarch who wears the crown. Closure and synecdoche describe similar processes, and because I am discussing art as a language, borrowing language terms seems appropriate.

It is not unusual in the Ice Age art of France and Spain for animal figures to be partial representations. Often, no legs or feet are shown, and sometimes only sections of animals appear. For mammoths, in particular, it seems to have been sufficient for the artist to outline the head and the configuration of the spine. If the dorsal line was made according to the accepted schema for the species, it brought (and still brings) the entire animal to life. Some animals are headless, and some consist only of a head. Michel Lorblanchet has estimated that 40 percent of the animal figures in Cougnac (Dordogne) and Pech-Merle are indicated only by the outline of the back, the mane, or a set of horns.[16] There are also headless bodies and isolated animal parts. Possibly these animals, which seem incomplete to us, were an accepted convention in the Ice Age, just as portraits, a genre with which we are familiar, do not appear to us as decapitated heads. Images very like portraits appear in the caves of Lascaux, Tito Bustillo, and Cosquer (Bouches-du-Rhône), to name only a few, in each of which a floating, disembodied horse's head appears somewhere high on a wall. This image appears so often that it seems to have had some special meaning.

The severely attenuated figure of a woman in a bent-over position is engraved or painted repeatedly in the Ice Age caves of France, such as Pech-Merle, Labastide (Hautes-Pyrénées), and, in Dordogne, Les Combarelles, Cougnac, Fronsac, Gare de Couze, and La Roche de Lalinde (fig. 3.6). It also appears in the cave at Gönnersdorf, Germany. The few lines of which this image is composed leave out the head, feet, arms, and sometimes breasts. The line of the buttocks and back is enough to evoke a generic woman. Some sculpted female forms, such as the steatite female figure from Peterfels, Germany, are realized with a similar minimal treatment and seem to embody the same succinct approach to the female figure as that of twentieth-century artists such as Constantin Brancusi and Jean Arp.

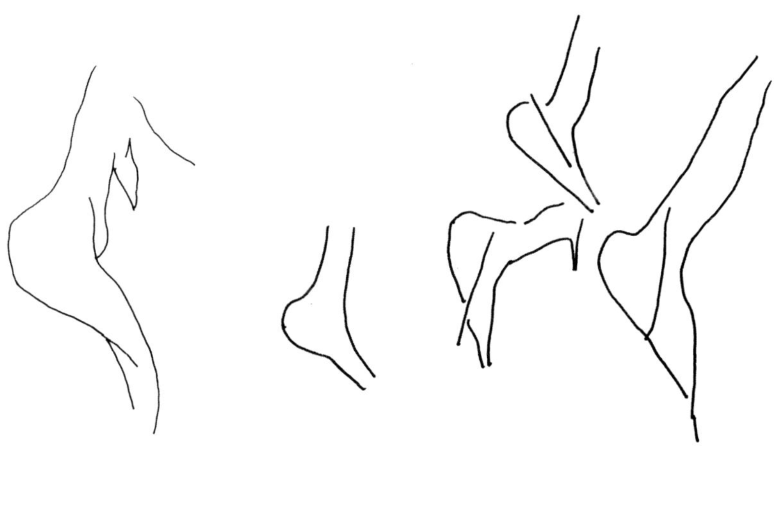

Figure 3.6. Schematic female figures. Left: La Gare de Couze (one figure). Right: La Roche de Lalinde (four figures).

Our minds want to fill in what is missing. In Chauvet, only 11 of 36 horses depicted actually have eyes.[17] Without our being aware of it, our minds supply the eyes that are not there. Perhaps this is what was meant by the ancient

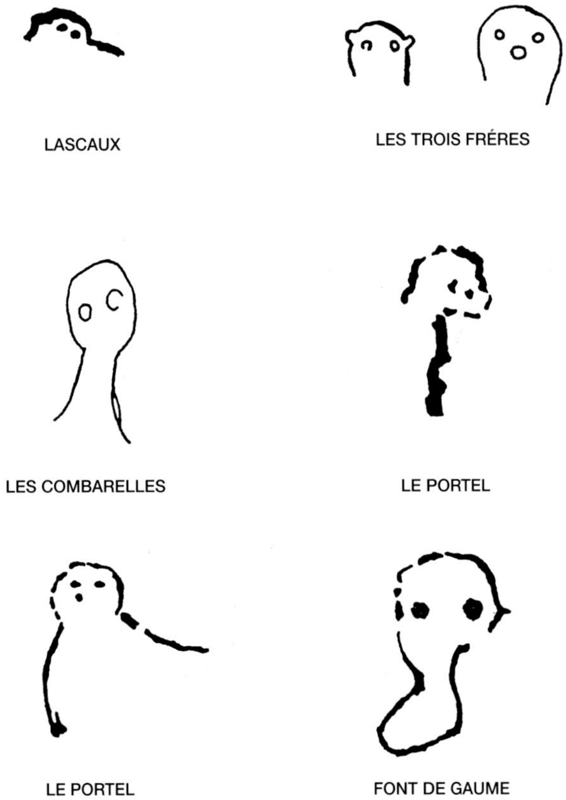

Figure 3.7. Schematic images called "ghosts" from Ice Age panels.

Chinese artist's dictum, "A figure painted without eyes must seem to look; without ears must seem to listen."[18] In several caves in France—Cougnac, Les Combarelles, Le Portel, Lascaux, Trois Frères, and Font de Gaume—there are marks that range from a nearly completed circle to a mere loop or the barest arc. Common to all these abbreviated figures are two dots side by side within the completed or implied circle (fig. 3.7). Prehistorians believe these schematic images represent some sort of presence, which they refer to as "ghosts." In such contexts, two dots placed side by side cry out to be read as eyes.

It takes very little to suggest a face. On the top of Black Mesa, near the Tewa-speaking Pueblo of San Ildefonso, New Mexico, a boulder called Tunjopin has two large sockets, unavoidably viewed as eyes, and another, smaller hole seen as a nose or a mouth. To complete the face, the boulder has been partially carved. It has been said that the people of the pueblo think of it as an upward-staring face whose eye sockets fill with water when it rains. Perhaps the carver who completed the face felt that its fixed regard was imploring rain.

On a larger scale, one sees the face that people have long pieced together from the shadowy spots on the moon, creating "the man in the moon." More recently, in photographs beamed back from the spacecraft *Voyager,* there appeared a distinct, mysterious, facelike configuration on Mars that, although we know it is only the light and shade from rock formations, insists on haunting us as a face. Picasso was one of many artists who recognized the human tendency to see a face if given the merest suggestion. "Two holes," he said—"that is the symbol for the face, enough to evoke it without representing it."[19] Rocks are peopled with faces.

Human infants appear to be born with a few basic responses: the desire to suck, a fear of falling, the need to turn toward a sound, and a fascination with faces. An innate response to faces, especially to eyes, continues in us as adults. The ability to read the expressions on faces must have been an important survival mechanism in human history.

The tendency to see faces appears to go back even farther in our lineage. In South Africa, the archaeologist Raymond Dart found an ironstone cobble believed to have been picked up by a distant Australopithecine ancestor 3 million years ago and carried to Makapansgat Cave, Limpopo, South Africa, from a place at least 32 kilometers away. It seems that the cobble was carried this distance because, with two depressions that might be seen as eyes, it appeared to be a face.[20] Such concern with faces may extend beyond our lineage as well. In recordings of a monkey's brain, it was found that a specific group of brain cells became active when confronted with a face.[21] In humans, information that might pertain to faces is sent to an area of the brain called the inferotemporal cortex, consisting of three regions of the temporal cortex in which neurons have been found that seem to respond solely to stimuli representing faces or parts of faces. Each face is distinguishable because it presents a unique pattern of firing over the many neurons responsible for face recognition. The specific area most involved in recognizing faces seems to be the fusiform gyrus, especially the right hemisphere fusiform gyrus.[22] With minimal suggestion, Ice Age artists often saw faces and often made them more complete. This use of closure results from the human propensity to make sense, to find meaning.

The Brain Constructs What It Perceives

From earliest times, humans have looked into the night sky at the stars and planets, pinpoints of light that seem to have no recognizable meaning. But our minds are programmed to fill in the blanks—in this case, literally to connect the dots—so that all over the world, in disparate cultures, humans have found animals and gods in the heavens. The figures differed from culture to culture, but the process was always the same. Our brains are constructed to make meaning from the seemingly random sense impressions that bombard us. We are driven to transform what appears as inchoate sensation into meaningful information because that is the only way we are able to respond rapidly. As it is for other animals, speed is essential for us to survive in real life. Therefore, we often must react on the basis of only partial information, which we interpret as if it were complete.

Each of us has an empty space on the retina that does not respond to light. It is the proverbial "blind spot" where the optic nerve passes through the retina and where, consequently, there are no photoreceptors. Unless its existence is demonstrated to us by examination, we are unaware of it. Although information arriving at the retina is interrupted by the gap in the visual field, we do not notice it, because our minds automatically fill in the empty space. The filling in of this information by the mind is another kind of closure.

Vilaynur S. Ramachandran, of the University of California's Center for Brain and Cognition, has discussed a neurological condition that he refers to as the Charles Bonnet syndrome. First described by the Swiss naturalist Charles Bonnet in the eighteenth century, it is a condition causing visual hallucinations. Patients with damage somewhere in their visual pathway replace the missing reality with vivid visual hallucinations. The cartoon artist James Thurber lost the sight in one eye at the age of six when he was accidentally shot with a toy arrow fired by his brother. Sight was poor in his remaining eye. Thurber wrote to his ophthalmologist describing images that he was hallucinating: a blue Hoover vacuum cleaner, an old woman with a gray parasol walking right through the side of a truck, a cat rolling across a street in a striped barrel, bridges rising lazily into the air like balloons. Thurber called these surreal images, resulting from flawed vision, "daydreams." Rather than being disturbed by them, he made use of them as stimuli for his drawings and stories.[23]

Beyond the eye, farther along on the visual processing pathway, holes can occur in the brain's perceptual field. In one example, a woman suffering from an arteriovenous malformation in her brain had it treated with a laser in order to prevent a dangerous hemorrhage. The procedure left scar tissue on part of her visual cortex, with the result that her visual area had a large blank spot, called a scotoma. Without her being aware that what she apparently saw was her own invention, her brain filled in the blank area with hallucinations, in this case cartoon characters. She seemed impelled to fill in the blank rather than to accept that there was a void in her vision.[24]

The term "filling in" is further qualified by scientists such as Andy Clark, who stresses that even normal vision is partly an act of imagination colored by experience and expectation.[25] In this view, perception itself is seen as a creative process.

Priming, or Expectation

Anyone who can handle a needle convincingly can make us see a thread which is not there.
—E. H. GOMBRICH

The images we use to fill up the voids in our visual perception are not arbitrary. When Greeks or Arabs or Indians looked up at the night sky to draw imagined lines between stars, they were influenced by their myths, which predisposed them to see certain animals or heroes or gods. Beliefs, suggestions,

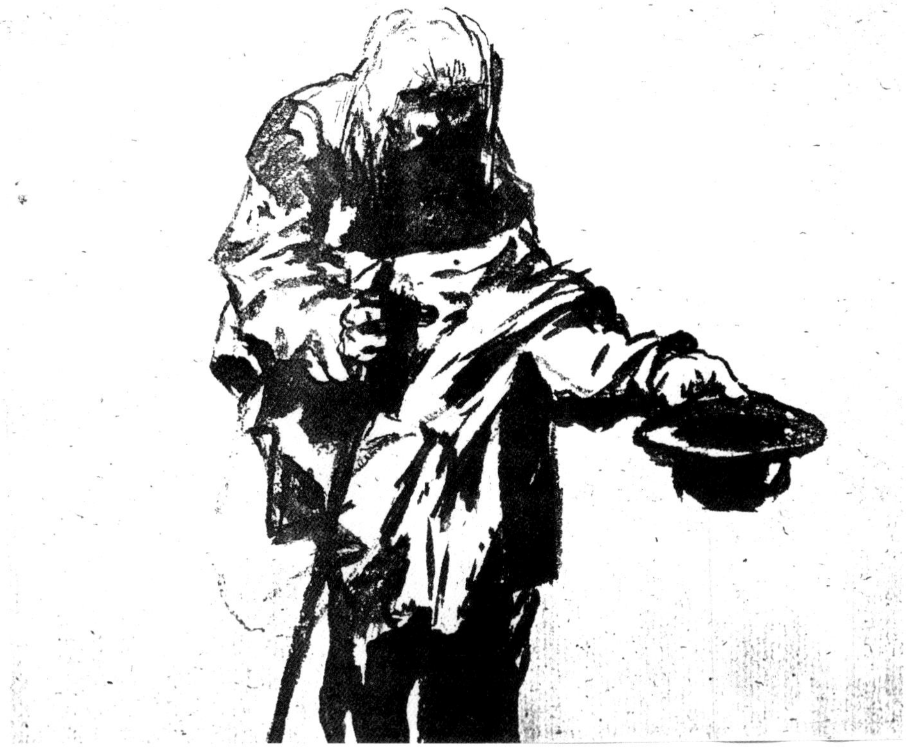

Figure 3.8. Francisco Goya, *Beggar with a Staff in His Right Hand,* undated but done between 1792 and 1828. Brush and ink, 14 by 20.3 cm. ©The Metropolitan Museum of Art

and hints set the stage for the interpretation of data in one way or another. Psychologists call such stage-setting "priming." Endel Tulving and Daniel Schecter described the process as "creating a context within which our expectations may work. One gives clues and a push in a specific direction. Then the imagination takes off."[26] Our imagination completes the partial image.

When imagery is arcane and inaccessible, such as one finds in cubist or abstract expressionist art, then the title of the work is important for priming the viewer about what to find. Representational art may be self-priming. For example, in a drawing by Francisco Goya (fig. 3.8), enough graphic information is given, especially when the viewer is primed by the hat and cane, for the viewer to know that this is a person, in fact a person in rags. In this late work, a quick sweep of the brush and a few ink strokes suggest only an eye, a cheek, and a nostril. Yet convincingly the subject becomes a real person who has a history and a highly individual character.

What we believe to be direct experience is not simple or seamless, for our perception of the world, which seems so smooth and inevitable, is really the assembling of a collage of fragments. These fragments are composed of interactions between the objective world and our mental modes of reaction. The neuropsychologist Karl Pribram said that perception is not direct but rather is a construction.[27] The more that is left out, the more we ourselves must supply to flesh it out, and the more we then project our own thoughts onto it. It is a seeming paradox that images that require the most work on our part in their construction are also the most powerful, because as they become a part of us, we literally become a part of them. Perception may be conceived of as a kind of detective work. To assemble an image we must use all our past experience and all our new experience and then collate all this information. When we interpret Rorschach inkblots, we are merely letting our minds do what they always do—draw conclusions from incomplete information. When the data are inconclusive, the brain makes the best guesses it can.

Sometimes the conclusions we draw seem startling. Ramachandran's brain hemorrhage patient filled in the blank spot in her perceptual field with seemingly arbitrary images. Although the imagery her brain used seemed to be random, the randomness itself might have been significant. The psychiatrist and dream specialist J. Allan Hobson wrote that "randomness seems to be an intrinsic aspect of brain function."[28] He expressed the belief that the images that appear in dreams might be random but that while we are dreaming and immediately afterward we create a narrative that provides the dream images with a story line. We may judge the importance of this aspect of brain function by the fact that the neuroscientist Francis Crick believed that as much as 90 percent of our gray matter is, in addition to any other function, wired to make interpretations or tell stories.[29] Again, our minds seem to be compelled to uncover meaning whenever the intrinsic meaning of an image is not apparent. In such instances we have wide scope to invent. Hobson said that "our creativity and our freedom [to create] both depend upon randomness." When our minds fill in the empty spaces, either in our perception or in our understanding, new and startling discoveries may take place, and the result is one aspect of what we call creativity.

PROJECTION, OR THE RORSCHACH EFFECT

> *You can't depend on your eyes when your imagination is out of focus.*
>
> —MARK TWAIN, *A Connecticut Yankee in King Arthur's Court*

There is no more intense black than the black of deep caves. To enter them is all the more daunting because of our natural dread of darkness. Geologic formations stirred the imaginations of the Ice Age artists who were the first humans to explore and leave their marks in these inaccessible places. By flickering tallow lamp, objects take on other presences, and we project onto suggestive formations some of the images that haunt our imaginations. This is the principle of the Rorschach test, in which psychologists devise amorphous shapes onto which viewers project images that are meaningful to themselves. It was in this frightening context of barely subdued darkness that most of what remains of the great Ice Age art was made. Here our senses are alert. Adrenalin flows, sensations are heightened, memories are imprinted. Our experiences at such times are committed to vivid, long-term memory.[30] This would have been a compelling reason for subjecting young men in tribal societies to frightening situations during ceremonial rites, times when important information was conferred on the initiates. Fear has a perverse attraction for modern humans, just as it might well have had for our Paleolithic forebears.

The viewer looks at a chance configuration and sees in it what is already in his mind. In some instances, the undulations of cave walls suggested to Ice Age artists almost an entire relief sculpture. Among the most striking examples is the ceiling of Altamira (see illus. p. 40). There, a standing bison was modeled on an outcrop, with a fissure forming the contours of its forehead. Another natural relief inspired a hunched bison. In one remarkable painting, a recumbent bison, head turned backward, juts out from the rest of the animal on a rocky outcrop (fig. 3.9). The outline of the animal's forehead and muzzle made use of the exact edges of this bulge in the ceiling. Further, the artist managed to make the bison's thigh correspond on a rocky ledge. An embossment on the ceiling was transformed into another recumbent bison by painting its limbs folded within the protruding bulk. Only the horns and tail were painted outside the natural stone embossment. A wild boar was painted in a similar manner on another outcrop.

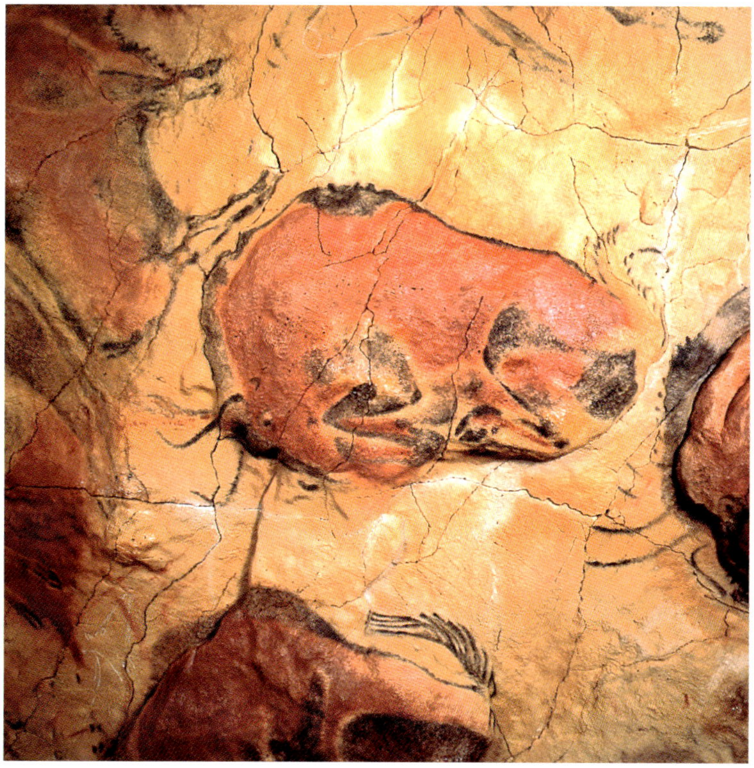

Figure 3.9. A bison on the ceiling at Altamira shows the use of natural rock projections to create animal figures with painted additions of horns and tails. 1.85 m. About 14,500 B.P.

Fortuitous stone configurations make the caves rich with suggested figures. A twisted stalagmite at El Castillo was seen as the hindquarters of a vertical bison. The animal's head, front legs, and ventral thigh were drawn into the preexisting shapes on one side of the formation (fig. 3.10). Another bison head

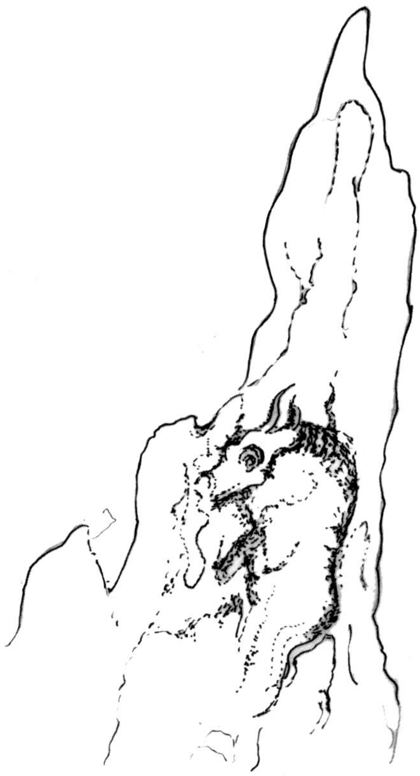

Figure 3.10. Above: Bison on a stalagmite at El Castillo. The artist used the natural formation to create the back tail and hind legs of a standing bison and completed the figure with black paint. Length of animal 80 cm. Below: On the other side, the curved tip of the stalagmite is the horn for the head of another bison.

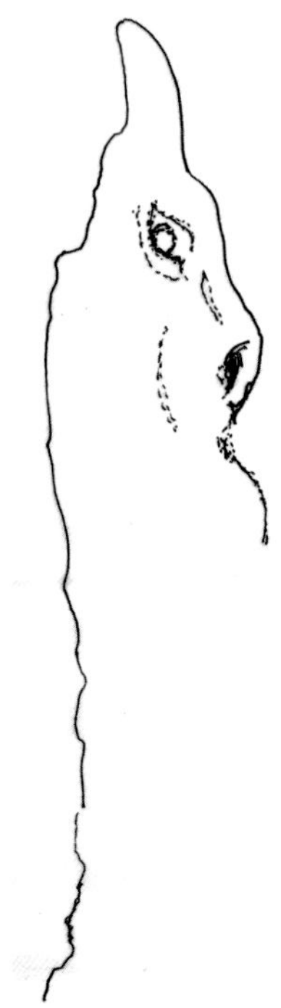

with horns upthrust appears on the other side of the stalactite, almost entirely using its natural formation, with only a small number of added marks. In some cases such formations were points of departure for figures that were then further delineated. Font de Gaume has many such examples. In one, a natural rocky relief was utilized for the figure of a bison. In the Lateral Gallery, the hindquarters, rump, and tail of a horse were formed by use of strands of dripped stalactites. The silhouette of a horse was partly formed by the natural rock. At Pech-Merle, a rocky formation was turned into a mammoth, and the creator of one of a pair of horses made use of a stalagmite for its modeling (the other horse is painted). In the same cave, stalactites became the hind legs and tail of a leaping horse and the long coats of woolly mammoths.

At Cougnac, a stalagmite formation was used for the back, legs, and pelt of an ibex, and stalactite formations became the pelt and legs of another animal. At Ekain, in the Spanish province of Guipúzcoa, stalactites formed a bison's back and tail, and at Altxerri, in the same province, stalactites were seen to form a bird. At Teyjat a stalactite that suggests a human head has eyes scratched on it. At Bernifal a small stalactite served as a nose for what was made into a human face; the same thing appears on a larger scale at La Colombière (Ain). At Le Portel, about 12,000 years ago, the outline of a man was painted around a small stalactite in such a way that it became a penis, on the tip of which the artist added a red dot. At Covalanas, a ledge was utilized to form part of the back and hindquarters of a large red deer. At Niaux, another stone relief formed an inverted horse's head and an up-ended bison. At Mas d'Azil, a naturally rippled rock surface suggested scales, and a fish was drawn around it. At Pergouset (Lot-et-Garonne), a natural bulge in a rock with a knob in the middle of it was seen as a belly with a navel. To complete the figure, an engraved vulva was added. Other examples of carved and engraved vulvas occur at myriad sites, including Marsoulas, Les Combarelles, Sireuil (Dordogne), Marcenac (Lot), Mas d'Azil, Tuc d'Audoubert, Pindal (Asturias), Covalanas, Hornos de la Peña, El Castillo, and La Pasiega. Natural formations served to make at least part of a figure in almost all the caves of France and Spain.

Natural holes, as we saw earlier, have been used as eyes with great frequency in rock art throughout the world. One of the most dramatic examples occurs in Niaux in the French Pyrénées, where a cup-shaped depression made by water dripping from a stalactite onto the cave floor was used by an artist to indicate the eye of a bison. The artist saw the hole as an eye and around it projected the bison's body. Other, similar holes nearby were read as wounds on the body (fig. 3.11). A horse at Gabillou has an eye formed by a pebble imbedded in the cave wall. A preexisting flint nodule was used to form the eye of a bison at Rouffignac. The more realistic head of the right-hand spotted horse at Pech-Merle is formed by a natural rock shape that might have inspired the horse images to begin with. An Ice Age artist at Niaux saw a rocky edge as the dorsal line of a vertical bison. The shadowed area behind this edge gave an illusion of the bulky bison. The mere addition of a few red lines to outline the head, belly and legs allow us once to witness the process of projection at work (fig. 3.12, see also illus. p. 118).

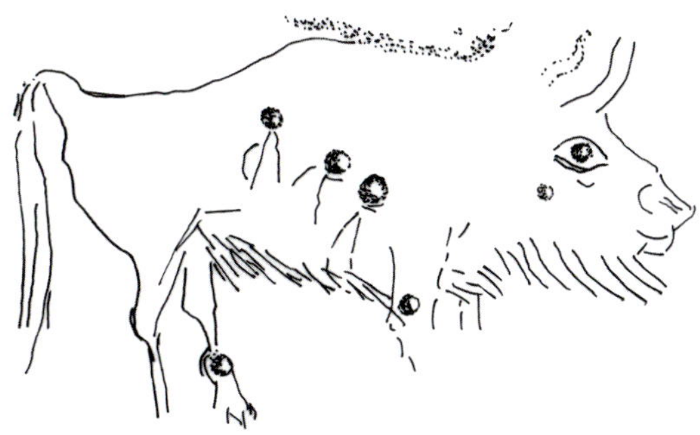

Figure 3.11. Bison incised on the clay floor at Niaux. The engraving was conceived around preexisting stalactite drip holes. One hole was made into the eye, and the other two were seen as wound marks. Width 57 cm, length 60 cm.

The same imaginative process took place in the use of three-dimensional artifacts. A small stone from Les Eyzies had a natural head shape. Recognizing this, someone added an eye, a nostril, ears, and a line for the mouth. Similar examples have been found in Spain at El Castillo and Pindal and in France at Niaux and La Croze à Gontron.

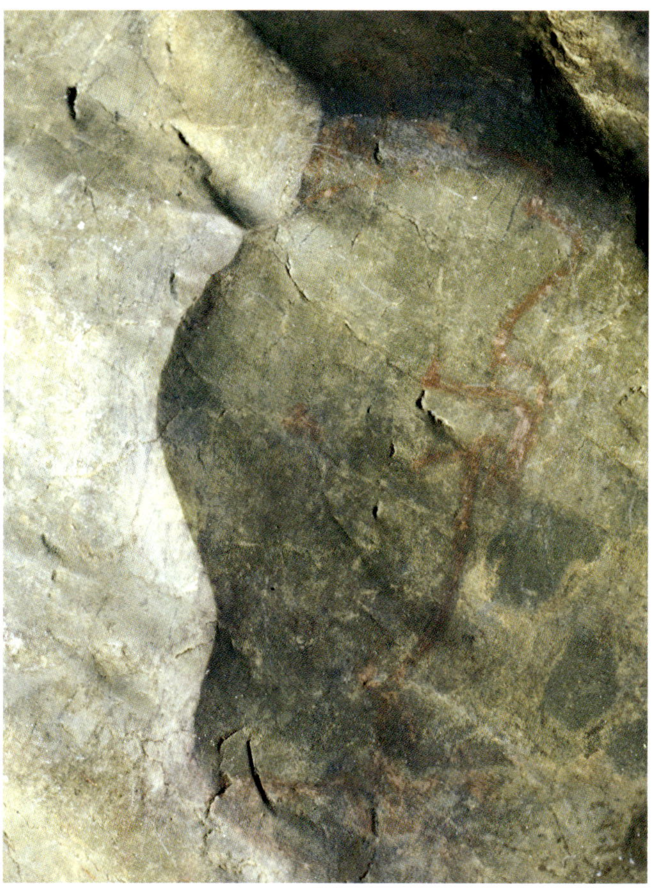

Figure 3.12. A bison at Niaux was created by using shadow to indicate form, making use of the convex-concave illusion. Drawing in red ocher on the farther wall completes the animal.
Photo: J. Clottes

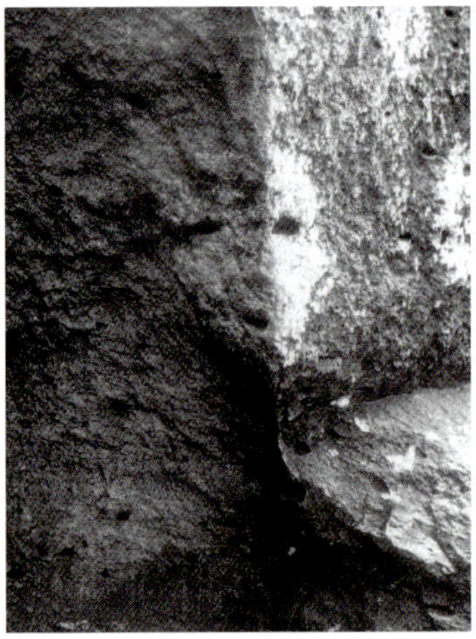

Figure 3.13. Petroglyph head at Cieneguilla, New Mexico. The artist observed what appeared to be a ready-made face and selected it by abrading around the face.

Examples of Projection in the Art of North American Indians

Projection is a human phenomenon that occurs in art everywhere. Other than Ice Age art, I am most familiar with the petroglyph art of the native people of the American Southwest, and so I compare the ways in which these two cultures, so distant from each other in space and time, used projection. Native American artists, too, projected images onto natural forms, but they did so less dramatically than did artists in the European caves, perhaps because they saw the surfaces in sunlight rather than under evocative lamplight. Chumash people in what is now California, for example, spoke of a sacred place in the Sierra Madre called Sapaksi, the House of the Sun, where eagles, falcons, bears, and ravens could be recognized in rock formations.[31] At Zuñi Pueblo in New Mexico, a bird was engraved on the edge of a rock face that juts out into space, so that the bird seems to be flying off the rock.[32]

In the Rio Grande area, many art panels are on escarpments of volcanic basalt studded with holes formed by gas bubbles in the once molten rock. The ubiquitous natural holes that remain in the hardened lava are seen as the eyes and mouths of faces or masks. Some of the innumerable examples in the Pueblo rock art of New Mexico are found at Comanche Gap and San Cristóbal in the Galisteo Basin, at Three Rivers in the southeastern part of the state, and at Piedras Marcadas in Petroglyph National Monument near Albuquerque. At La Cieneguilla, near Santa Fe, a striking little face appeared when bubble holes were imagined to be eyes and an open mouth (fig. 3.13).[33] At Zuñi, a natural break in a rock served as a mouth around which a face was engraved. Three natural slits in sedimentary rock were used to create three grinning faces at Pueblo Blanco, New Mexico (fig. 3.14).

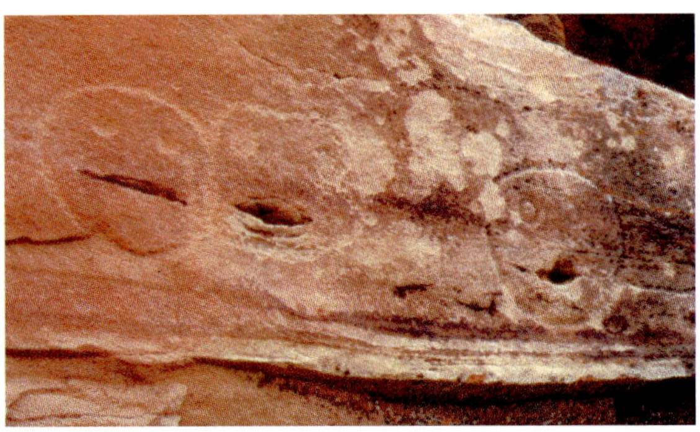

Figure 3.14. Three grinning faces making use of natural rock slits for mouths, Pueblo Blanco, New Mexico.

Holes were also used for vaginas—for example, at Rochester Creek, Utah. In Peterborough, Ontario, the creator of a five-foot-high female figure in the Northern Woodland style made use of a natural hole for a vulva. There is a granite boulder at Peninsula Range, Canebrake, Washington, near Agua Caliente Springs, where a natural formation was seen as a vulva. In the desert of southern California, the Kumeyaay people sought out certain cracks in rocks that were then enhanced into vulva symbols. Some can be seen at Anza-Borrego Desert State Park in California. All these graphic manipulations create a double entendre in which the forms are read both as morphological configuration and as image.

Projection and Creativity

Projection was used and written about in early historic times. The first-century Roman writer Pliny the Elder wrote of how the artist Protogenes and others dashed sponges saturated with paint at a wall to give the illusion of foam and to make suggestive shapes that could be used in their paintings.[34] Similarly, a ninth-century Chinese treatise described a group of artists called "the untrammeled," who "excelled in splattering ink to paint landscapes." The author wrote of one Tang dynasty artist, Wang Mo, saying that "when sufficiently drunk, he would splatter the ink onto the painting surface. . . . [Later] he would follow the shapes, making these into mountains, rocks, clouds and water."[35] In the eleventh century the Chinese artist Sung Ti wrote advice to a colleague in order to help him improve his landscape technique:

> You should choose an old tumbledown wall and throw over it a piece of white silk. Then, morning and evening, you should gaze at it until, at length, you can see the ruins through the silk, its prominences, its levels, its zigzags, and its cleavages, storing them up in your mind and fixing them in your eyes. Make the prominences your mountains, the lower part your water, the hollows your ravines, the cracks your streams, the lighter parts your nearer points, the darker parts your more distant points. Get all these thoroughly into you, and soon you will see men, birds, plants, and trees, flying and moving among them. You then ply your brush according to your fancy.[36]

This technique, using a silk covering, has been known as "Chinese occlusion." Four hundred years later, Leonardo da Vinci wrote of his own process for stimulating the imagination:

> You should look at certain walls stained with damp, or at stones of uneven colour. If you have to invent some backgrounds, you will be able to see in these the likeness of divine landscapes, adorned with mountains, ruins, rocks, woods, great plains, hills and valleys in great variety; and then again you will see there battles and strange figures in violent action, expressions of faces and clothes and an infinity of things which you will be able to reduce to their complete and proper forms. In such walls the same thing happens as in the

> sound of bells, in whose stroke you may find every named word which you can imagine.[37]

Leonardo's words inspired Alexander Cozens, the eighteenth-century artist and drawing master, to make use of inkblots to stimulate the artistic imagination. Cozens described the use of what he called "blottings" in a book published around 1785. The method consisted of making inkblots to produce chance shapes. He wrote: "To sketch . . . is to transfer ideas from the mind to the paper. . . . to blot is to make varied spots . . . producing accidental forms . . . from which ideas are presented to the mind. . . . To sketch is to delineate ideas: blotting suggests them." We know the mind is eager to make its own sense of these suggestions. As Cozens put it, his method "may yet be of considerable service in opening the mind and putting it upon the scent of new thoughts."[38] The art historian E. H. Gombrich saw a link between the fashion started by Cozens and the diagnostic tool developed by Rorschach 150 years later.

Without knowing of the ideas of Leonardo, much less Protogenes or the Chinese "untrammeled" painters, artists have continued to devise similar techniques to stimulate creativity. Apollonius of Tyana is said to have been inspired by looking at cloud formations. Mantegna also used clouds to find forms, specifically faces. Botticelli is said to have thrown colored sponges at his canvases.[39] Goya, in masterpieces of his old age, made intense little paintings by dropping water onto ivory plaquettes that were prepared with wet black paint. He would then manipulate the resulting shadowy blots into the lights and darks of forms. Henry Moore collected beach stones to derive inspiration from their sea-eroded forms. Jean Arp threw cut-up pieces of paper onto a background paper, using the aleatory result almost as he found it. The sculptor Jacques Lipschitz threw handfuls of soft clay on the ground and then examined them to find shapes that interested him. There was even an artist, briefly in vogue, who selected and enlarged for his sculptures the shapes made by well-masticated chewing gum. Jan van Goyen, Joseph Mallord William Turner, and Willem de Kooning used streaks or other randomly made marks on the canvas before they began painting. A number of artists have looked at the suggestive potential of fire by scorching, smoking, and using the marks left by an explosion. Such techniques have continued to be used to stimulate the artist's imagination.

In 1945, after the end of World War II, a group of artists met regularly in a little bistro in Paris called Le Catalan. They were Max Ernst, Alexander Calder, Balthasar Balthus, Jean Cocteau, and Pablo Picasso. While they talked and caroused they drew on the paper tablecloths, incorporating in their drawings stains from wine and coffee, lipstick and mustard, using these as points of departure for their improvisations. Someone saved these tablecloths, and many years later they were exhibited as *Jeux de Nappes,* or *Tablecloth Games.*

Many artists have sensed that there is some basic link between the origin of art and the process of projection. More than 500 years ago the architect Leon Battista Alberti, now famous for his treatise on Renaissance linear perspective, hypothesized about the origin of representational art:

> In a tree trunk, a lump of earth, or in some other thing were accidentally discovered one day certain contours that needed only a very slight change to look strikingly like some natural object. Noticing this, people tried to see if it were not possible by addition or subtraction to complete what still was lacking for a perfect likeness. From that day, man's capacity to create images grew apace until he was able to create any likeness, even when there was no vague outline in the material to aid him.[40]

This art origin myth seems made to order to explain the process of projection.

Picasso was familiar with many caves in his native Spain and his adopted France. Although he vowed that he would never return to Spain while Franco ruled, he did return clandestinely and incognito to view the cave art that had been newly discovered in the Cantabrian region.[41] Picasso well understood the ancient roots of his work, and he devised an origin story of his own: "If it occurred to man to create his own images, it's because he discovered them all around him, almost formed, already within his grasp. He saw them in a bone, in the irregular surface of cavern walls, in a piece of wood. . . . One form might suggest a woman, another a bison, and still another the head of a demon."[42] He described projection as he imagined it to have occurred in Ice Age art, at the same time revealing the cognitive process involved in his own creativity and making clear a link uniting his art-making process with that of the Ice Age artists.

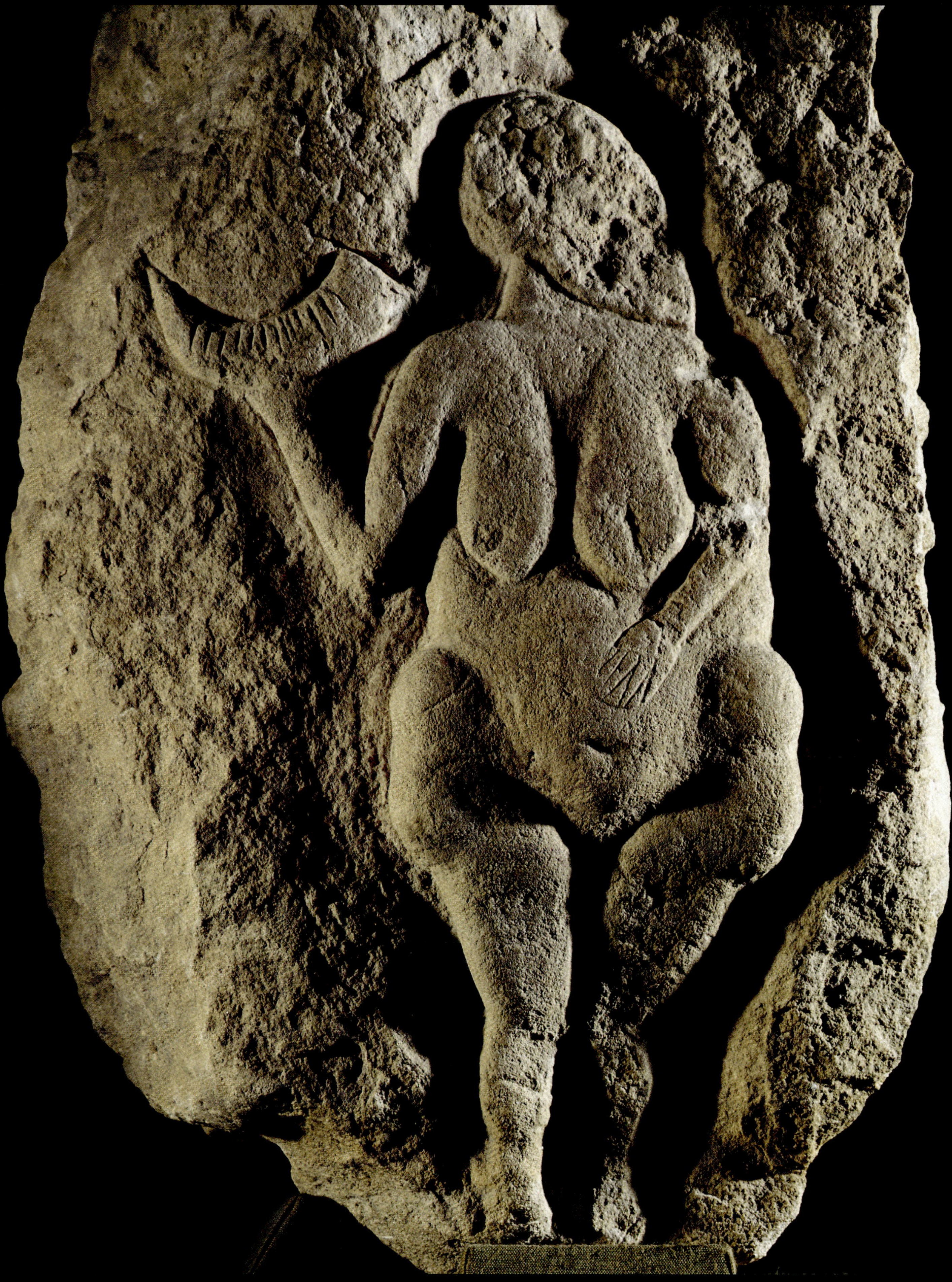

4

ANALOGY

Finding Likeness in the Unlike

An idea is a feat of association.

—ROBERT FROST

HUMANS ARE ALWAYS SEARCHING for likeness between things that are unlike. This is especially clear in the utterances of children, who make surprising, often poetic comparisons, because they are just learning how to relate things to one another. As an example, my son, Jedidiah, at the age of four, likened the sound of crickets to that of "hundreds of freshly oiled scissors." The search for analogy is frozen into language.

Anecdotal evidence suggests that analogy making is an inborn human trait. The "Wild Boy of Aveyron" fared for himself from the time he was deserted in childhood until the age of about 11 or 12. In January 1800 he was found wandering naked in the woods, eating acorns and roots. Brought to Paris, he was placed in the care of the psychologist Jean-Marc Gaspard Itard, who gave him the name Victor and attempted to teach him to speak, all the while using him as a subject of research. Because of his age, Victor was never able to learn to speak more than a few words, but by combining these with gestures he was able to communicate with his mentor. Commenting on Victor's organization of reality, Itard said, "When considering things from the point of view of their similarity or of their common qualities, Victor concluded that since there was a resemblance of shape between certain objects, there ought in certain circumstances to be an identity of uses and functions."[1]

Victor's belief may reveal a universal thought process. Among traditional people this thought process might be seen in sympathetic magic. For example, the Pueblo Indians of the American Southwest are in perpetual need of rain. Smoke, with its analogy to clouds, was traditionally thought to induce the formation of rain clouds. Keresan and Zuñi rain priests whipped the roots of yucca plants into suds in terrace shaped bowls to imitate rain clouds.[2] The froth was lifted off, cast to the four directions, and placed on altars.

Opposite: Carved bas-relief on limestone from Laussel (Dordogne) called 'the Venus of Laussel'. The horn in right hand may have metaphoric meaning. C. 27,000 to 22,000 B.P. Height 54.5 cm. Photo by E. Lessing / Art Resource, N.Y.

Such concepts, applied to healing, have been called the "law of similars," most recently by proponents of homeopathy, a school of medicine founded by Samuel Hahnemann at the end of the eighteenth century. But similar ideas go back much earlier, to the "doctrine of signatures," which expresses the belief that plants have been marked by a creator with signs indicating their medicinal purposes. Such ideas first came to light in ancient China. Similar beliefs were codified in Europe during the Middle Ages and further popularized by Paracelsus during the Renaissance. A plant or animal, it was believed, resembled the part of the body whose ills it could cure. Hahnemann, in his 1810 treatise *Organon of Rational Medicine,* expressed this concept as "like cures like." His followers affirm that the Greek physician Hippocrates, known as the father of medicine, expressed the idea in almost the same words 2,400 years ago.

Examples of uses of plant and animal products according to such beliefs can be found in various parts of the world. In ancient Europe, a hairy-looking lichen was used as a hair strengthener, and another lichen, parts of which resembled a dog's teeth, was used to treat rabies. Lungwort was prescribed for chest ailments because its spotted leaves seemed to resemble diseased lungs. Rhinoceros horns were thought to be aphrodisiacs because of their phallic shape, and even today rhinoceroses are slaughtered for their horns, which are sold primarily in Africa and Asia.[3] The same kind of thought was seen in the curing beliefs of North American Natives who thought a red plant was good for purification of the blood and a yellow plant for treating jaundice.[4] So widespread was the belief in the link between appearance and healing power that it may reveal a universal analogy-making process in the human mind.

Graphic artists sometimes use analogy to create a subtle reverberation between shapes, tying together unlike forms in an underlying unity. Degas did this in his painting *Dancers Practicing at the Bar.* An unlikely similarity of form is drawn between the young ballet student, hand on hip, one leg raised high, and a watering can used to wet down the studio floor, its handle echoing the dancer's arm and its long spout like the dancer's raised leg. This analogy was no accident; Degas used the device at other times as well. In *The Dance Class,* from the previous year, the watering can is turned so that the spout is hidden. The dancer nearest to it, wearing a ribbon of the same green as the watering can, stands watching the dance master with hand on hip, a position that mimics the way the bent handle meets the can.

Analogy making is part of a systematic ordering of the world based on finding similarities and then describing one system of phenomena in terms of another system. It is related to what the ethologist Desmond Morris was thinking when he defined art as a taxonomic urge, an urge to classify so as to find analogies.[5] Artists use each of two opposed mental processes—specifying and generalizing—to give themselves and then, vicariously, the sensitized viewer a thrill of discovery. The discovery itself might be reward enough, because it allows us to see deeper similarities beneath the varied and transient world of the senses, but it does more than that. New links give us hope that events and objects are not entirely isolated but rather form part of an underlying and unsuspected unity to our world.

An example of the power of analogy is an incident that occurred during the Cold War. Vladimir Engelhardt, the leading biochemist in the Soviet Union in the 1960s, told a visiting scientific delegation the following story. A newly designed airplane kept losing first one wing and then the other in trial runs. Finally, the manager of the factory consulted the oldest and wisest aircraft designer in the country. After pondering the problem, the designer advised drilling small holes through both wings at 10-centimeter intervals along the line of cleavage. That solved the problem. The plane flew successfully. Surprised, other engineers asked him how he knew that the holes would balance the forces and strengthen rather than weaken the wings. "Such problems," he explained, "are too complex to solve by logic." He had been inspired when he made a comparison between the airplane's wing and Soviet toilet paper, which never tore along the line of perforation. "Such problems can be solved only by analogy."[6]

In this chapter I delve into three aspects of analogy making that Ice Age people first used in creating art and that have reappeared around the world throughout human history. They are metaphor, exaggeration (or hyperbole), and use of found objects. I treat exaggeration as analogy because in the instances I discuss, the exaggerated form is considered to be essentially similar to the normal form and is universally recognized as such. I classify found objects under analogy because the art maker sees in the object an underlying likeness to something quite different, and by the maker's action, the found object reveals its transformed meaning. Metaphor is related to analogy because it is another, more poetic way of signaling likeness.

Metaphors have a way of exploding the bounds of perception, of making plain the essential unity of nature.

—CHET RAYMO, *The Virgin and the Mousetrap*

METAPHOR

The animals in Ice Age art, especially the majestic painted animals in caves such as Lascaux, Niaux, and Chauvet, convey an almost palpable physical presence. Yet we come away from viewing them with the feeling that they embody meanings just beyond our grasp. From the first glimpse of this art, prehistorians and other viewers have formulated theories about that hidden meaning: that the art represents hunting magic, animal rebirth, clans, totems, and a host of other suggestions. Each theory dominated until a new one emerged, superceding and negating the previous one.

Rather than speculate about overarching meanings, I want to mine a different vein and try to find clues to specific associations in small, seemingly insignificant details. These are more akin to often overlooked evidence called "Morellian details" by art specialists who investigate forgeries. In a Rembrandt print, for instance, these detectives find the most rewarding evidence not in the figures themselves but in marks made in neglected corners, in lines indicating, say, grass or shadow, made without the care given to the more important images. With this in mind, I look closely at some seemingly incidental lines in a larger composition at Lascaux and find a possible Ice Age metaphor.

Water and Snakes

The Chamber of the Felines at Lascaux is extremely difficult to reach, even by cave explorer standards. One must stoop, crouch, crawl, and worm one's way into a narrow crack to see a tangle of engravings. On one panel is an engraving of three lions (fig. 4.1). One male lion, claws unsheathed, nostrils enlarged,

Figure 4.1. Lions confronting one another in the Chamber of the Felines, Lascaux. The one on the right appears to be urinating, possibly to claim territorial ownership by spraying his scent. Right, 100 cm; left, about 75 cm.

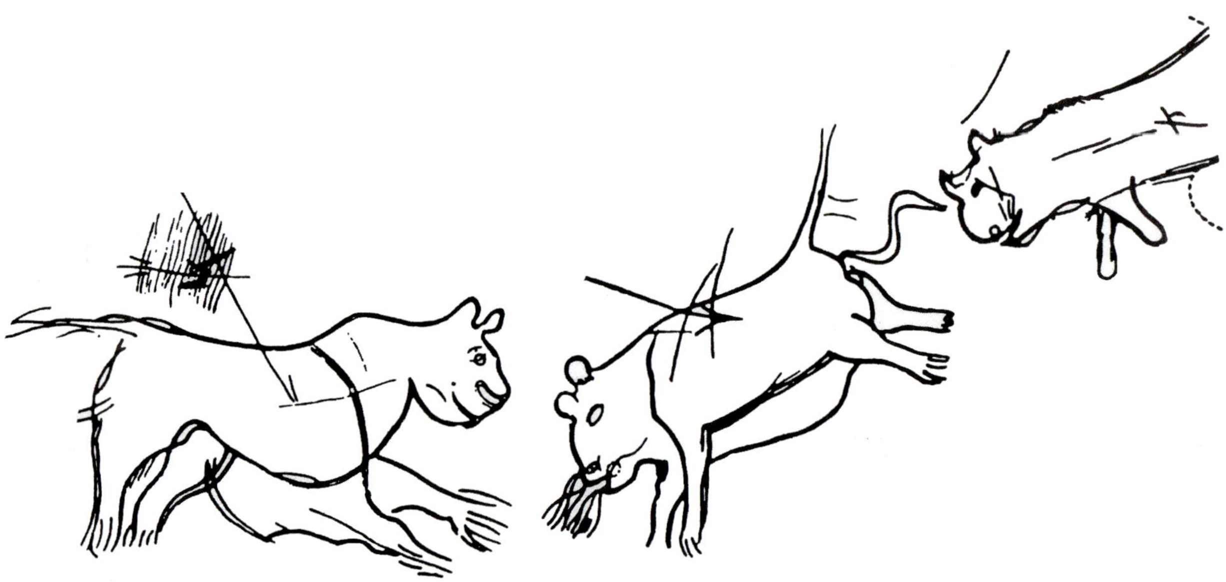

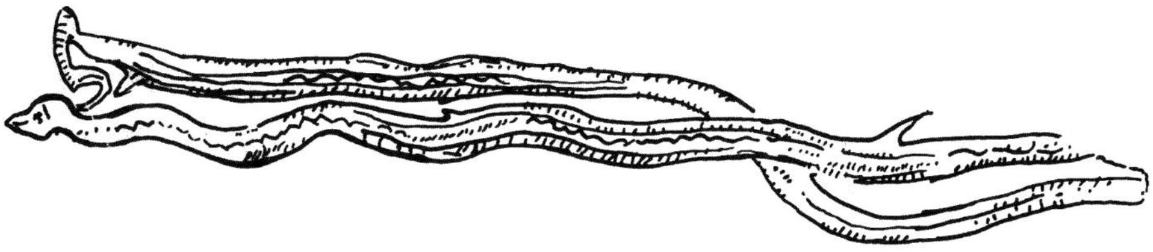

Figure 4.2. Engraved snakes on a baton of reindeer antler from Montgaudier. Length 37.2 cm.

seems to be demonstrating territoriality. Facing it is another lion, possibly growling. "Its tail lashes the air above it and it shoots out a jet of urine, marking out its territory."[7] Two parallel wavy lines emerge from its hindquarters. For their survival, Ice Age hunters had to study the habits of animals carefully, so they must have known that cats mark their territorial boundaries with urine.

Such a sinuous line was used metaphorically in ancient Egypt as well as in China and the Americas to mean water. The lines emanating from the Lascaux lion give suggestive evidence of a liquid meaning for the sinuous line at least as far back as 17,000 years ago. Ice Age people would have observed that water does not flow straight but rather moves in eddies and meanders, following a fixed pattern of elliptical integrals, a wavy line. In the absence of topographic irregularities, great rivers, like small trickles, take on the same form. To the Ice Age mind, as to us now, the sinuous line probably was associated with flowing liquid.

In another example from about the same period and culture as the Lascaux lions, a baton from Montgaudier (Charente) features two clearly engraved snakes. One of them, especially, shows the curving snake body and a smaller curving line within it (fig. 4.2). People would have observed that the snake, whose sides alternately contract and extend as it moves, leaves just such a trace in the earth. By association we can conclude that in at least some instances, this line meant serpent. Lines similar to it are seen at Altamira, La Pileta, Hornos de la Peña, and Ardales, all in Spain. In France, examples are at Rouffignac and Trois Frères. That the same undulating line was used for both snake and water strongly suggests that people made an association between the two.[8]

Figure 4.3. Engraved plaquette from Mal'ta, Siberia. Left: Side depicting three snakes. Right: Side with cupmarks in spiral formations.

Perhaps the oldest known depictions of snakes are three engraved creatures wriggling across one face of a plaquette made of mammoth tusk from Mal'ta, Siberia (fig. 4.3). It has been given a wide range of dates, from 15,000 to 26,000 years ago. On its opposite face is

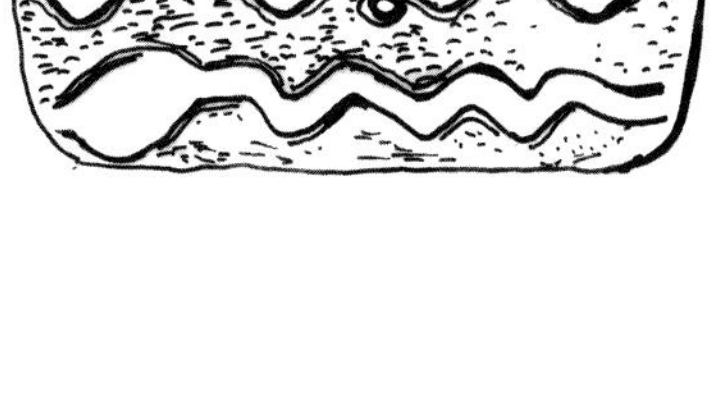

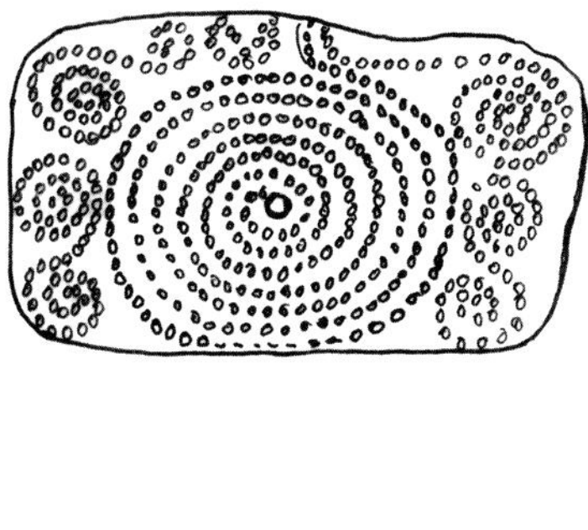

an intricate composition of spirals that could indicate snakes in the coiled position but could also have water signification.

Much confirming evidence of a serpent-water-rain metaphor comes from later societies of the Eurasian Neolithic and of Australia, Africa, and the Americas. One North American example of the association of rain with serpent deities can be seen in the famous Hopi Indian snake dance, during which dancers collect venomous rattlesnakes to carry during the ritual. The snakes are then carried in the dancers' mouths. In the end they are set free to carry the message of the people's need to the powers that dispense rain.[9] In the desert of the Hopi country and throughout much of the U.S. Southwest, rain is always desperately needed, and pleas for rain have always been prominent in the prayers of the people there.

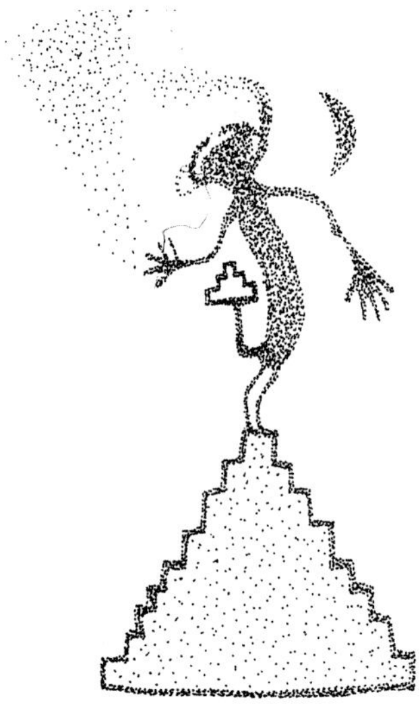

Figure 4.4. Pueblo petroglyph in New Mexico showing a horned figure standing on a cloud terrace, a metaphor for rain and fertility. A small cloud terrace appears on the figure's penis.

Metaphors can be enriched with multiple meanings. The snake has been associated not only with water but also with the penis. Hueco Tanks, New Mexico, is named for a deep natural cistern where Native Americans, probably Apaches, left white-painted pictographs of figures with enlarged penises with tips that appear to double as snakes' heads.[10] A horned figure with a penis that is an actual snake is found in a petroglyph in New Mexico's Galisteo Basin.

Among the Indians of the Southwest, from prehistoric times to the present, the image of a stepped pyramid, or even the steps alone, refers to clouds.[11] In a petroglyph from Arroyo del Macho, New Mexico, that meaning is particularly clear, for the pyramid is filled with pecked dots, most likely indicating potential drops of rain. A figure stands atop the pyramid. On his erect penis is a tiny version of the cloud terrace (fig. 4.4). This glyph permits us to glimpse the associative process in the artist's mind and probably in the minds of the society as a whole. The rain potential of the cloud is being compared to the liquid potential of the penis. And in a larger metaphor, the rain, which fertilizes mother earth, is likened to human semen, thus linking individual and cosmic fecundity.

Spirals

The spiral is another form fraught with metaphoric meaning. The oldest known spirals are those on the mammoth-tusk plaquette mentioned earlier, found in a Siberian grave (fig. 4.3). They are made of circular indentations called *cupmarks.*[12] From a large central spiral radiate connected spirals also made of cupmarks. Early people could easily see, as we do, the profusion of spirals in nature: in vines, ferns, shells, horns, tusks, coiled snakes, whirlpools, and waves. The webs most spiders spin contain a beautiful and easily discernible spiral laid over the silk spokes that anchor it. Early people must also have known of some of the spiral forms in the bodies of game animals and in their own bodies—the intestines and the umbilical cord.

Spirals have been favored markings in prehistoric art all over the world, with the surprising exception of the European Ice Age. A few examples on batons of antler from Arudy and Isturitz (Basses Pyrénées), Lespugue (Hautes-Garonne), and Lourdes (Hautes-Pyrénées) seem to be primarily decorative. We do not know if they conveyed any meaning. Spirals seem to have had different meanings in different societies. Even for one society, that of the Zuñi Indians of the U.S. Southwest, they had multiple meanings. The anthropologist Frank Cushing wrote that the Zuñis equated spirals with marks made by the whirlwind. M. Jane Young, another anthropologist, wrote that the most frequent interpretation she heard at Zuñi was that the spiral stood for a journey in search of the center, a journey that is part of the Zuñis' origin belief.[13] Among other tribes of the North American Southwest, the spiral is also often a metaphor for a mythic journey. One Hopi has been quoted as saying, "The spiral is the migration symbol. The center is the emergence and the turns of the spiral are the migration path."[14] Depending on context and line direction, the spiral is associated with a journey away from the center or back to the center at life's end. We can muse on the suggestive fact that it was a grave in which the Ice Age mammoth tusk with the spiral was found.

Male and Female

An example of a visual pun with metaphoric overtones is seen on a bifurcated baton from Gorge d'Enfer, Dordogne (fig. 4.5). It is *V* shaped around a circular central form. Each of the two projections of reindeer antler is worked to look like a phallus. Alexander Marshack described it: "One phallus is marked on both sides as though it were a fish, with eyes and head at the tip and a fish tail in the rear. The other projection is phallic on both phases of the tip, but it has double 'eyes' in the rear as though they served as testes. The composition seems to be an example of symbolic play, of visual punning, a crossing of comparative images."[15]

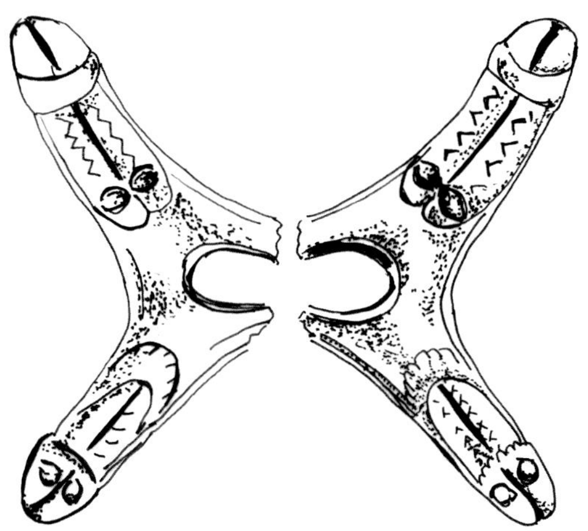

Figure 4.5. Bifurcated baton of reindeer antler found at Gorge d'Enfer, with a phallus shown on one branch and a fish on the other. The baton is then flipped to show the reverse side.

Marshack believed this piece depicted phallus, fish, and liquid, which could be water, urine, or semen. He cited as a further example of this relationship a baton from Bruniquel (Tarn-et-Garonne) in the form of a phallus decorated with fish. Another phalliform staff decorated with fish comes from Isturitz. If these observations are correct, then the Ice Age artists were creating metaphors relating penis to fish. In a suggestive parallel, a stone club discovered in a prehistoric cache on the American Northwest Coast has a phallus at one end and a toothed, fishlike creature at the other, possibly also a vulva (fig. 4.6). In many more recent tribal societies, the image of a fish is associated with fertility.

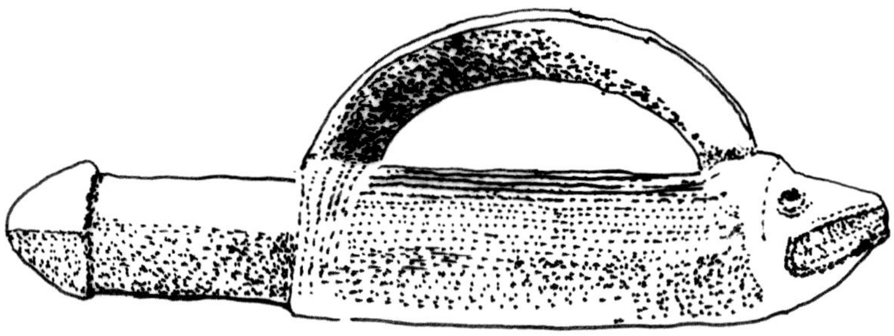

Figure 4.6. Phallus-fish stone club from Alaska, originally painted. The fish end has also been interpreted as a toothed, vulvic mouth.

That appears to have been the intent of an Ice Age mammoth ivory piece found at Dolní Vestonice (fig. 4.7). The figure is highly abstract, consisting of a rod with two lobed appendages. At first it may seem to be a highly stylized female figure with torso and breasts. Then again it seems to be a penis with testicles. This might be considered only a visual pun, but the repeated occurrence of the theme in other, similar artifacts leads one to believe that it was a commonly understood Ice Age metaphor as well. Another female figure, from Grimaldi (Liguria) in northern Italy, dated to about 20,000 years ago, has a clearly formed penis for a head (fig. 4.8). A 15,000-year-old figure from the cave of Le Placard (Charente), carved out of reindeer antler, has a long, unmistakably phallic neck and a prominent vulva (fig. 4.9). A similar, tiny calcite figure from the cave of Weinberg (Bavaria), dated to 23,000 years ago, also has a phallic neck and a vulva.[16]

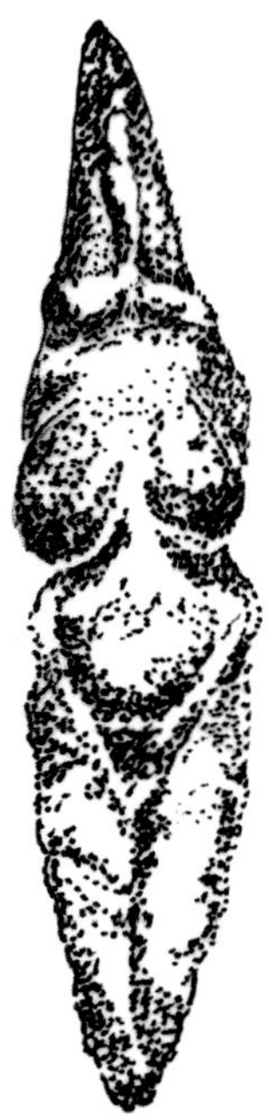

Figure 4.7. Carved mammoth ivory with two lobed appendages, from Dolní Vestonice, Czech Republic, about 26,000 B.P. This piece is thought to be a highly abstract figure combining male and female.

If these Ice Age sculptors intended to convey the unlikely similarity between male and female sexual organs, then they find good company with others who made what seems to be the same analogy in later times. From Lepenski Vir on the lower Danube, a group of carved figures dates to the end of the Ice Age. Upright phallic shapes at the bases of some of the torsos can be seen as penises, yet they also have vulvar attributes. There is a similar Neolithic piece from Hungary and a 6,000-year-old Chalcolithic piece carved of steatite from Cyprus. This androgynous image persisted throughout the ages. A clay figurine found in Iran, approximately 3,000 years old, depicts a female with a stalklike torso and neck, small pointed breasts, large tapering thighs, and tiny stumplike feet.[17] But looked at sideways, the figurine is a phallus. The female's buttocks become the male's testicles (fig. 4.10).

Similar examples of sexual ambiguity come from much more recent times. A Brancusi sculpture called *Adam and Eve* and a painting by Joan Miró called

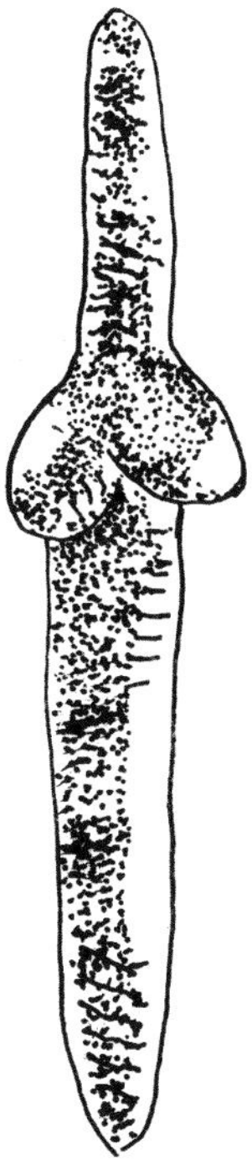

Man and Woman both combine male and female parts. The sculptor Louise Bourgeois produced an example of the same theme in latex in 1968 and called it *Fillette*. She said explicitly that she merged the imagery of "phallic breasts, male and female, active and passive."[18] It is likely all that these artists were saying that in terms of form alone, one can discover a similarity between male and female organs, so that by association these forms may be coupled.

Left: Figure 4.8 Female figure with penis head, carved in steatite, from Grimaldi-Savignano, (Modeno) Italy. Height 23 cm.

Woman, Horn, and Crescent Moon

Female figurines and carvings from the Ice Age have survived in relative abundance. One of the best known and most intriguing is a limestone relief carving from Laussel, in Dordogne (fig. 4.11, see illus. p. 86). It depicts a large, possibly pregnant woman with her left hand on her belly and a horn upheld in her right hand. It seems natural to wonder, as many have, whether the horn might have served as a metaphor for the moon in its crescent phase. It would not be difficult to associate the cyclical waxing and waning of the moon with the menstrual cycle. The horn in the Laussel figurine is engraved with 13 marks, the number of days from the crescent to the full moon and the number of crescent moons in the lunar year.

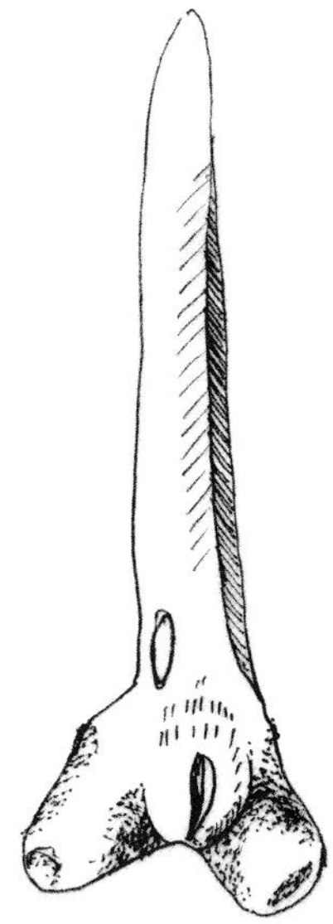

Figure 4.9. An androgynous carving from Le Placard combines vulva and phallus. Height 15 cm.

The moon has long been associated with women and often with goddesses. About 15,000 years after the Laussel figure, a Babylonian goddess, Astarte, was depicted with a crescent moon on her head. In Ice Age art, bison horns are frequently shown as crescents. The association of horn, crescent moon, and gestation in Ice Age art is impossible to prove, but it is also too suggestive to be ignored. That the moon is cyclical, dies, and is reborn seems a likely metaphor for female fertility and human procreation. If this were a general, universally understood concept, then it would explain another female figure, this one from Gxalingenwa Rock in KwaZulu-Natal, South Africa. She, too, holds a crescent-shaped object (see fig. 5.17).

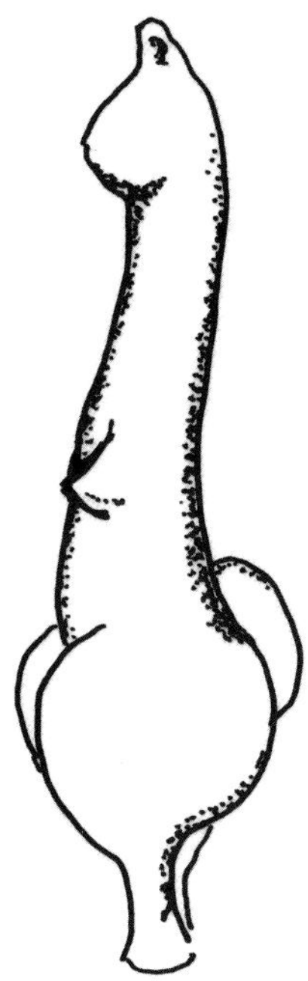

Figure 4.10. A clay figurine from Iran shows both male and female characteristics.

Layered Meanings

Jane Young, a student of Zuñi Pueblo culture, says that Zuñi verbal expression abounds in wordplay and metaphor, expressing layer upon layer of meaning. She writes of a Zuñi "aesthetic of accumulation": "Zuñi ritual symbols,

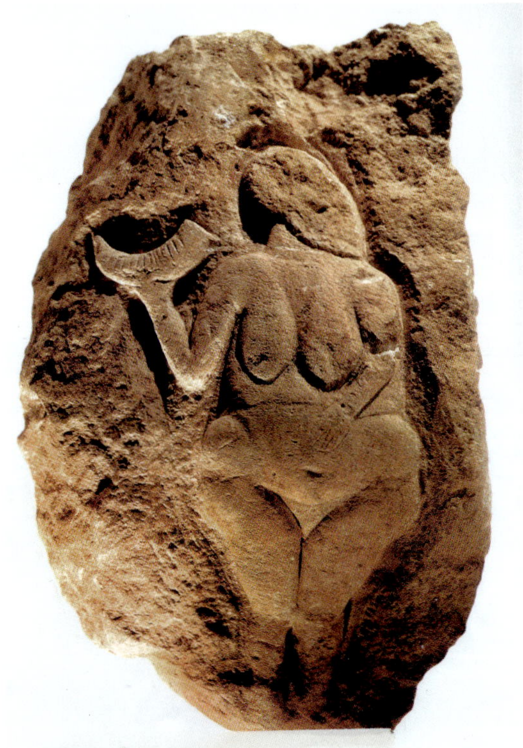

Figure 4.11. The "Venus of Laussel," carved in low relief on a convex limestone block, 27,000–22,000 B.P. Height 54.5 cm. The woman holds a horn or possibly a crescent moon with 13 incised marks. Photo: E. Lessing/Art Resource N.Y.

whether expressed verbally or visually, are frequently multivalent or multireferential, standing for both themselves and something else at the same time."[19] Perhaps only a culture so accepting of syncretism as that of the American Indian could encompass two such different religions as their own and that of their conquerors in what appears to be a workable unity. The seventeenth-century mission church at Zuñi is painted with *kachina* figures. Jesus is depicted as a Zuñi rain priest standing on a traditional Indian cloud terrace. The artist, Alex Seowtewa, seems to have been able to join these two belief systems effortlessly; he likens a Zuñi four-day fast to Christianity's Lent and Judaism's Passover.[20] This ability to layer metaphor upon metaphor probably increases a symbol's power and mystery.

Throughout history, painters and sculptors have made use of visual metaphors. Rembrandt's hanging animal carcasses are strongly associated with human mortality. Later, Chaim Soutine's paintings of the same subject were even more painfully attentive to the ironic beauty of fleshy putrescence. Van Gogh's cypress trees are also flames reaching to burning and incandescent skies. We have already seen the analogy Degas made between the ballet dancer with lifted leg and the watering can. He also modeled the flanks of his racing horses to recall the hips and rumps of the women he so often drew as they bathed and dried themselves. Georgia O'Keeffe appears to have used flower forms as metaphors for the vagina, despite her claims to the contrary. Later, Judy Chicago did this blatantly in her series of flower plates in *The Dinner Party.*

The Evolution of Metaphor

Metaphor making, like so many of the other conceptual and aesthetic tools we work with, is a gift from earlier stages of evolution. It goes back at least to our primate ancestors. Washoe, a chimpanzees who was brought up by human foster parents and was taught to communicate in American Sign Language, created metaphors, puns, and even rhymes. Washoe described a swan as "water, bird." Another chimp, Lucy, called radishes "cry, hurt, food."[21] The chimp Moja invented a combination sign for Alka-Seltzer: "listen, drink."[22] Sometimes the chimps used words in a different context, in a manner akin to the metaphoric process. Washoe decided that calling people "potty" and "dirty" could be insults.[23] A bonobo, named Panbanisha told her trainer in sign language that a certain woman with a bouffant hairstyle had "hair like a mushroom." The trainer, Sue Savage-Rumbaugh, related this and added that Panbanisha was right.[24]

A female gorilla named Koko learned to communicate with her human trainers by the use of sign language and combined signs that she already knew in order to yield new meanings, thus creating metaphors, puns, and even, occasionally, rhymes. Like the chimp Washoe, she independently arrived at the word "potty" as an insult. When confronted for the first time with a mask, Koko put together two signs, calling it "eye, hat." To express the idea of death, she combined three words she knew and arrived at "comfortable, hole, 'bye."[25]

Human children begin to use metaphors almost as soon as they can play with speech, and it is for this reason that the language of children is full of natural poetry. Humans seem to delight in looking at unlike things and finding something they share. We are always generalizing, connecting, simplifying, and finding the similar in the dissimilar. Sometimes this process appears to yield a hidden order. Science, as much as art, can be enriched by it. The astronomer Chet Raymo wrote: "Even the sturdiest of scientific concepts is rooted in metaphor. Philosophers of science insist that science is metaphorical. They cite, for example, Newton's 'clockwork' solar system and Robert Boyle's elastic 'spring' of air. Christian Huygens, a Dutchman who lived by the water, first thought of light as a 'wave.' Alfred Wegener, a meteorologist who traveled in the frozen Arctic, conceived of continents drifting like 'rafts' of ice."[26]

The cognitive linguists George Lakoff and Mark Johnson, who have studied metaphor, believe that most of the normal human conceptual system is metaphorically grounded. They go so far as to assert that people cannot function as humans without metaphor.[27] Psychologists help explain how the human mind is able to make metaphors. Studies with month-old babies have shown that they can recognize by sight pacifier nipples that they have felt but never seen. Infants seem to have an innate capacity to transfer information from one sensory mode to another, and it may be this generalizing function that causes humans to generate metaphors.[28]

Metaphors are linkages of seemingly unrelated things. Neuroscientists give us a possible explanation for their formation. Firing neurons have a natural tendency to forge links with other neurons, making new connections. This capacity to achieve seemingly unrelated interconnectedness is called "cross-modal abstraction." The neuroscientist V. S. Ramachandran suggests that such ability is explained by the progressive and explosive enlargement, during primate evolution, of the part of the brain where three areas of differing brain function come together. Known as the temporal-parietal-occipital junction, it is involved in abstraction. Another associated brain area is the angular gyrus, which has also been enlarged enormously during primate evolution. Ramachandran finds that people with left angular gyrus lesions have difficulty with metaphor. This finding confirms his belief that the angular gyrus is involved in cross-modal connections and that these new, sometimes unexpected connections are what create metaphors.[29] Scientists use metaphors to show how our brains make metaphors. For example, the neurologist Antonio Damasio described two varieties of gray matter in the brain: in one variety, the neurons were "layered as in a cake," and in the other, they were "like cashew nuts inside a bowl."[30]

EXAGGERATION, OR HYPERBOLE

Nothing produces laughter more than a surprising disproportion between that which one expects and that which one sees.

—BLAISE PASCAL

Exaggeration is common in Ice Age art. Analogy is made between a figure with which we are familiar and an unexpectedly distorted one. Exaggeration was particularly used in depicting parts of animal and human anatomy. In the rare instances in which they are depicted, men generally have erect penises that are much exaggerated in size. An example is from the cave of Le Cirq, Dordogne (fig. 4.12). The purpose of this exaggeration might have been to suggest fertility, masculinity, and concomitant testosterone-associated secondary features such as ferocity and bravery.

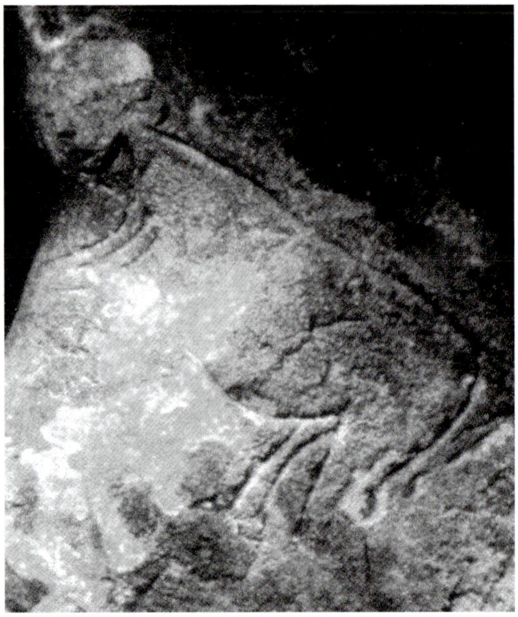

Figure 4.12. Male figure with exaggerated penis, Le Cirq.

Perhaps exaggeration serves an aesthetic role. Or it might serve to fulfill fantasy—in the case of the Le Cirq engraving, it might represent wishful thinking. There seems to be something universally compelling about exaggeration of the male reproductive organ. In South Africa, at Prentjiesberg, Ugie, San artists also used such exaggeration. In Arnhem Land, in Australia's Northern Territory, several figures on one panel have greatly exaggerated penises, each painted a little differently from the others. One man's is so elongated that he wears it wrapped around his waist, perhaps to illustrate a story about Ngulick, a Mimi spirit figure who is known for his lecherous behavior. Ngulick is said to consummate his seductions by taking over the body of a mortal man who becomes the vehicle for his indiscretions. The man is therefore not responsible for his actions. When chastised, the man whose body has been used for this scandalous purpose can reply innocently: "It wasn't me. It was Ngulick."[31]

In North America, the "trickster" is a ubiquitous, complex, and often lecherous figure. In one story his penis, like Ngulick's, is long enough to be carried wrapped around his body. The Wakdjunkaga of the Winnebago people carries his coiled up in a box on his back. The American Indian trickster is often a humpbacked flute player, first seen among the Hopi people.[32] In one petroglyph at Holiday Mesa, New Mexico, the flute player's preposterously elongated penis extends around a corner to another rock face, where it is shown in coitus with a female (fig. 4.13). A clue to the meaning of this petroglyph may lie in a Hopi story that tells of a beautiful young woman who rejected the advances of all young men. Coveting her and challenged by her desire for chastity, the flute player discovered where she went to relieve herself. He dug a trench to this spot and made a continuous pipe of reeds, which he hid by covering it with earth and grass. When she was in a vulnerable position, he extended his penis inside the pipe so that it could enter and impregnate her from this great distance.[33]

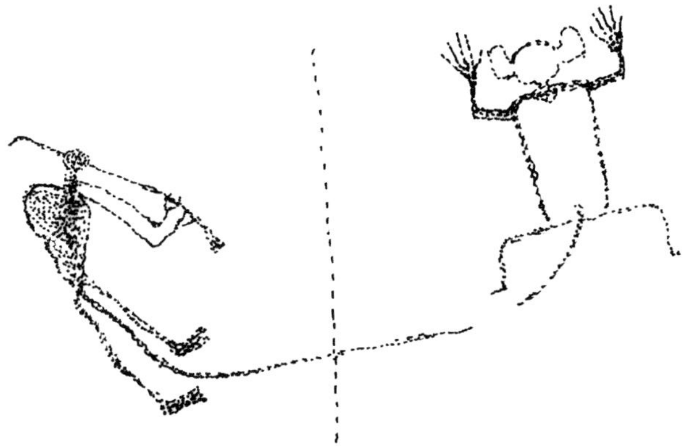

Figure 4.13. Flute player in coitus, Holiday Mesa, New Mexico.

Exaggerated Animals

Animal necks were favored subjects for Ice Age exaggeration. Even when necks were extensively distorted, there seems to have been no trouble in accepting the distorted animals as analogous to those with more normal proportions. Examples of animals with elongated necks appear at Les Combarelles, Le Portel, Pergouset, Labastide, Gabillou, and Cosquer in France and at Altxerri in Spain. A bird from Montrastruc, Bruniquel has a neck so preposterously long that it loops back on itself and may be mistaken for two necks intertwined. At La Cauna, Belvis (Aude), a strange bird-headed quadruped also has a ludicrously long neck (fig. 4. 14).

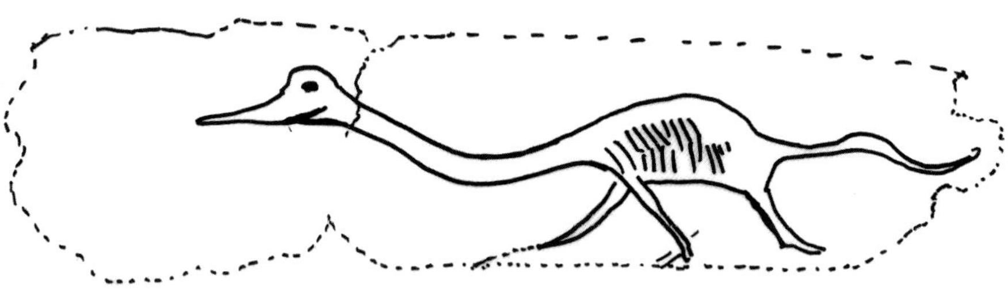

Figure 4.14. Birdlike animal with an exaggerated neck at La Cauna. 13.5 cm.

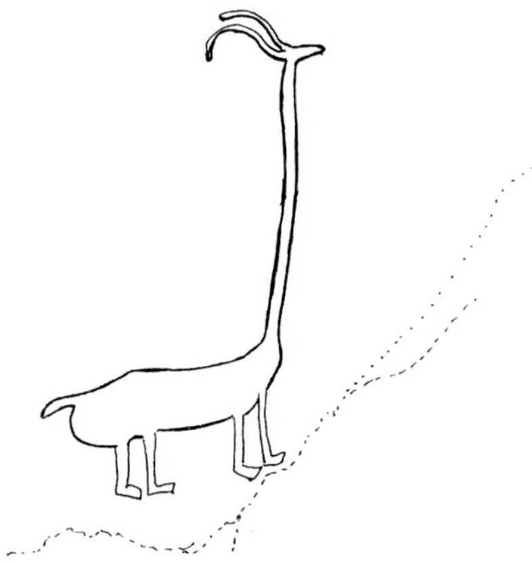

Figure 4.15. Long-necked animal at Nine Mile Canyon, Utah.

Prehistoric artists in other cultures used similar kinds of neck distortions. In South America, one of the monumental earth sculptures at Nazca, Peru, is formed into a bird with an elongated neck. In North America, there is an extremely long-necked animal at Nine Mile Canyon, Utah (fig. 4.15). The elongated neck was a favored device of the extraordinary Mimbres pottery painters in what is now New Mexico. One Mimbres painter depicted a crane with a neck so exaggerated that it loops back and forth three times (fig. 4.16). Another, even more spectacular example places a crane's body in the center of the bowl. Its neck curves in sinuous waves, like water, completely around its body for more than 360 degrees. Fish cling to the undulating neck as if it were simultaneously meant to be water waves.

Fred Kabotie, an artist and member of the Hopi tribe, attempted to interpret a number of Mimbres works with the rationale that the Hopis shared kinship with these ancient potters and possibly carried in their oral tradition some inheritance from them. One Hopi legend, he recounted, was about a long-necked crane. Kabotie said it was one of the children's favorite stories: "Every time it was told the children laughed about the crane and his long neck."[34] If he was correct, then the exaggeration in this instance was meant to be humor-

Figure 4.16. Mimbres pot depicting a crane with an exaggerated neck. Height 12,4 cm, diameter 17,7 cm.

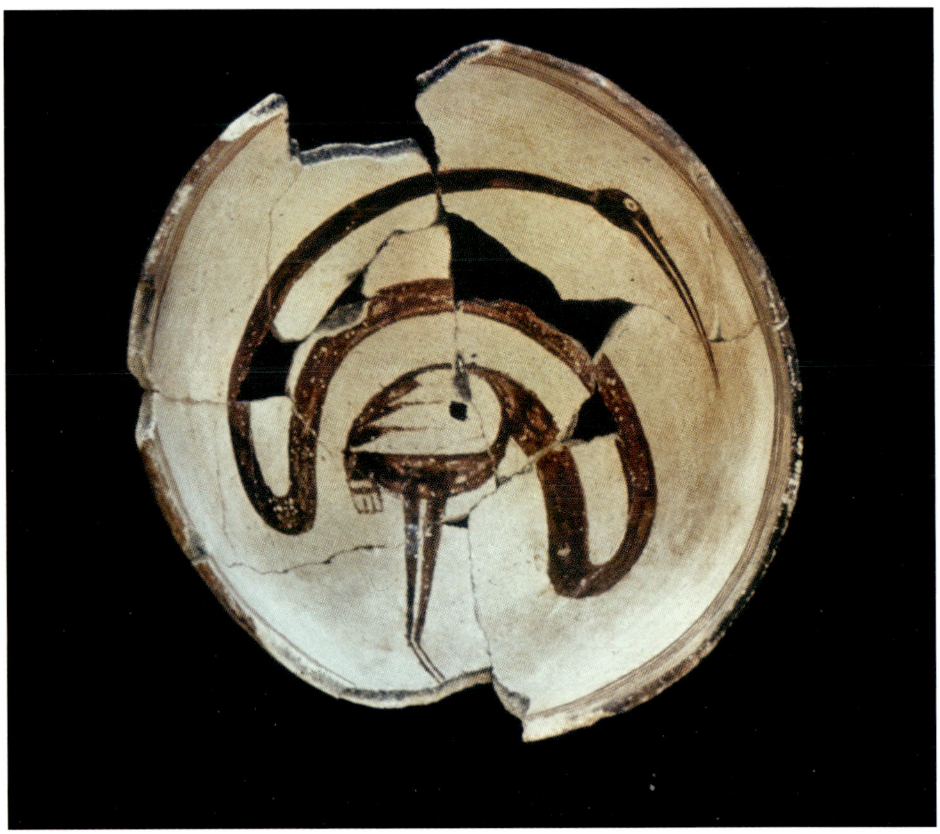

ous. This should not surprise us, because exaggeration has a humorous aspect for us when it is used in cartoons. However, hyperbole was probably used in prehistory primarily for purposes other than humor.

Besides necks, antlers and horns have been favored subjects of exaggeration in art. Antlers on one of the stags from Lascaux, painted about 17,000 years ago, are like none ever seen. The animal itself is carefully and realistically depicted, but its antlers are pure fantasy, conveying a feeling of joyful inventiveness (fig. 4.17). In Ice Age Siberia, artists portrayed deer with exaggerated antlers (fig. 4.18). Scythian artists crafted animals with antlers that were often even more outrageously extended, luxuriantly branching or coiled in a spiral, as in an extravagantly decorative example wrought in gold (fig. 4.19).

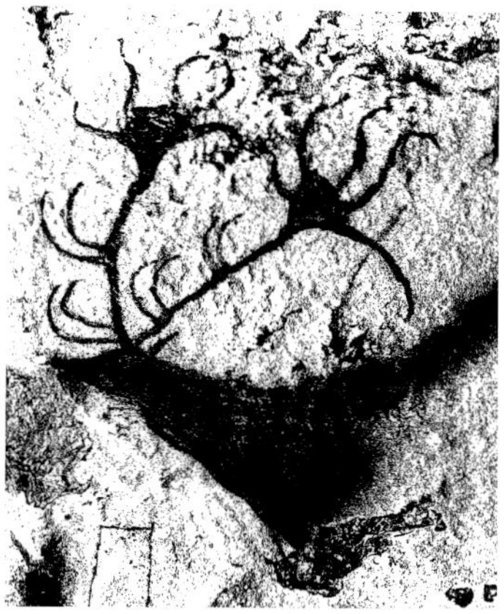

Figure 4.17. Painted stag with fantastic, exaggerated antlers, Lascaux. Height 1.40 m.

Horns, too, were exaggerated in Ice Age art, although with somewhat less panache. An ibex with exaggerated horns was found on a stone plaque at La Mouthe. Many of the horns on a group of rhinoceroses at Chauvet are flamboyantly elongated. In addition, one of the horns points forward instead of backward. In South Africa, San artists made a rhinoceros with exaggerated horns at Keurfontein, Vosburg, and several others were similarly made at Thaba Sione, Mmabatho, where one animal was given three horns instead of two.

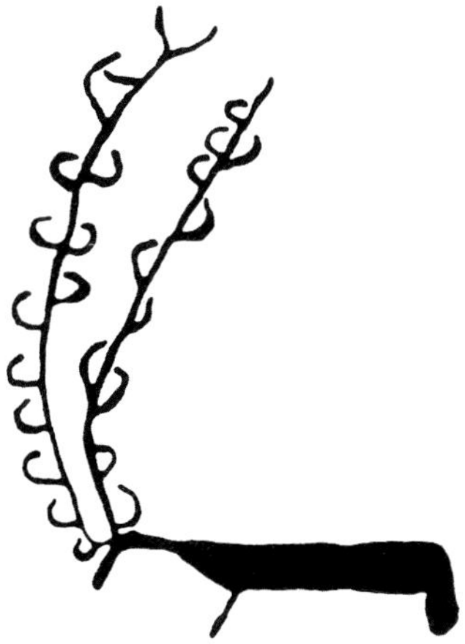

Figure 4.18. Pictograph of deer with luxuriantly branching antlers, Altay, Yelangash, Siberia, from about 2,500 years ago.

It must have been with the same mindset that elephant and mammoth trunks were subjects for exaggeration. At Les Combarelles, a mammoth has an exaggerated trunk. Another appears at Gargas, where there is also an elk with a very elongated snout. At La Baume-Latrone, an odd, finger-painted mammoth has an elongated trunk with a hook-shaped flourish at the end (fig. 4.20). On the other side of the world, in South Africa, an extremely elongated elephant trunk is seen in the ancient San rock art site at Barnes' Shelter, Giant's Castle, in the Drakensberg Mountains of KwaZulu-Natal (fig. 4.21). Other San elephants with exaggerated trunks are found in South Africa in Britstown District, Wepener District, Orange Free State, and Aliwal North.

Tails were exaggerated in some Ice Age caves. Most of the animals in the Axial Gallery at Lascaux have unrealistically elongated tails. The four "Chinese" horses have tails that reach their feet (see p. 144). In some other examples, tails go below the feet. The cow with a black head has a tail that sweeps the ground. A leaping horse has a long tail that sweeps out in an arc, and a leaping cow has a tail that curves back in an enormous *S*. There are examples of such huge tails in Font de Gaume, La Mouthe, and Gabillou—all in the same geographical area, where the tails may have been a preferred style. But

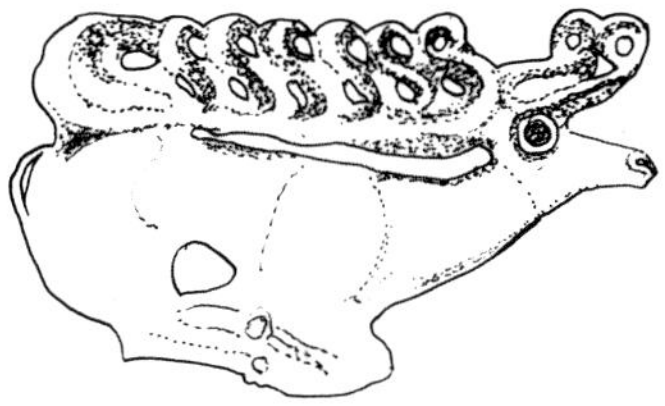

Figure 4.19. Scythian gold figure dated to the end of the ninth century B.P.. Length 31.75 cm., width 19 cm.

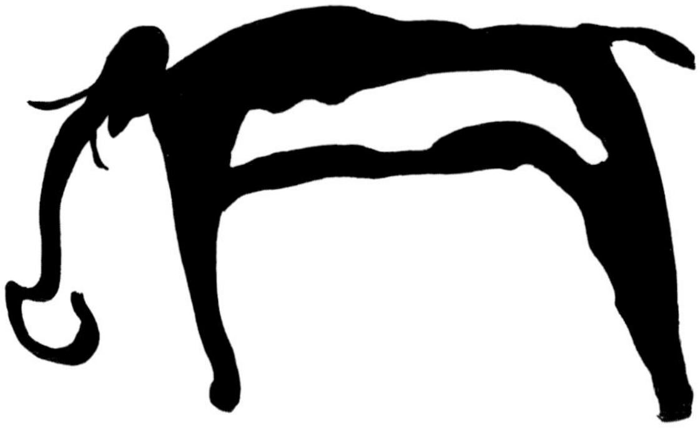

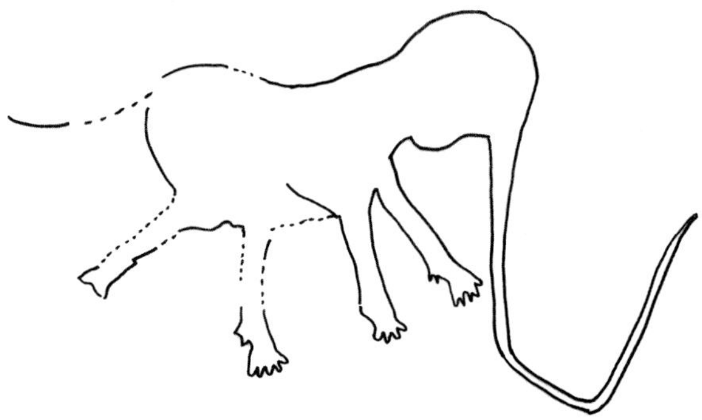

they are occasionally found in other areas, such as Candamo in Spain, and in more widely separated prehistoric art. On a Mimbres pot, a coyote has a tail so long that it winds completely around him three times in ever widening circles (fig. 4.22). In Cottonwood Canyon, Utah, there is a petroglyph of a quadruped whose enormously elongated tail curves in ever smaller circles (fig. 4.23). A similar figure appears in the Woodland area at La Moille Cave, Minnesota. A mask from Burkina Faso, central Africa, presents a chameleon with a tail similarly coiled. And many more examples of animals with elongated, coiled tails exist worldwide.

An important animal in Native American lore is the mythic underwater panther, commonly depicted in symmetrical pairs with elongated tails joined in a knot. Long-tailed panthers are particularly spectacular in the rock paintings of the prehistoric people who lived along the conjunction of the lower Rio Grande and the Devils River. One, especially, known as the curly-tailed panther, was placed in a rockshelter that looms over a section of Devils River and can be reached only by inching dangerously along the cliff face above a sheer drop. This panther, occupying the entire space at one end of the shelter, measures about 2.75m from nose to base of tail. The tail itself curls in the form of a spiral for 3.6m, making the whole animal an impressive 6.4m long.

(top) Figure 4.20 Mammoth at La Baume-Latrone with an elongated trunk made by fingers dipped in red ocher clay. 1.2 m.

(bottom) Figure 4.21. Elephant with elongated trunk and fantastic feet at Barnes' Shelter, South Africa.

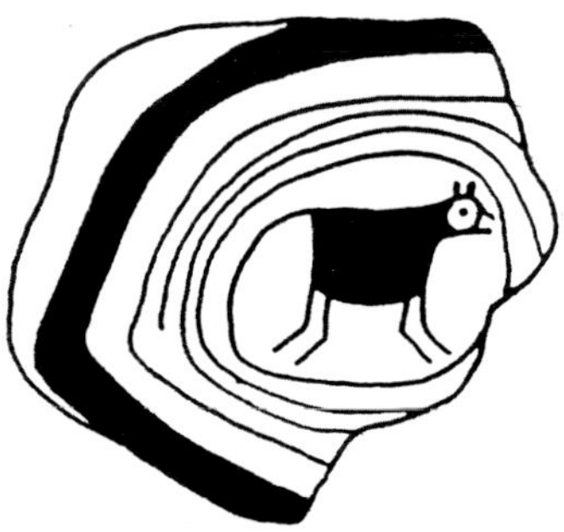

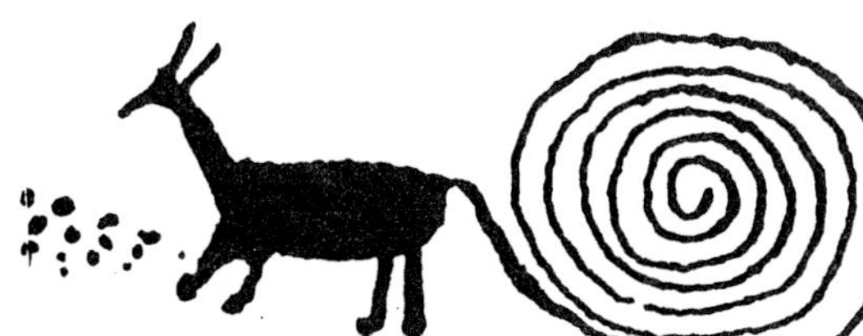

(left) Figure 4.22. Mimbres pot depicting a quadruped, probably a coyote, with an exaggerated tail that winds around its body four times. About 1,000 B.P.

(right) Figure 4.23. Quadruped with an exaggerated tail wound into a spiral, Cottonwood Canyon, Utah.

Caricature

The most common form of visual hyperbole occurs in caricature, which requires both exaggeration and simplification. We tend to think of caricature as humorous because it involves, as Pascal put it, a "disproportion between that which one expects and that which one sees." We carry a mental model of a subject's normal size, and we are startled and sometimes amused when an image deviates too far from that norm. But I think the exaggeration we see in Ice Age and subsequent prehistoric art was not meant primarily for humor. Some of it had a darker side, to surprise and to frighten. I cannot improve on Art Spiegelman's remark that caricature creates compressed icons that can "burrow deep into the brain." Moreover, caricature may be a graphic change that artists are almost impelled to make, even when they attempt to capture a subject, with its neck, antlers, and horns, as realistically as possible—like an added flourish on a signature.

Caricature is by definition a charged or loaded image. . . . its wit lies in the visual concision of using a few deft strokes to make its point. The compression of ideas into memorable icons gives [it the] ability to burrow deep into the brain.

—ART SPIEGELMAN, "Drawing Blood and the Art of Outrage"

The prehistorian Ann Sieveking referred to a "jokey" style on Ice Age plaques from Lortet (Hautes-Pyrénées), Gourdan (Haute-Garonne), Isturitz[35] and a small number of other sites. Although animals predominated as subject matter in the European Ice Age, a relatively small number of humans are seen. Many of these faces seem close to animals, with noses that resemble snouts. Leaving out the faces that appear to be bestialized, what is left are caricatures of eccentric humanity. Indeed, they resemble studies done by Leonardo da Vinci, that appear to investigate and elaborate extreme facial variation. Protuberances are often enlarged, the nose and chin for example. We cannot be sure these graphic changes were meant to convey the witty and slightly derisive meaning they have for us. The only thing we can state with assurance is that faces are simplified and exaggerated. Simplification and exaggeration are the hallmarks of caricature and these engravings are surely caricatures. Were it not for the discoveries at the site of la Marche one would say there are few if any real portraits, but discoveries at La Marche have yielded a large number of human faces depicted on plaques dated to about 14,000 years ago. These bear an astonishing resemblance to drawings by Breughel or Daumier whose portraits reveal hints of the mind behind the face. (fig. 4.24)

Caricature over the ages has remained extremely consistent, with both simplification and exaggeration of facial features. In a head of Cardinal Scipio Borghese by the consummately realistic Renaissance sculptor Bernini, we see nearly the same treatment as in petroglyph heads from Marsoulas and

Figure 4.24. Caricature heads from Ice Age sites.

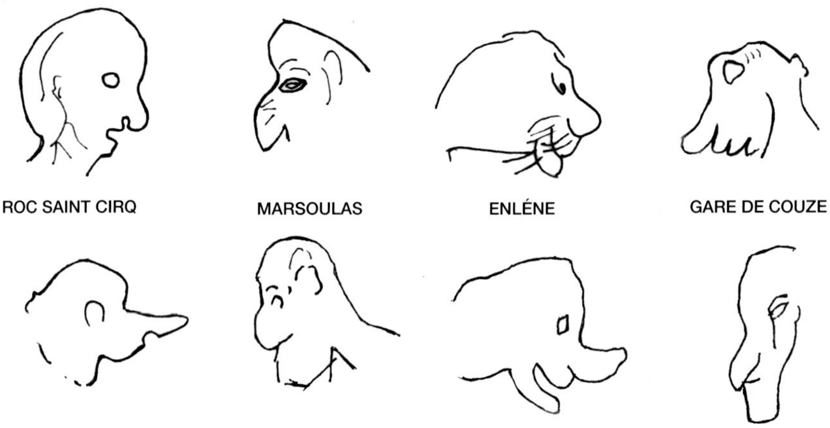

Labastide (fig. 4.25), although the images are separated by roughly 15,000 years. Recently, archaeologists discovered a face that is even more starkly simplified and more than 10,000 years older in a cave near Vilhonneur (Charente). The artist used the facelike shape of a stalagmite and turned it into a face by means of only three painted black lines (fig. 4.26). We see, therefore, at the very beginning of art the impulse to simplify and exaggerate.

Shamans and Monsters

Sometimes exaggerations appear to have ominous intent. The enlarged horns on the rhinoceroses at Chauvet may make an already intimidating animal even more frightening. At Altamira, a human head confronts intruders from deep within the recesses of the cave. It is made of a projecting angle of rock. The sharp corner becomes the exaggeratedly large nose in an hauntingly long, thin face. On either side of the rock angle, two large, wide-open painted eyes stare out with frightening intensity (see fig. 4.30).

In Inuit art, heads are sometimes carved with greatly enlarged ears. Contemporary carvers who have made these say that exaggerated ears represent the

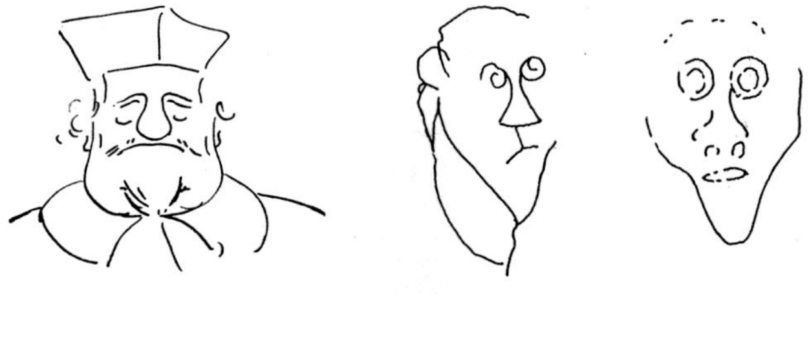

Figure 4.25. Left: G. Bernini, head of Cardinal Scipio Borghese, done in the style of a caricature. Center: Caricature head from Marsoulas. Height 20.3 cm. Right: Caricature head from Labastide.

heightened sensitivity of *angakqu* (shamans) to everything around them.[36] Exaggerations in vastly differing societies may seem to share darker intentions. In Arizona's Petrified Forest National Park, for example, a petroglyph of a mountain lion with enormous open jaws and sharp claws effectively emphasizes the fearful aspects of the animal (fig. 4.27). A similar attempt to alarm by exaggeration is found in the use of "False Face" masks by members of the Iroquois Confederacy in northeastern North America. Bering Sea Eskimos, too, made distorted masks, theirs depicting Tunghak, the old man who lives in the moon and controls game animals. East Greenland Eskimos made masks depicting Tupilak, a spirit of ill omen. In all these masks the enlarged nose appears to be twisted as if broken and never reset. Often the mouth is skewed as if the victim had suffered a paralyzing stroke or Bell's palsy, and the tongue often protrudes.

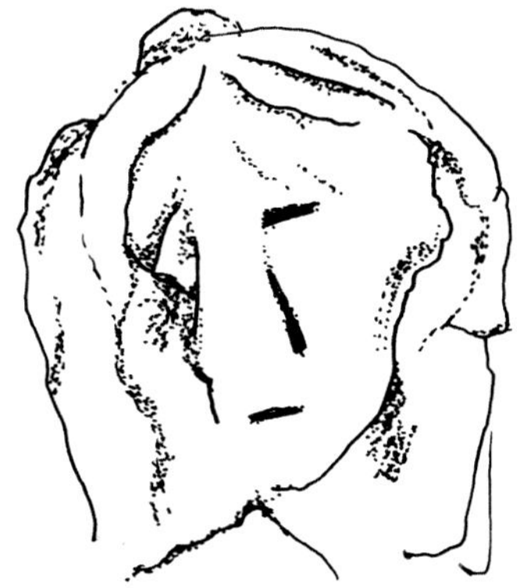

Figure 4.26. Face created on a stalagmite in a cave near Vilhonneur.

Some masks of the Western Pende people of Congo have a twisted quality and similar distortions, as does an Ibibio mask from Nigeria. There is even an ancient Aztec mask similarly distorted.[37] We do not know the motivation behind many of these masks. However, the English painter Francis Bacon often twisted features in his portraits, such as those of the shrieking popes, in a manner analogous to the False Face masks. He explained his motive: "In a painting that's even worth looking at, the image must be twisted if it is to make a renewed assault upon the nervous system."[38]

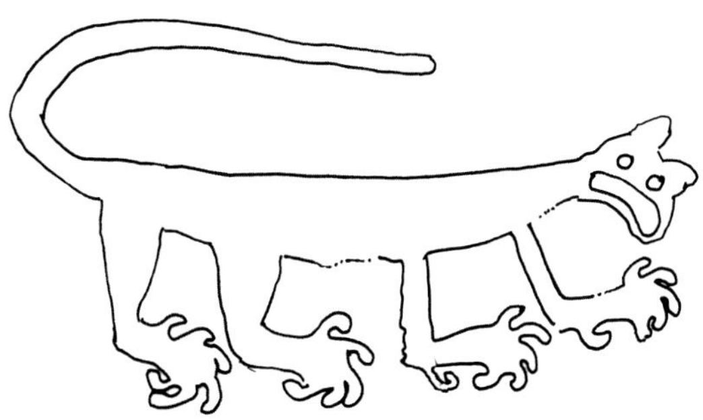

Figure 4.27. Mountain lion petroglyph, Petrified Forest, Arizona.

Hyperbole in Recent Art

Artists throughout history have made use of the same kinds of exaggeration, to the point of caricature, that Ice Age artists first employed. Anonymous medieval carvers join Bosch, Brueghel, Daumier, Dubuffet, and Picasso among the many examples. John Singer Sargent, the consummately skilled, very realistic nineteenth-century portrait and landscape painter, seemed uncharacteristically fascinated by a particular cartoon face, which appears in one of his early notebooks (fig. 4.28).[39] It looks much like one engraved on rock that Colonel Garrick M. Mallery attributed to the Hopi Indians of Arizona (fig. 4.29).[40] Sargent drew similar cartoon faces several other times, much later in life.[41] It is as if he had found access to some basic, severely simplified, universal linear figure that may be similar to and perhaps derived from children's experimentation.

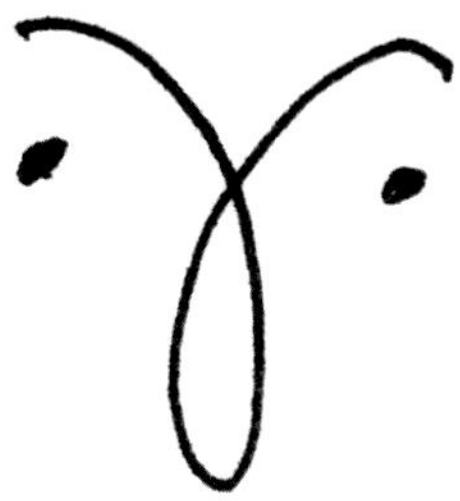

Figure 4.28. A sketch by the American 19th century artist John Singer Sargent.

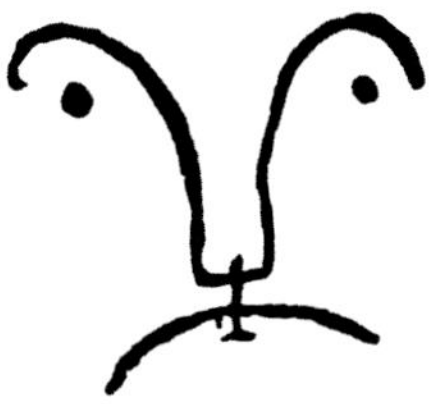

Figure 4.29. Hopi petroglyph of a kachina.

Apparently this image hovered in his mind but was deemed inappropriate for his professional work.

The twentieth-century artist Joan Miró, on the other hand, made use of his attraction to caricature from the beginning. Miro's iconography appears initially to be an abstraction but is actually based on caricature. Following the development of his art, one can see dogs, cats, roosters, insects, people, and body parts gradually simplified, distorted, and stylized until they become a personal vocabulary. More recently, the American painter Philip Guston achieved fame in the early 1950s as an abstract expressionist. At the peak of his career, in the late 1960s, he unexpectedly turned away from his popular past work and began to paint in a figurative style, creating cartoonish images with angry and despairing messages.

The Neuroscience of Hyperbole

Why is caricature such a persistent feature in art from the Ice Age to the present? V. S. Ramachandran explains caricature by means of the psychological concept of "peak shift," which derives from animal learning experiments with birds. In a mammalian example he gives, a rat is taught to discriminate between a square and a rectangle in order to gain a food reward. If the rat finds that the food is always at the rectangle, it will chose ever longer and thinner rectangles that are ever farther removed from the square.[42] Ramachandran believes that the rats have found the essence of the rectangle and that this ability may relate neurologically to human activities such as cartooning, in which the artist looks for the essence and then exaggerates it. But Ramachandran provides no example of primate use of this "peak shift," and so it must await evidence from a species biologically closer to humans to be more meaningful in casting light on human art making.

How far can we push exaggeration before we lose recognition? It seems that certain images can be highly distorted without losing their recognizability. Ironically, caricatures may not make recognition more difficult; very young children who are just starting to understand that drawings refer to objects in the real world can identify distorted cartoon animals even though the cartoons look nothing like the animals as they appear in life or in photographs. Indeed, it seems that exaggeration, up to a certain point, aids recognition. Computer scientists have found important evidence to confirm the efficiency of cartoon imagery in conveying information to the brain. They have discovered that when computers are used to simulate human perception, they recognize cartoons before they recognize photographs.[43] It might seem counterintuitive, but researchers have found that caricatures require less time for correct recognition than do more realistic pictures.[44]

A computer can do even more than interpret cartoons. One has been devised that can scan photographs of a face and then use the information to create a cartoon. Paul Churchland, who specializes in cognitive philosophy, discussed this computer, called the "Face Bender."[45] In this instance artificial intelligence may suggest reasons for the universal appeal of graphic hyperbole, or cartooning. Examining the working process of our perception, scientists have found that a good likeness is one that evokes the same early neural response in the visual system that the real object evokes.[46] They have concluded from all this information that exaggerations may accurately simulate the way our brain encodes representation of a face during normal perception.[47]

Many artists have known this all along. It is one aspect of the use of exaggeration and distortion in art making. Paul Bonnard wrote: "There is a formula that perfectly fits painting: lots of little lies for the sake of one big truth."[48] Vincent van Gogh wrote to his brother, Theo: "I should be desperate if my figures were correct. . . . my great longing is to make these very incorrectnesses, those deviations, remodelings, changes in reality, so that they may become, yes, lies if you like, but truer than the literal truth."[49] Degas and Delacroix wrote much the same thing, as did Picasso: "Art is a lie which lets us see the truth."[50] Shakespeare expressed this idea 400 years earlier: "The truest poetry is the most feigning."[51]

FOUND OBJECTS

The first "found" art object may have been a small piece of black basaltic tuff that appears to have the shape of a woman. It was excavated at Berekhat Ram in the Golan Heights from layers dated to the Middle Paleolithic.[52] This means that some early man recognized it as a figure at least 230,000 years ago and perhaps as much as 800,000 years ago, long before the emergence of *Homo sapiens sapiens*. This piece of stone, born in a volcanic eruption, had the appropriate protuberant shapes to suggest, by analogy, the ample female form that early prehistorians called a Venus figure. The only way one can be sure that a natural formation was viewed this way in the prehistoric past, however, is to find evidence of some deliberate modification. Using microscopic analysis,

I don't design my work. I don't carve it. I just make what I see from found objects. . . . I think that God is the artist in my work. I'm just the hands that he blessed.

—Bessie Harvey,
Tennessee folk artist

the meticulous researcher Alexander Marshack found non-natural grooves around what would be the neck and the arms of the figure. For some archeologists that confirms the hypothesis that the long-ago maker of these grooves also saw in this stone the female figure that we now see.

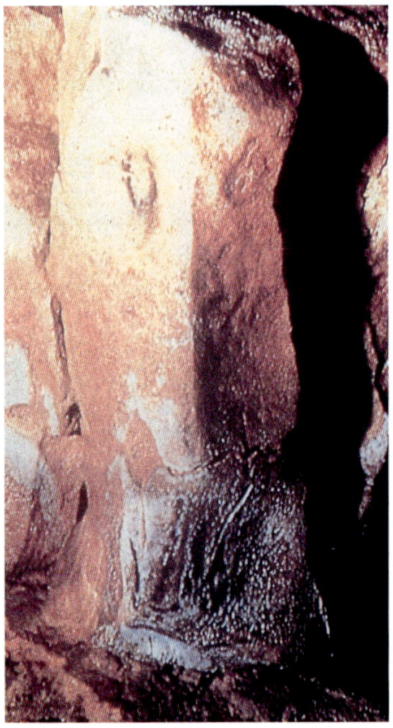

Figure 4.30. Found face with eyes added, Altamira. © Museo de Altamira

Found objects are figures that are generally recognizable in their existing form. The object may be left unaltered, or it might be somewhat modified (also called *rectified*) to enhance the likeness. The fewer changes made to the found object to transform it into the analogous image, the more we can appreciate the artist's symbolic mental leap.

Modern humans left many clear examples of the use of found objects, generally of stone or bone, to represent subjects that those objects were perceived to resemble. With regard to Ice Age artists, the caves themselves might even be thought of as giant found objects. They were secret spaces, often with jewel-like, calcite-covered ceilings and walls and almost always with tantalizing formations. A chance formation or surface irregularity might strongly suggest an image, such as the face at Altamira that needed only eyes to be completed. Two other natural stone formations at Altamira were also recognized as potential faces or masks. Augmented by eyes and possibly other minimal markings, they were transformed into arresting presences in the cave (fig. 4.30).

The use of found shapes is a prime characteristic of the Ice Age art of France and Spain. And these hunting people tended to find what they were already most concerned with—animals. A bison on the cave wall at Bernifal was left as found, with the mere addition of painted red circles for the eyes and a painted half circle for the nostril. Deeper into the same cave, a second natural rocky bison was modified by the addition of a single black circle for an eye. Similar, almost entirely formed bison have been found at Mas d'Azil and Le Portel. Not long ago, Claude Archambeau, a guide at Bernifal, found a naturally formed bear with a faint painted circle where the eye would be. At nearby Les Combarelles, Archambeau discovered another tiny bison, also made entirely of a natural rock formation.[53] One can accept that prehistoric people recognized these formations as bison because a few faint, confirming lines are carved or painted onto their surfaces, serving to further describe the animal.

In Ice Age Spain, at Hornos de la Peña, only an eye and a nostril were added to augment the face of an animal, possibly a deer, on a hanging stone formation. A comparable rock was similarly animated at Trois Frères, and there are also examples at La Pasiega and Montespan (Haute-Garonne). At Tibiran (Hautes-Pyrénées), a stalactite has the shape of a bear's head. At Arcy-sur-Cure, 18 engravings borrow lines from natural surface formations. In one example, only the eye and some strokes to indicate hair were added to create a horse. At Bernifal, a small stalactite serves as the nose for what seems to be a human face, and the same thing appears on a larger scale at Abri du Colombier (Ardèche).

A pebble unearthed at Les Eyzies must have appeared to its prehistoric finder to have the shape of a human head, to which was added an ear, a nostril, and the line for a mouth. A horse phalange found at Mas d'Azil was seen as a horse's head, with the addition of an eye and a nostril (fig. 4.31). Mammoth metacarpals became, with little change, the five little human statuettes found in Przedmost, Moravia. The same cognitive process used on similar material is seen much later on other continents. An early Haida sculptor on the Northwest Coast of North America transformed a whale vertebra into a bird's head (fig. 4.32).

The Sinagua people in the American Southwest took the symmetrical shells of Pacific Ocean brachiopods and, with minor changes, turned them into toads. One of the earliest pieces of art found in the Americas is a fossil vertebra from a llama dated 12,000 to 14,000 years ago and found at the site of Tequisquiac, Mexico.[54] The natural holes through which muscles and nerves passed have been used as eyes, the shape has been slightly modified, and holes have been cut for nostrils. The result is a coyote's head (fig. 4.33).

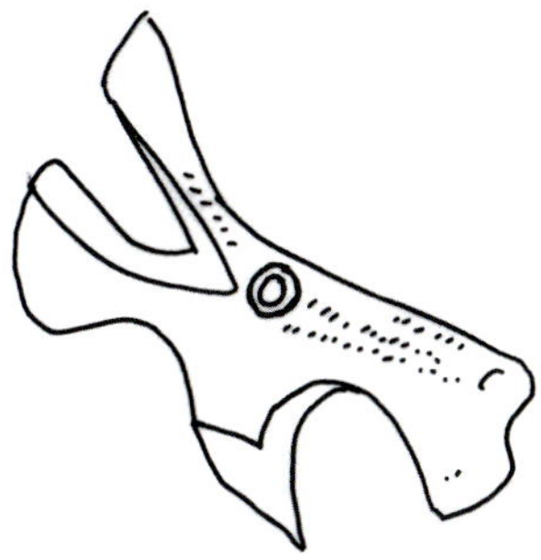

Figure 4.31. Horse phalange made into a horse's head, Mas d'Azil.

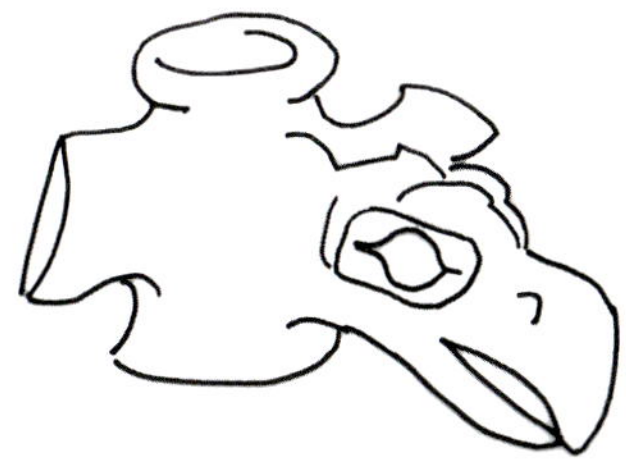

Figure 4.32. Whale vertebra made into a bird's head by a Haida artist.

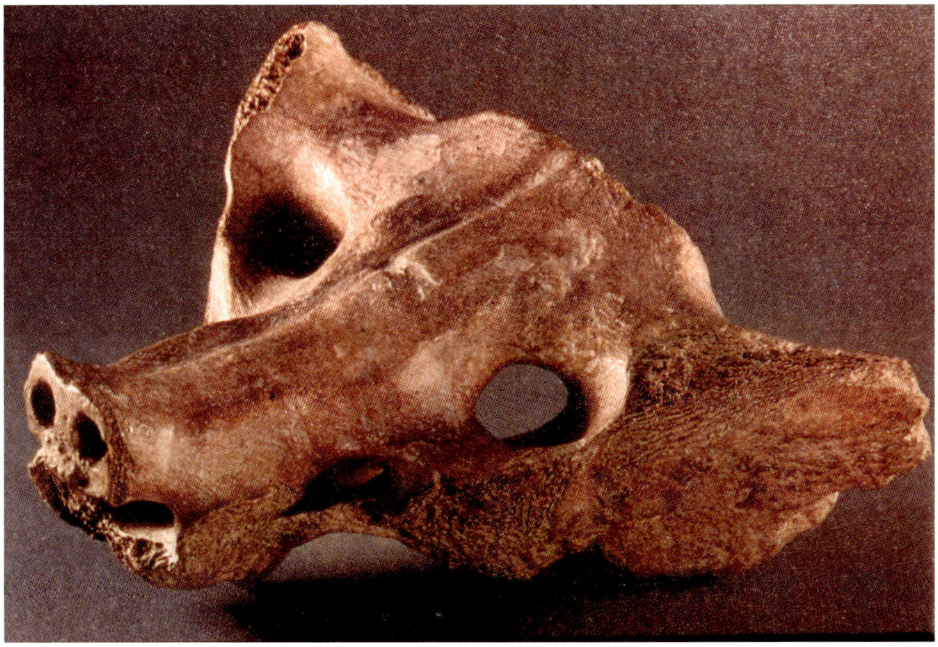

Figure 4.33. Fossil vertebra of a llama made into a coyote's head. 13 cm. About 12,000–14,000 B.P.

One of the most spectacular examples of the use of found figures in Ice Age art occurs in the little-known Spanish cave of Ekain. A large natural rock formation in the center of one of the chambers startles the viewer because it bears the unmistakable form of a horse. It is unmodified except for the likely addition of a single nostril. Horses played an enormous role in European Ice Age art. We can imagine that the serendipitous discovery of this massive horse shape, occupying a central spot in a small cave, had a powerful effect. This ready-made form speaks eerily even to cave visitors today. To people for whom the horse apparently had mythical and spiritual meaning, this natural formation might have confirmed the belief that there was a deeper order to their world.

Double Entendres

Sometimes we know that Ice Age artists recognized found objects because they placed on or within them smaller engraved or painted images of the same animal as that from which the bone or antler was derived. We saw earlier that a horse phalange found at Mas d'Azil was seen as a horse's head, with the addition of an eye and a nostril. We can suppose that a piece of antler from El Pendo (Cantabria) was recognized as being deer shaped because it was decorated with smaller deer heads, similarly shaped.

A particularly suggestive and complex example of the interplay between the natural and the man-made is the large wall painting of the spotted horses from Pech-Merle (see fig. 1.1). As the archaeologist Denis Vialou analyzed it: "The horse on the right is placed at the edge of a natural cutout surface in the rock, the top of which outlines with a striking resemblance a horse's head and neck. It is within this purely natural horse's head that the artist has placed the abstracted head of his own artwork. The realistic and the stylized images confront one another in a symbolic artifice of great profundity."[55] The result of these graphic manipulations is a double entendre in which the forms are read both as natural, geological, found configurations and as man-made figurative art.

In North America, in a similar vein, an Eskimo artist from the Cape Dorset area took a bear tooth with an evocative bear shape, smoothed it, and added dots for nostrils and ears, making of it a tiny bear's head. Near Cross River, New York, are two large rocks with uncanny resemblances to bears' heads, and in fact bears were engraved on them by members of one of the many northern tribes that passed through this land.

In a rockshelter in the Kimberley area of South Africa, an engraved ostrich with lowered head was placed next to a natural hollow in the rock.

When the hollow fills with water, the impression is that the bird is drinking from a waterhole.[56] By contrast, in the rock art of the Spanish Levant, believed to date to the Neolithic or possibly up to the Bronze Age, artists seem largely to have ignored the figurative possibilities of the natural rock formations. In the rare instances when the characteristics of the stone surfaces were used, it was to suggest a landscape setting for painted animals and human figures. At Cingle de la Mola (Valencia), painted hunters with bows and arrows hide behind a jutting rock, ostensibly out of view of the game they are stalking. An unusual use of natural formations occurs at Cuevas de Araña (Valencia), where natural holes suggested beehives, and bees were painted flying around them.

Australian Aboriginal art, too, was less sensitive to the possibility of the found object and its potential for double entendre. Such objects and natural formations seem not to have had the same visual resonance for Aborigines as for European Ice Age artists. The anthropologists Baldwin Spencer and F. J. Gillen wrote, "We have never met in Central Australia with any attempt to take advantage of natural peculiarities in the material out of which the object is fashioned."[57] In many ways the landscape itself seems to have been the object of focus, but it evoked stories more often than images. Special landforms were, and still are, viewed more as the sites of ancient Dreamtime events and thus as reminders of what took place rather than as visual icons. An exception is that holes in rocks are often viewed as body orifices, usually vulvas.

Modern Use of the Found Object

The artistic use of found objects largely disappeared from the official art of the sophisticated European world until it was revived with bravura by the Surrealists, who carried the process to an outrageous conclusion. Marcel Duchamp distinguished between objects that were usable as art just as he found them, which he called "readymades," and objects that needed some addition or modification, which he called "rectified" objects. The most notorious readymade was the work entitled *Fountain* that Duchamp entered in the famous "Armory Show" for the Society of Independent Artists, held in New York in 1917. In fact this piece was a common commercial urinal. It was submitted under a pseudonym, was never in fact exhibited at the show (although Alfred Stieglitz showed it briefly at his 291 gallery), and ultimately it was lost. Previously Duchamp had shown a bicycle wheel mounted on a stool, and later a hat rack, objects taken from hardware stores or junk heaps. Selected by the artist, the fountain-urinal was wrenched from its normal environment to appear in a gallery setting. Selection was the key. Despite its rejection by the Armory Show, this piece had enormous influence. The statement it made, in a nose-thumbing fashion, was that art has to do with the artist's intent. Today, following in Duchamp's tradition, much art is considered to be whatever the artist calls "art."

A famous example of finding analogy in art is Picasso's *Bull's Head.* We are aware that the head is a bicycle seat and the horns are handlebars, but with minimal rearrangement these objects have been transformed into a bull's head. Much of the magic of such metamorphosis comes from the exposure of the conceptual process. Even as the artist reveals to us the secret of his trick, he is able, like a consummate magician, to bewilder our senses. For the fullest effect the viewer must be made aware of the double meaning. Picasso understood this completely. Speaking of his bicycle-bull sculpture he said: "If one was only aware of the head of a bull and not of the bicycle seat and handlebars of which it was formed, this sculpture would lose its interest."[58]

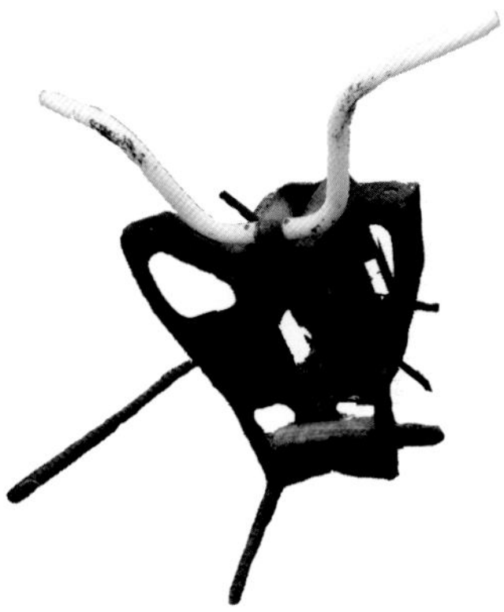

Figure 4.34. Joe Minter, *Bull's Head,* 1999. Handlebars, automobile air conditioner, chain, shackle, and rebar.

The Alabama artist Joe Minter, best known for his political art, made a bull's head of his own with recycled industrial materials. A cast-off machine part reminded him of a bull's head, and like Picasso, he used bicycle handlebars for the horns (fig. 4.34). Minter worked as a factory welder until he retired and decided to make objects for his own purposes. He had no art background and had not looked at books showing reproductions of Picasso's work, but he, too, noticed the similarity between handlebars and horns. He was working in a tradition called at various times folk, grassroots, primitive, backyard, visionary, outsider, vernacular, *naif* or *brut.*

For some folk artists in contemporary times, found objects seem to be signs from the supernatural. Bessie Harvey, a descendant of slaves, lived and worked in eastern Tennessee. She took gnarled and twisted pieces of wood and found already hidden in them the figures she would bring forth. In speaking of the use of found objects in her work, Harvey said:

> I don't design my work. I don't carve it. I just make what I see from found objects. The wood—the insects has already created what it is, and time. Time rots away a lot of wood, and inside that wood, these little people hide. I just go to them and find what I see and bring it out. I think that God is the artist in my work. I'm just the hands that he blessed to do and the mind and the eyes that he blessed to do it for a purpose, and the purpose is to reassure the people that God's

love is real and it's true. It's the only way that we're going to survive here. . . . Most artists, our kind, especially the black ones, say they work for God.[59]

Dealing with such materials, found by chance, the artist often feels that the object's serendipitous appearance and the intuitive sense he or she feels about how the material must be used are a spiritual communication. Bessie Harvey voiced what might have been a common feeling for artists working with such materials—those in Ice Age Europe and later ones in traditional societies everywhere.

Assemblage

Frequently art is made with groupings of found objects. It may be that any one of the objects is neutral, but together they resonate with meaning that creates new analogies. The process and result is called assemblage. In 1975, at a site in France known as La Roche-Cotard, an enigmatic Neanderthal "assemblage" was discovered and dated to at least 32,000 years ago (fig. 4.35). Twenty years later the prehistorian Michel Lorblanchet, finding the piece in a museum, interpreted it as a mask.[60] The object consists in part of a flint nodule that could have been seen as a mask or face. A splinter of bone appears to have been deliberately placed in the natural hole under a projection of the flint that looks like the bridge of a nose, where it could have been understood as eyelids for the face. If this combination of objects is indeed an assemblage, then it is a simple construction made by the friction fit of one piece into another.

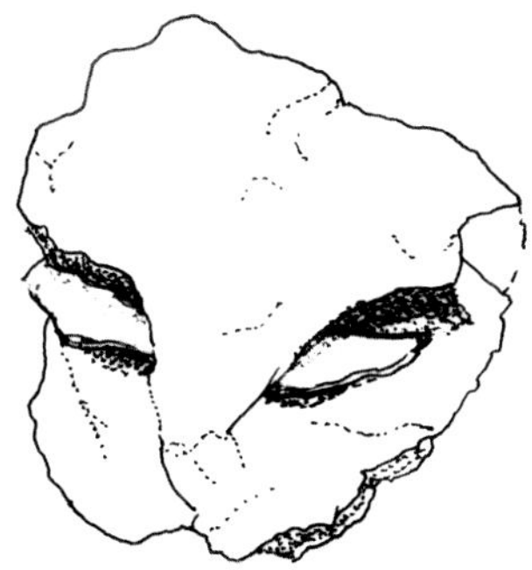

Figure 4.35 "Assemblage" from La Roche-Cotard. Friction fit of stone into bone.

We know that the people of the European Ice Age had the technology for assembling objects by more complex means. In bead production, materials such as shell, stones, bones, and teeth were assembled to be sewn onto leather clothing. In the burial at Sungir, Russia, mentioned in chapter 1, the two boys' leather clothing had disintegrated, but thousands of beads of ivory and of arctic fox canines survived. At Grotte les Enfants on the Italian Riviera, large clusters of decorated shells had been attached to the long-disintegrated clothing of two children. Nearby, an adult wore a shell headdress. People of the Ice Age were able to haft tools; small stone points were shaped to be inserted into wood or bone handles. We know that Ice Age artisans had knowledge of available natural adhesives such as mastic, bitumin, and asphalt, beginning with the Neanderthals and increasingly in the Late Paleolithic.

A transitional society known as Natufian appeared in what is now Israel, still partaking of some Paleolithic attributes but also incorporating some that are considered Neolithic. In the excavation of Jericho, the archaeologist Kathleen Kenyon uncovered a group of nine human skulls that had been modified by being plastered with clay and then colored with red oxide. Cowrie shells were inserted in the eye sockets, giving the impression of lidded eyes. A variety of types of shells appear to have been used as well.[61] These macabre assemblages have been dated to roughly 8,000 years ago. The shells, brought from distant places, carried a precious and exotic aura, and the skulls surely carried their own emotional associations.

Many contemporary artists use found objects, frequently the cast-off detritus of our throwaway society, to create assemblages. Found objects bring with them a history and a penumbra of meaning. Joe Minter uses found materials exclusively. Tony Price, a New Mexico artist, collected metallic discards from Los Alamos National Laboratory, which is closely associated with nuclear weapons. He used these ominous materials to make sculptures with analogous prehistoric and indigenous American themes. An example is his *Hopi Nuclear Maidens*. The reference appears to be a melding of the Hopi Corn Maidens and the Hiroshima Maidens. Even further, this piece reminds us that many American Indians were employed to dig uranium in the large open-pit mine near Laguna and Acoma Pueblos without adequate protection or, in many cases, any protection at all. Many still suffer from exposure to this toxic material. Another artist who uses junk from the nuclear industry with sinister implications is Woody Vasulka. One of his pieces is built around a celestial navigator, a piece of military hardware designed to deliver a deadly bomb load.

Using natural cast-off material, the contemporary sculptor Deborah Butterfield became known by assembling clay-rich dirt, twigs, brambles, and wood scraps into life-size horses. In her more recent work she has used scrap metal as well, but the resulting assemblages still read as horses. In this respect her work has obvious analogies to that of the Ice Age artists. They often had horses in their heads and as a result found them everywhere they looked. Butterfield, too, has horses in her head, and so, as one reviewer said, she can take almost anything and make a horse out of it.

One of the most original and dedicated of the contemporary artists using found materials is Holly Hughes. She creates large, site-specific art with the collaboration of the communities in which the art is requested. These are not always the usual art patrons but often small towns, trailer parks, old age homes, and American Indian pueblos. Hughes invites the willing help of anyone who wants to participate and uses as material only the indigenous trash found in each area. The theme of the piece is devised by Hughes, who relates each piece to the site in which it is being made. The bison's head shown here is made of ranch trash more clearly seen in close-up details of the head (fig. 4.36).

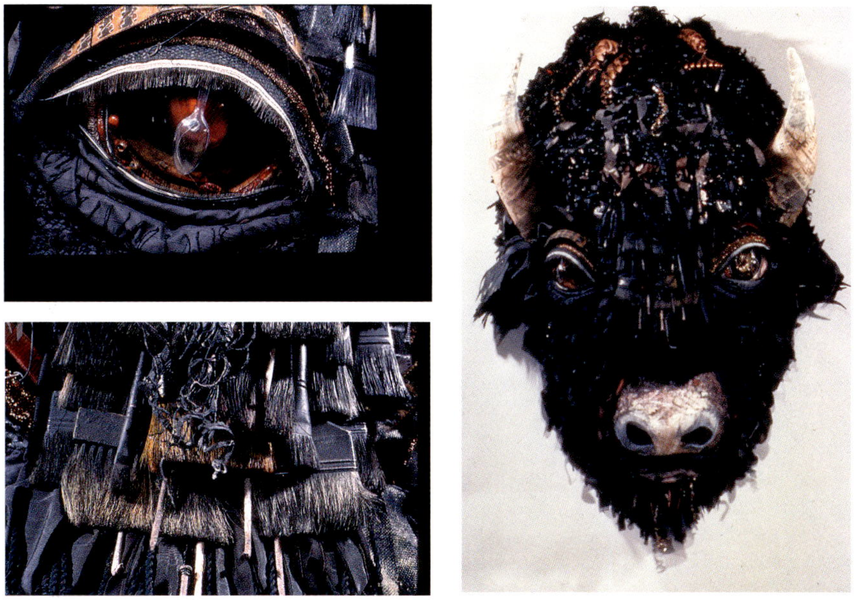

Figure 4.36. Holly Hughes, *Buffalo,* 1992. Found ranch trash, including paint brushes, rusted nails, fishing reel, horseshoe, plastic spoon, and pottery shards. Height: almost 2 meters, width 1.27 meters, depth 63.5 cm. Details show the eye and the bridge of the nose. Photo: H. Hughes

Art itself has been recycled to make other art. Indeed, one of the puzzling aspects of much Ice Age art is the frequent superpositioning of paintings or carvings over one other. One sees recarving in bas-relief and sculpture. In some of the elaborate caves such as Lascaux and Altamira, there are multiple layers of paintings. In one peculiar instance of a painted bison at La Pasiega, Spain, some prehistoric dabbler at a later time added lines that seem to change the bison's head into a human head. To our uninitiated eye it suggests Dalí's well-known painting of Leonardo's *La Gioconda,* in which Dalí changed everything by adding a moustache to the woman's face. *Appropriation* is the current term given to the blatant use of complete works of someone else's art for one's own purposes.

Sometimes changes are made to earlier icons to undermine or even change their meaning. Early Christian missionaries superimposed their own imagery, often consisting of crosses, on American Indian petroglyphs to mitigate their power and even change what they considered to be diabolical pagan imagery. Sometimes ancient imagery was appropriated in order to take over its aura and power for new purposes. Churches frequently are built on ancient religious sites, just as Chartres was built over a Druid temple. In a like manner one can believe that Paleolithic artists made use of even earlier Paleolithic art to incorporate into their own work the potency of the image as well as the now special, perhaps even sacred, quality of the site. This might explain the superpositioning of some images, which one sees in much early art. In the Aboriginal rock art of Australia, for example, paintings are layered over one another in a manner similar to that of the cave art of Europe. In both cases the art making might have been a performance involving the resanctification of an older site.

Found Music

Musicians may have their own kind of found art. Mozart, it is said, once heard a starling singing in a street vendor's cage and used the song as the theme for the last movement of his *G Major Concerto* for piano and orchestra. Indeed, he was so struck with the starling's song that he obtained a starling as a pet. Beethoven, Bach, and Vivaldi used birdsong in instrumental works. Ottorino Respighi, as we have seen, as well as Olivier Messiaen, incorporated birdsong in their music. Gustav Mahler used cowbells, and Tchaikovsky used church bells and cannons. Many composers, including, notably, Bela Bartok, have used folk tunes. George Crumb used the sounds of wolves and whales. Charles Ives and other musicians used street noises. John Cage used the sounds of the audience itself in the concert hall.

We have seen "appropriation" in visual art, but musicians, if anything, lead the way. Composers have always taken themes from their predecessors. Two of the most famous are Brahms's *Variation on a Theme by Haydn* and Rachmaninoff's *Rhapsody on a Theme of Paganini.* In contemporary popular music, appropriation is known as "sampling." Certain kinds of music—rap, for example—almost invariably use recycled scraps of jazz, soul, and pop. One of the newest musical art forms, "soundscape art," documents everyday sounds, arranges them into collages, and transforms them electronically.

Nature's Use of Found Material

With the use of found objects, artists are imitating in the closest possible way the archetypal methods of the "Grand Designer." More and more, in explaining the evolution of increasingly novel and complex structures, biologists are finding that nature and their own bodies used what was at hand but used it in an analogous way that might become a new way. The ossicles of our middle ear are appropriated from small bones in an earlier version of the jaw. Our bodies make use of the proteins found in the body using them over and over again—for example, as hormones in the body as a whole and then as neurotransmitters in the brain. Evolution has recruited material called crystallin, already available in the body globulins, to make specific receptors used by eyes.

The eye has evolved dozens of variations in insects, fish, and mammals. Each of these has a different structure adapted to the specific animal's needs. The uses are analogous, but in each case the eye consists of crystallin used in different mixes for differing light sensitivity. And this chemical, crystallin, which was once thought to be highly specialized and unique to the eye's lens, has been found to exist throughout the body, performing quite different tasks in other places. So even entire, incredibly complex structures such as the lenses in our eyes are made from material that once served a different purpose—one might say, from found material. The developmental biologist Margaret McFall-Ngau said:

> The lesson is that there is nothing new under the sun. The genome is resourceful, and when posed with the question, "How do I achieve the development and evolution of this new structure?" there's more and more evidence that it just goes back to itself and says, "Let's rearrange these genes in a different way in a different place to come up with what would appear to be something completely novel."[62]

Nature's use of preexisting structures for new purposes is called *preadaptation* or *exaptation*. Reptilian feathers are a commonly cited example. Feathers evolved from scales because they were useful for temperature regulation. Then nature found they could be useful for flight. The artist, like nature—or nature, like the artist—makes use of existing materials by appropriating the same substances and structures that were there all along to produce the strikingly new and original.

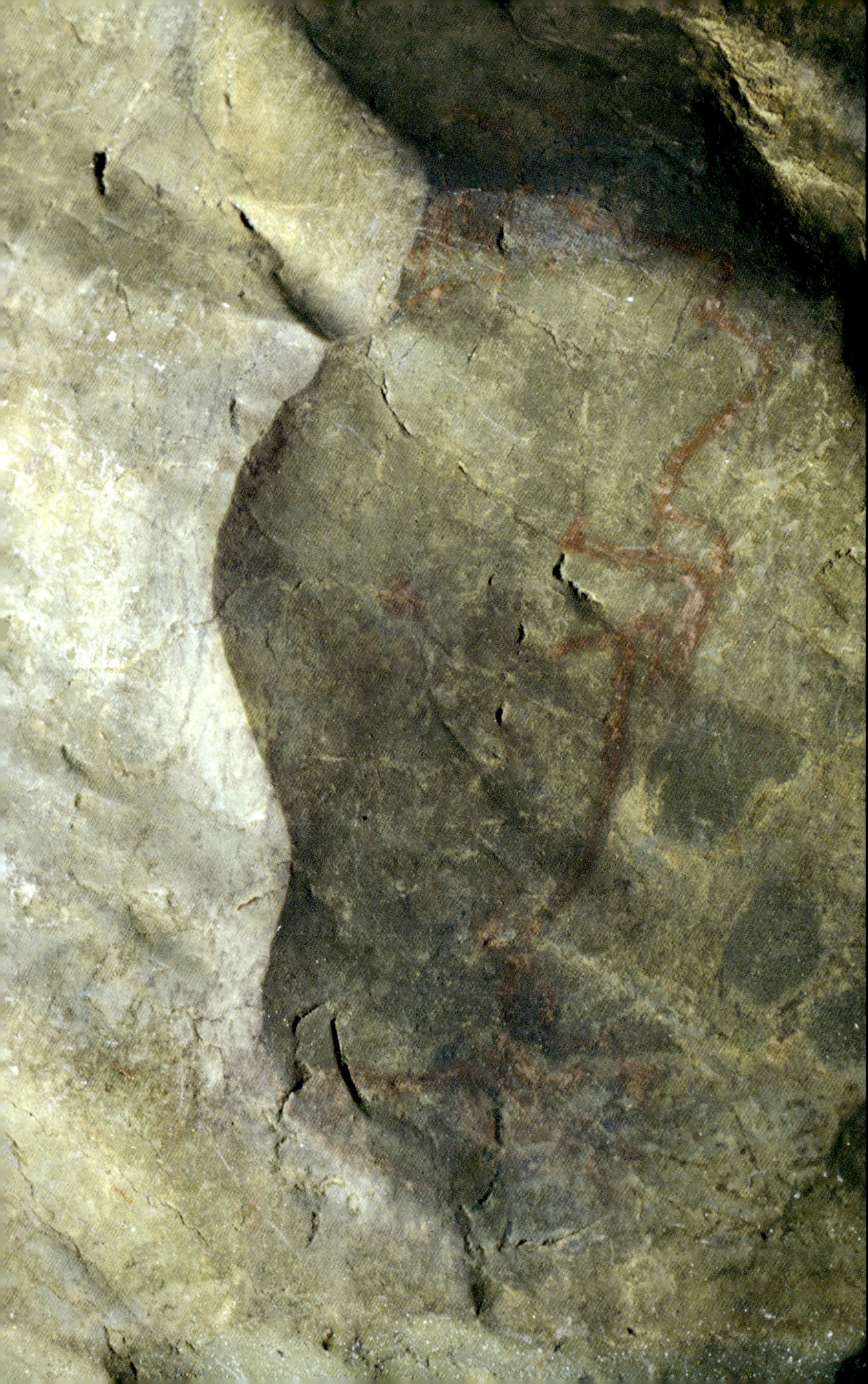

5

AMBIGUITY

Playing with Multiple Meanings

The "discovery of appearances" is really the discovery of the ambiguities of vision.
—E. H. GOMBRICH, *Art and Illusion*

IN COMPARISON WITH COMPUTERS, our brains are poorly designed for precision. That may be our saving grace. Computers are not designed, as we are, for ambiguity. To put it another way, we are well designed to make inferences with minimal and often uncertain input. Our brains are able to scan vast amounts of information very quickly. We are also able to take incomplete and confusing, sometimes barely comprehensible sensory data and make informed guesses from it. Often we can draw more than one interpretation from the information that we continuously absorb. The physician and philosopher Lewis Thomas contends that our capacity to use ambiguity is a major source of our creativity.[1] When a quick response is needed, we are able to select among alternatives and then, if necessary, act rapidly. But when a swift reaction is not required, we can take the time to stand back and observe the workings of our own minds. Psychologists have set up ambiguous situations in which we can experience ourselves vacillating between two or more equally plausible interpretations; they call this *equivocation.*

Sometimes neither of two interpretations is more probable than the other, but we cannot simultaneously accept both because we cannot give our attention to two displays of neuronal activity simultaneously. We may make a decision that seems reasonable for a few moments and then, without volition, find ourselves able to see only the alternative possibility. When an image presents a choice of two equally plausible interpretations, psychologists call it an *unstable figure.* Neurologists call it *multistable.* Kurt Koffka, one of the group of Gestalt psychologists, preferred to use the term *stimulus constellation,* referring to the creative potential such images offer the viewer.[2]

Opposite: Vertical bison from Niaux Cave (Ariège) uses ambiguity between concave and convex. The dorsal line is the stone edge. An illusion of relief is formed by the shadow of a hollow in the wall enhanced by a red line to show head and belly. C. 13,000 B.P. Photo by J. Clottes.

Many artists have relished multistable figures. Odilon Redon, the twentieth-century French painter, is known for a mysterious quality that suffuses his work. Describing this quality, he wrote: "The essence of the mystery is to preserve a state of ambivalence through double and triple possible interpretations, through mere hints of interpretations."[3] Ambivalent figures can also be sources of pleasure, of humor, and sometimes of laughter. Puns, both verbal and visual, use the confusion inherent in language or in vision. They tease our mental loopholes; they toy with the Achilles' heels of our cognition. One part of our mind can sit back and watch the bizarre results with fascination.

Uncertainty about how to interpret confusing perceived information creates ambiguity and leaves us perplexed. One way to deal with this perplexity is to defuse our uncertainty by playing with it. Often this results in puns. Perplexity may be likened to a foreign body in an oyster. The oyster resolves the irritation by encapsulating it with nacre and produces a pearl; we humans take our disturbances and produce puns. We are most familiar with verbal puns, which are based on aural confusion. Sometimes two words sound the same but are spelled differently, sometimes the same word has more than one meaning, and on occasion the sounds are not exact but close enough to lead to ambiguous meaning. In all such instances someone deliberately manipulates the phonic components of language to arrive at a pun. There are also visual puns, in which the confusion is not of sounds but of lines and forms.

Puns are most often sources of humor. Verbal humor and visual humor are processed in different parts of the brain, but there is a central location in the right frontal lobe where information from throughout the brain is integrated with emotional responses. In documented medical cases in which tumors exist in this central location, patients burst into spontaneous laughter with no apparent cause. The role of this central area in humor is even more suggestive because serious damage there destroys the normal humor response.[4]

Sometimes the use of visual illusion in art appears to be directed toward a kind of game playing, making use of optical puns to trick the viewer and to rivet attention. Punning, used in the service of art making, is one way to satisfy the artist's ever-present urge to execute a tour de force. Ice Age humans apparently were familiar with many of the most common visual illusions and reacted to them much as we do. This seems evident because we find puns in Ice Age art that are similar to those made in our own day.

In this chapter I look at some of these visual puns, especially at three aspects of visual ambiguity that have played a major role in art making from as far back as there is any record. They are figure-ground reversal, the ambiguous perception of convex and concave surfaces, and spatial ambiguity.

FIGURE-GROUND REVERSAL

A contour line between two interlocking figures has a double function, and the act of tracing such a line therefore presents a special difficulty. On either side of it a figure takes shape simultaneously.
—MAURITS C. ESCHER

While he was photographing a 15,000-year-old stone engraving from Les Eyzies, the philosopher-architect Siegfried Giedion made a discovery:

> In the Museum of Laugerie a triangular block of stone with incurving sides caught my eye because of its shape. I took it out into the sunshine to photograph it. It then became apparent as the engraved outline of a bovid. . . . At first glance it appeared as though the animal were grazing on a slightly convex ledge, with his strongly emphasized forelegs resting on a lower level. When I lifted up the stone to take it back, I turned it by chance through an angle of 180 degrees. This enabled me to see that the curve of this ledge formed the neck and chest of another animal . . . which, in our way of looking at pictures, would be described as standing on its head.[5]

Giedion used this discovery as a point of departure for a theory about the Paleolithic sense of space. He believed the carving confirmed his theory that adherence to a strict vertical or horizontal orientation was not a constraint for Ice Age artists.

I am struck by something quite different in Giedion's discovery. I believe it reveals the ability of these earliest artists to use sophisticated graphic manipulation to achieve what is known as *figure-ground reversal.* When looking at the first photograph of the stone Giedion described, the viewer is aware of one animal only (fig. 5.1). The lines that form the other animal are lost in the background. When the orientation is changed, the second animal comes into view, and the newly upside-down one becomes part of the background.

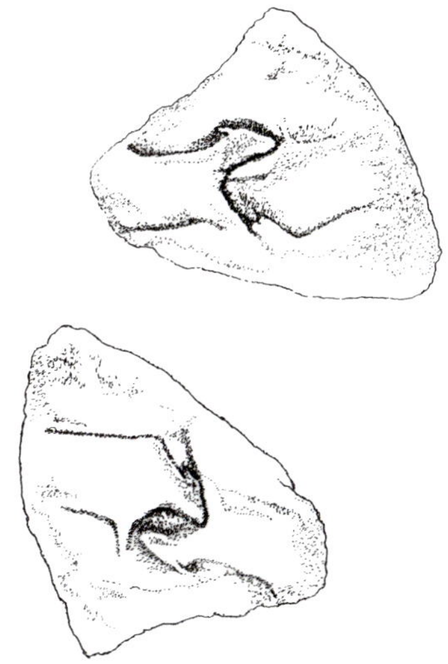

Figure 5.1. Figure-ground reversal occurs through inversion in an artifact from Laugerie.

Artists and psychologists refer to an object as *figure* and to the space around it as *ground.* The figure is meant to be read as nearer, and the ground is what lies behind it. A borderline between two adjacent figures is ambivalent if it can be seen to belong to either of two figures. The ambiguity that results can cause us to alternate between two different, equally plausible interpretations of what we are seeing.

Face-Vase

The Danish psychologist Edgar Rubin first described the phenomenon of figure-ground reversal in 1915: "One can then state as a fundamental principle, when two fields have a common border and one is seen as a figure and the other as ground, the immediate perceptual experience is characterized by a shaping effect which emerges from the common border of the fields and which operates only on one field or operates more strongly on one than on the other."[6] Rubin gave a vivid graphic demonstration of what he meant in his now famous "face-vase" figure. Its shapes can be seen alternately as figure and ground, so that it can be interpreted equally well as a vase or as two profiles facing each other (fig. 5.2).

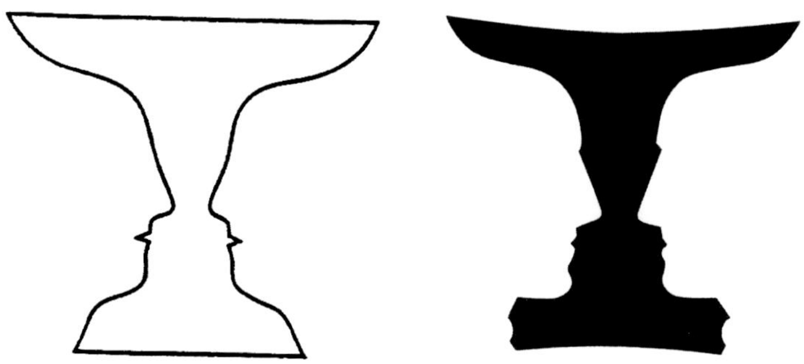

Figure 5.2. Face-vase figure. One sees the face or the vase, alternately. Left: Example using line. Right: Example using mass.

The terms *figure* and *ground,* used in this way, may have been new to the twentieth century, but there is increasing evidence that the optical effect was known long before then. A number of Ice Age figures on plaquettes and in caves appear first as one animal and then as another as the viewer's concentration shifts from figure to ground.

In the dark Ice Age caves, such effects might initially have been inevitable results of the flickering and changing light from the stone lamps the artists carried. As the angle of light changed, even slightly, figures emerged from the man-made lines and from the uneven shapes of the wall surfaces. As the light moved, those figures disappeared, and other, previously unseen ones emerged. Many of the Ice Age examples that I give later in this chapter under the heading of "spatial ambiguity" are, in the context of cave lighting, examples of figure-ground ambiguity. As the light changes, one part of the image may merge with the background until the light changes again and that part is brought to our attention, while the part we had been looking at recedes. Another cause of figure-ground ambiguity might be the changing position of the viewer. Sometimes images are seen and then never found again because a particular viewing position and illumination are never exactly duplicated.

Thousands of years after the European Ice Age, and on another continent, a small group of ceramic pot painters now called the Mimbres people achieved an inventive mastery of figure-ground inversion. Their relatively brief tenure, from about 900 to 1250, was still prehistory in the American Southwest. They lived along the Mimbres River, for which they are named, and were members of the larger Mogollon desert culture. The Mimbres people used their splendid, representational black-and-white pottery for ritual burial purposes, a sign that the vessels were much prized. The pots were vehicles for a florescence of artistic expression characterized by storytelling and fantasy. On a handful of them, painters made use of figure-ground reversal in pictures placed on the interiors of bowls. In one example, four birds alternate with four humans, all of them sharing a single head (fig. 5.3).

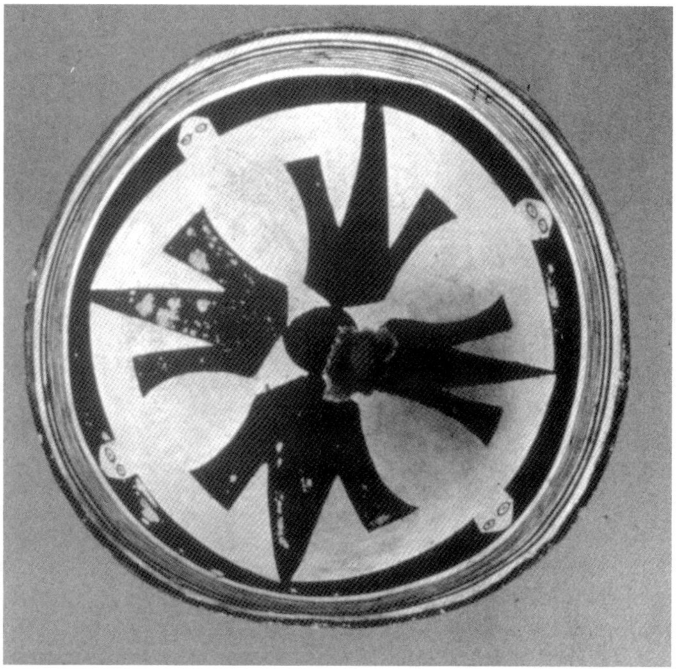

Figure 5.3. Mimbres bowl painted with white owl-like birds that reverse from figure to ground to become black humanlike figures sharing one head. Height 10 cm, diameter 25 cm. Photo: S.A. LeBlanc

The people of the prehistoric Jornada Mogollon culture were related to and contemporaneous with the Mimbres but lived east of the Rio Grande, primarily in New Mexico, in an area now known as Three Rivers. The work that survives from their hands consists mainly of engravings on rock. These engravings share the graphic playfulness seen on the Mimbres pots and occasionally a similar use of figure-ground ambiguity.

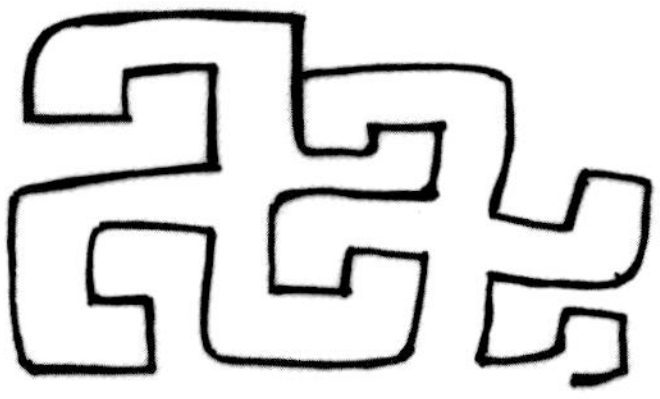

Figure 5.4. Pueblo rock engraving from the Little Colorado River basin, Arizona. Two images alternate as figure and ground. Although commonly termed a swastika, this design is technically known as a *sauvastika,* because its arms face left and not right like the arms of the European version made infamous by the Nazis. In China the symbol means "thunderbolt." Some North American Indian tribes call the image "rolling thunder."

Other uses of this visual device have appeared at other times and in other places. It seems to have been a rare independent discovery made intermittently by individual artists. Another North American example is found in rock art in the Little Colorado River basin area of Arizona, where two swastikas incised in the rock switch back and forth from figure to ground. This geometric exercise, reminiscent of Moorish tile designs, was probably carried out by an ancestor of the present-day Zuñi people (fig. 5.4).

Two of many pots made at Zia Pueblo, New Mexico, in the late 1880s—both apparently decorated by the same painter—made use of heart motifs. Only by means of a mental shift, again with figure-ground reversal, does one realize that the design alternately depicts four hummingbirds whose beaks meet

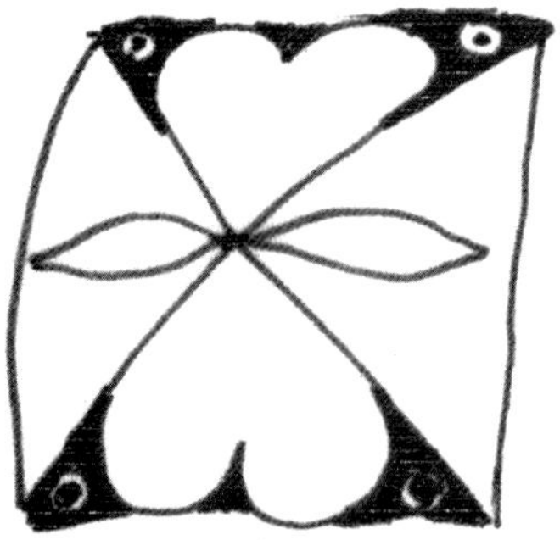

Figure 5.5. An abstract design on a Zia pot reverses to four hummingbirds whose beaks meet in the center.

at a central point (fig. 5.5). Sometimes figure-ground reversal is less strong, and although two figures share a line, both can be seen at the same time. An example appears in another Mimbres pot, on which a long-necked crane reverses to a face (fig. 5.6).

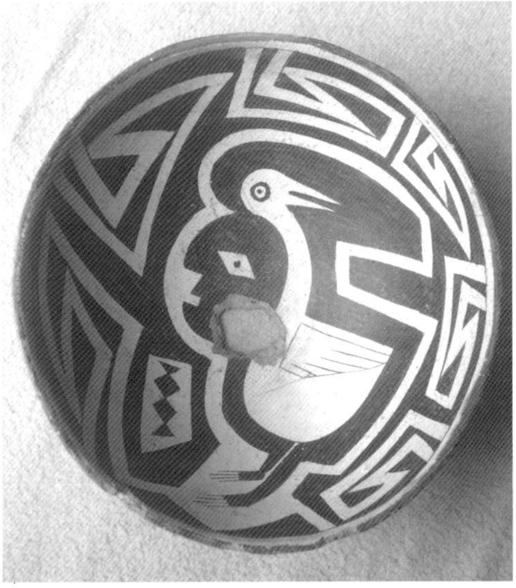

Figure 5.6. Mimbres bowl depicting a crane and a human head in near perfect figure-ground reversal. Height 10.5 cm, diameter 25 cm.
Photo: S.A. LeBlanc

John Clegg, an archaeologist and specialist in Australian rock art, has pointed out a figure in New South Wales at a place called the "fishman" site.[7] In the most prominent engraving there, the negative space, or ground, between the legs of a man has been made to form a fish (fig. 5.7). The man appears to be a bit discomforted. In modern times Picasso, a voracious explorer of graphic possibilities, made a similar etching. In this case the space between the legs of the standing nude became the torso for another,

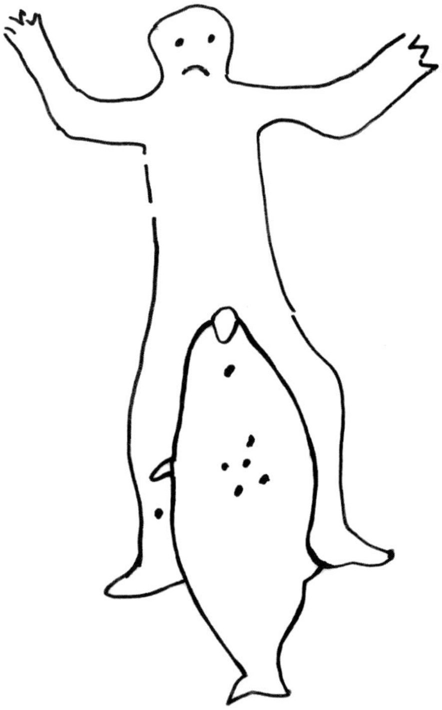

Figure 5.7. The "fishman," an Aboriginal engraving on sandstone from the vicinity of Sidney, Australia. Figure 1.65 meters high; fish 1.2 meters long.

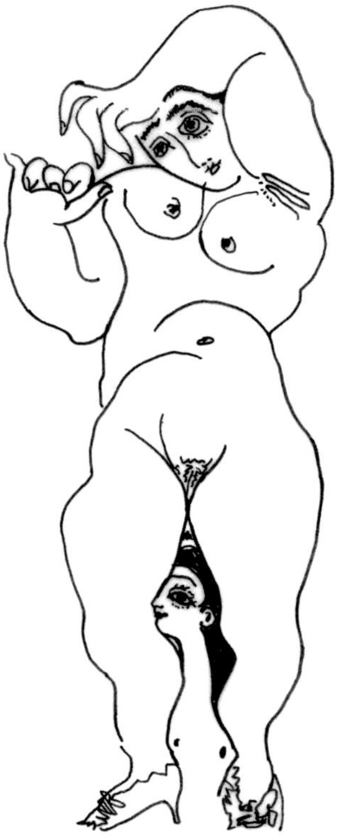

Figure 5.8. Copy after a section of a Pablo Picasso etching. This demonstrates partial figure-ground reversal, similar to that of the "fishman" image.

smaller nude woman (fig. 5.8).

Maurits Escher, whose impressions of Lascaux began this inquiry, has been almost synonymous with figure-ground reversal, which he carried to unparalleled virtuosity. He was directly influenced by Moorish geometric tile work.[8] In his *Study of Regular Division of the Plane with Birds,* we can see an example of interlocked, reversed figures (fig. 5.9). Escher described the problems involved in creating this kind of deliberate confusion: "The act of tracing such a line is a complicated business. On either side of it, simultaneously, a recognizability takes shape. But the human eye and mind cannot be busy with two things at the same moment, and so there must be a quick and continual jumping from one side to the other. . . . this difficulty is perhaps the very moving spring of my perseverance."[9]

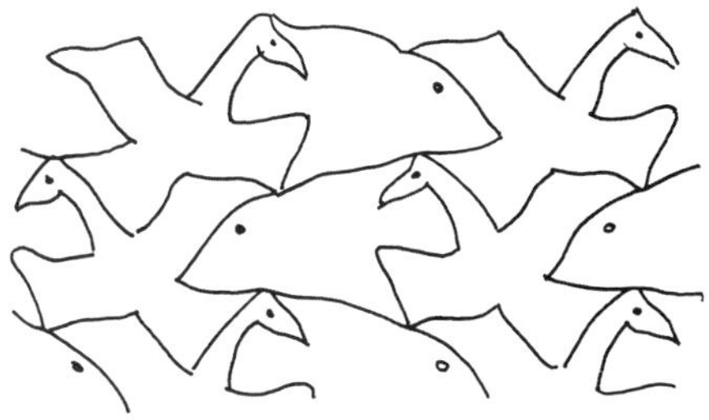

Figure 5.9 After Maurits Escher's study of birds and fish showing full figure-ground reversal.

In modern Europe, many artists have delighted in creating this kind of graphic pun. Salvador Dalí had an obvious love for optical tricks and based much of his work on them. He used the same principle of figure-ground ambiguity, but with much greater complexity, in making double images, compositions in which the graphic elements can have two or even three ways of being resolved. Whether deliberate or coincidental, Dalí's use of vase and face in *Apparition of Face and Fruit Dish on a Beach* echoes Rubin's vase-face diagram. Depending on how one sees it, the painting depicts a fruit dish with fruit on a table, a hallucinatory face, a dog, or, on a smaller scale, a landscape with many little scenes. Perhaps Dalí's most famous and most striking example of double imagery appears in his series incorporating the bust of Voltaire, done in 1940–41. In *Slave Market with the Disappearing Bust of Voltaire,* one sees alternately a group of figures and a ghostlike head of Voltaire (fig. 5.10).

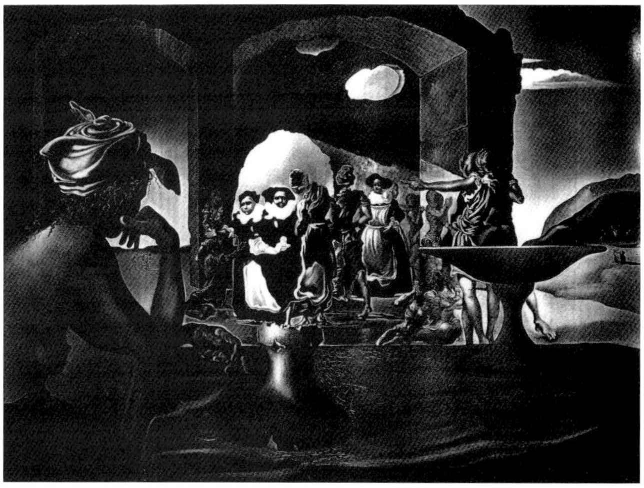

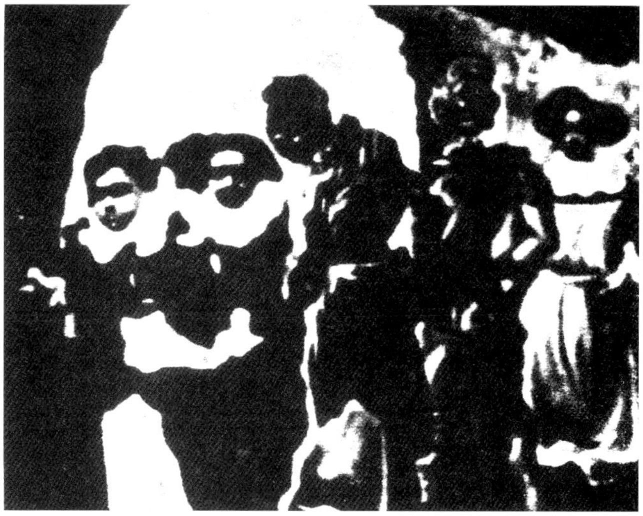

Figure 5.10 Salvador Dalí, Images reverse from *Slave Market with the Disappearing Bust of Voltaire*. Entire painting above and detailed below.

The Belgian artist René Magritte used alternation of figure and ground in two paintings done in 1927. In both *Les muscles célestes* and *Les jambes du ciel,* the "ground" of the sky, which dominates the upper half of the painting,

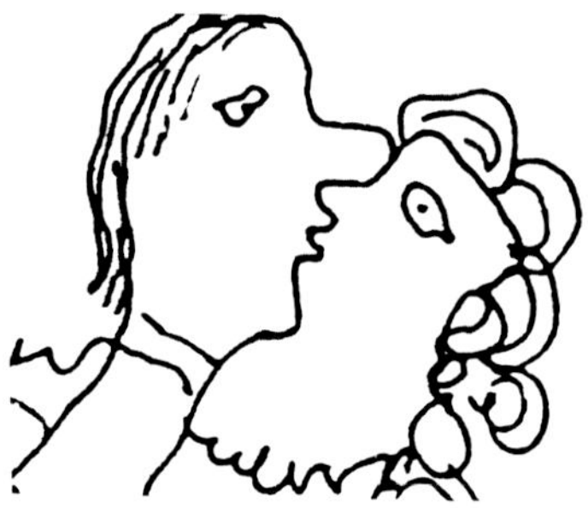

Figure 5.11 Copy after a section of a cartoon *Animal Magnetism* by William Steig, showing interlocking faces that can be reversed so that the viewer sees first one face and then another.

continues down into the lower half of the picture to become enigmatic, sky-colored "figures." The tour de force here is that at some imperceptible point, what is far back becomes close front. And yet it is impossible for us to pinpoint the exact place where the background shifts into the foreground.

In one deceptively simple cartoon drawing by the artist William Steig—*Animal Magnetism* (fig. 5.11)—we can almost feel the rapid series of mental shifts as we interpret first one way, then another. We can almost hear a click of gears changing somewhere in our head. The same graphic device was used in 1995 by the Australian Aboriginal art student Shaun Edwards (Injarr), of the Koko-per tribe on the Staaten River, Queensland. Edwards had been brought to Cairns a few months before to join an art program for Aborigines. He had never previously been off his tribal land. So meager were the funds available to train students that a volunteer teacher was able to provide materials only for inexpensive linoleum prints. The art library consisted of a few illustrated books containing fairly standard European art reproductions. One trip to an ancient Aboriginal rock art site near Cairns constituted Edwards's only other experience with art history.[10] He stumbled upon figure-ground reversal on his own while experimenting with line as he made his linoleum prints (fig. 5.12).

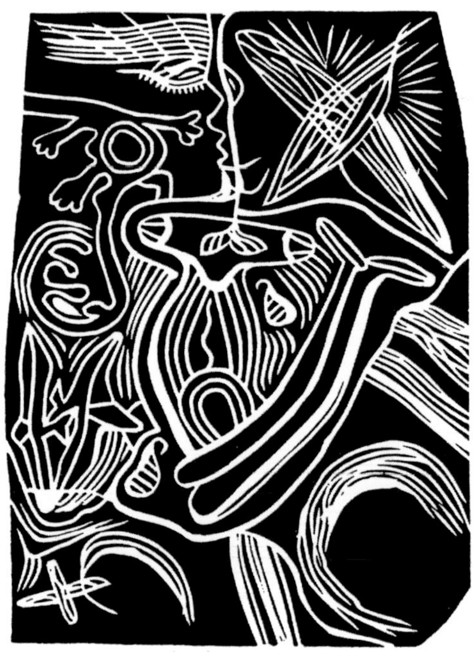

Figure 5.12. Shawn Edwards, *Rape at the Station,* linoleum print, 1995. This image also shows figure-ground reversal in interlocking faces.

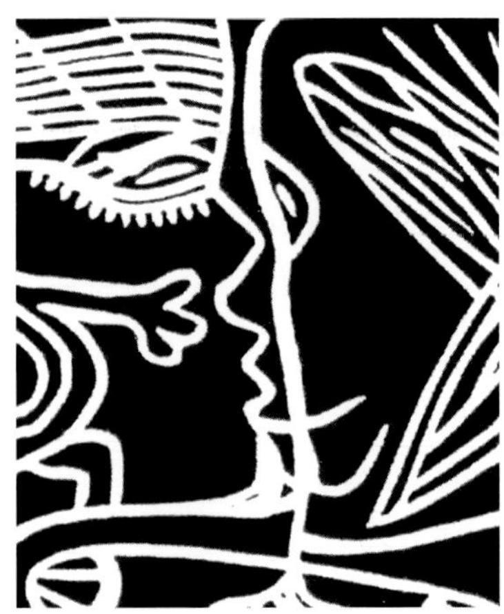

Detail from top center of print. Simplified below.

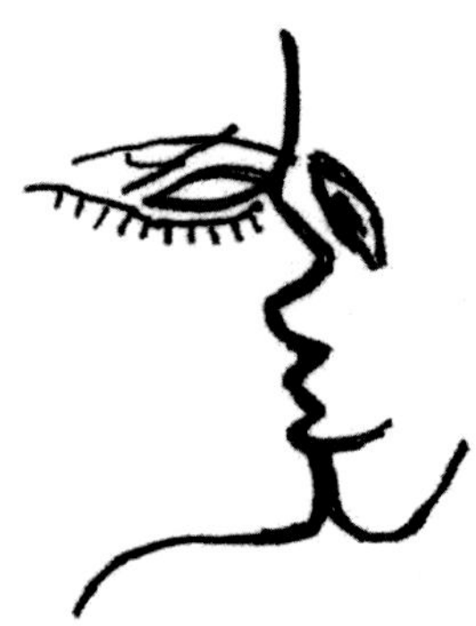

The Psychology of Figure Reversal

Figure-ground organization in graphics seems to be innate. As soon as a human being places a mark on a surface, that surface or pictorial field is automatically transformed into an imaginary space with one thing behind and one thing in front. The psychologist Irvin Rock wrote that "there is a universal tendency in looking at a drawing to perceive the region within certain contours as a solid two-dimensional object."[11] About the reversal of figure and ground, Rock said that "there is a general acceptance of the (Gestalt originated) hypothesis that figure perception entails an underlying process of neural events which is self-satiating."[12] He added that "figure reversal is based on a process of neural fatigue, inhibition or satiation, resulting in a change in the firing of cortical cells. The firing of one set of cells, which leads to one perceptual outcome, ceases, and the firing of another set of cells, which leads to another perceptual outcome, begins."[13]

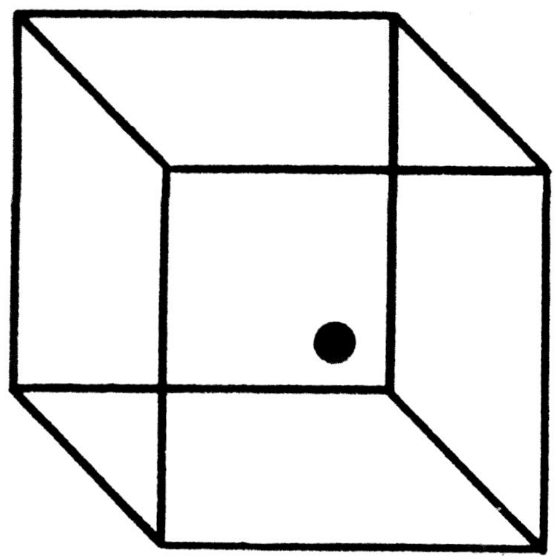

Figure 5.13. Necker's cube. When one regards it fixedly surfaces flip back and forth. The black dot sometimes appears on the front face and sometimes on the back face.

In essence, this is what happens when our brains process the optical illusion of Necker's cube, a figure described by the Swiss crystallographer Louis Albert Necker in 1832. It consists of 12 lines drawn to form a cube (fig. 5.13). There are no size differences among the sides, so the figure is without perspective cues. Necker's cube can be understood equally well as a figure viewed from above or below. This phenomenon occurs when two equally plausible interpretations exist. Neither position is more probable than the other, but we cannot simultaneously accept both views. Our brain makes a decision that is acceptable for a few moments, and then a sudden shift takes place and we see only the alternative interpretation.

Irvin Rock suggested that perceptual interpretation might be the result of a rapid-fire, unconscious process of problem solving. According to his view, "perceptual organization results from a 'decision'; reversals of ambiguous figures can be understood if one assumes that the process of decision is a continuous one, entailing constant trial and error or oscillation from one possibility to another."[14] In making sense of figure-ground reversals, our brains repeatedly and involuntarily shift back and forth from one alternative interpretation to the next. We have no control over the process. As we do now, Ice Age artists must have watched with fascination this bizarre reaction of their perceptual system and sometimes used it for their own graphic wonderment.

CONVEX-CONCAVE AMBIGUITY

Any one aspect of the visual information provided by your eyes is usually ambiguous.

—FRANCIS CRICK,
The Astonishing Hypothesis

Ice Age artists in France and Spain were aware of and experimented with the use of shading to give the illusion of convex form. Even as early as Chauvet cave, perhaps 30,000 years ago, artists produced impressive examples. At the same time, they were aware of the fine line of perceptual ambiguity that exists between convex and concave forms.

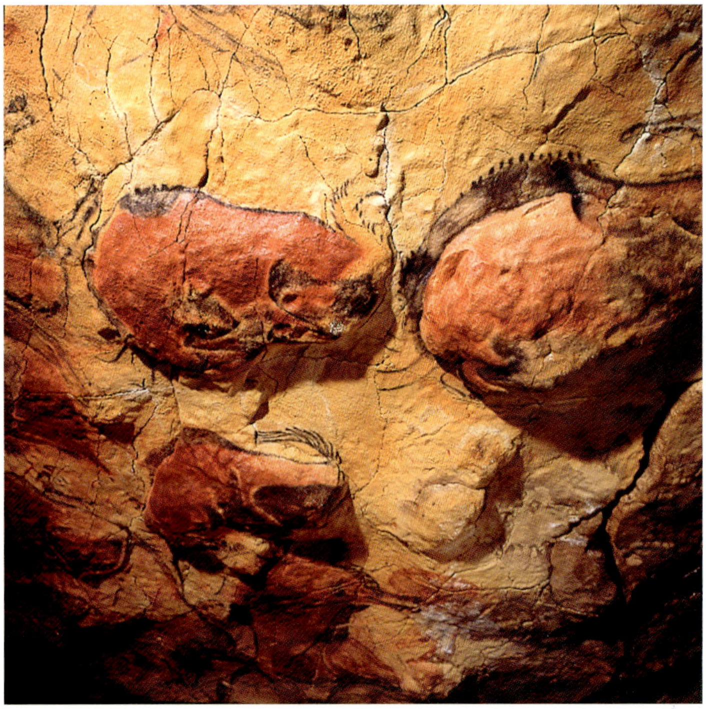

Figure 5.14. Ceiling of the Polychrome Chamber at Altamira, showing the use of natural rocky protuberances to form bison. Photo: P.A. Saura Ramos

On the ceiling of the famous Polychrome Chamber at Altamira, dated to approximately 15,000 years ago, an Ice Age painter used rock projections to create figures of bison on a naturally formed bas-relief (fig. 5.14, see illus. p. 40). This was an obvious way to make use of the surface irregularities. What is not seen well in photographs and cannot be appreciated unless one sees the Altamira ceiling firsthand is that often it was the depressions between the outcroppings of rock that were used to form the animals. Convex forms, which would normally be used in a bas-relief to give volume to protruding figures, became background. Concave forms, which would ordinarily recede into the background, were used to indicate the projecting figures. The "belling bison," for example, was painted in a concavity between swelling rocks on which two other bison appear. Another use of this ambiguity is at El Castillo, near Altamira. The bulk of the bison was placed on a portion of the cave wall that recedes—not, as one would expect, on the part that bulges forward. Many examples show that Ice Age artists used convex surfaces to portray three-dimensional forms. It is surprising to recognize their discovery that concavity, too, could give the appearance of volume in what is sometimes called "false relief."

Figure 5.15. Two bison at El Castillo appear similar, but the artist used concavity, or false relief, to suggest three-dimensional form in the larger one. For the other bison, convexity served the same end.

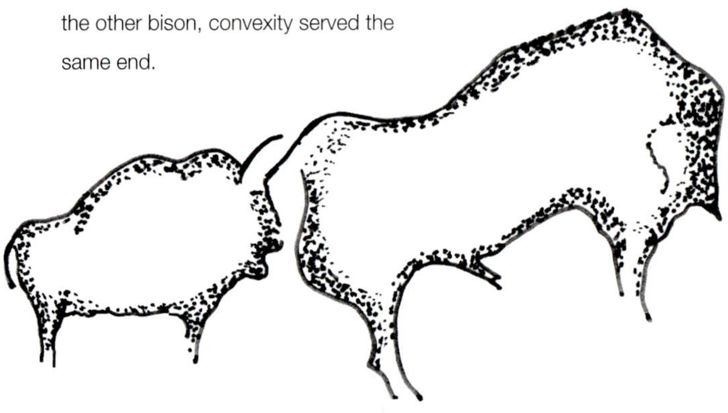

False Relief

Again at El Castillo, two black-painted bison, one behind the other, offer a clear example of false relief (fig. 5.15). These animals are situated in an alcove behind the ledge on which the artist probably stood to paint. The animal portrayed in front is larger and is judged to have been painted earlier than the one behind it. This more imposing bison was painted on a concave surface, and the rear animal, on a convex one. Use of a concave surface next to a convex one to achieve the same visual effect clearly demonstrates that the artist understood this ambiguity; indeed, the painter might have reveled in it. The Spanish scholar Reynaldo Gonzáles García believes that the decision to use convex or concave surfaces was made on the basis of the type of animal to be depicted,[15] but in this case the two animals are both bison. The limitations of available surface were not a factor here, either; there was sufficient space to place the first figure slightly to the right or left and avoid any surface irregularity. The decision to work with the concave surface was deliberate. When one steps back a certain distance and views the figures from directly in front, both bison give the appearance of being equally rounded and three-dimensional.

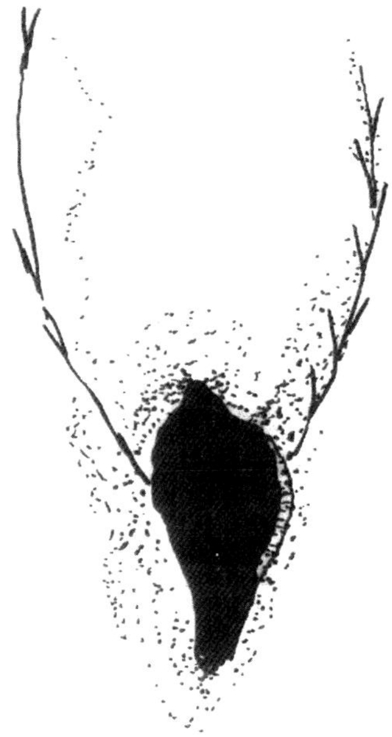

Figure 5.16. A hole in the wall at Niaux has been made to look like the head of a deer by the addition of antlers.

Another example of this visual trick occurs at Lascaux, where the "red cow with a black collar" in the Axial Gallery has a belly that appears convex from the normal viewing position but is actually concave. This illusion was used over and over again in the caves. At Font de Gaume, for example, where a dozen bison were depicted in similar false relief, the artists seem consistently to have preferred placing convex-appearing bison paintings on concave surfaces.

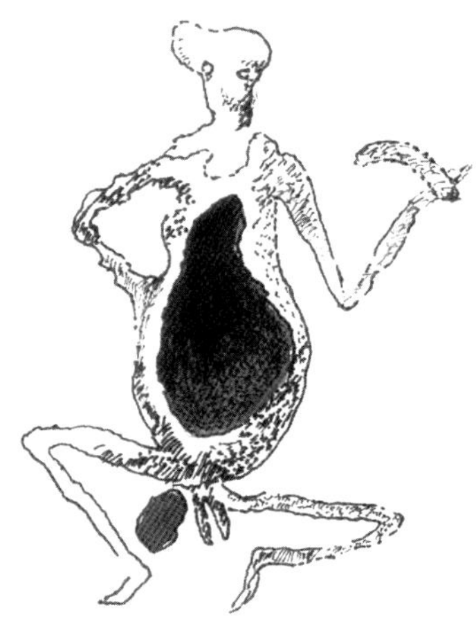

Figure 5.17. A hole in a rock face has been used as a female belly, South Africa.

I use the term *false relief* for images that give the illusion that a surface is convex when in fact it is concave. In the examples from El Castillo and Font de Gaume, artists made use of preexisting surface irregularities for this purpose. When, by removing some ground, an artist creates a convex carving whose high points are on what is left of the surface on which it is carved, we refer to it as *bas-relief*. In the more unusual instance, when the artist carves into the ground to make a figure that will be concave, or lower than the original surface, the result is technically called *champlevé* (raised ground). Ice Age sculptors sometimes mixed the two techniques in one carving.

An extreme version of the use of concavity can be seen at Niaux. Crowned with drawn antlers, the dark head of a deer faces toward the viewer, until one becomes aware that the head is actually the deep shadow of a hole in the cave wall. It has been changed into a deer's head by the simple act of placing antlers above it (fig. 5.16). Such play with concavity seems to have had universal appeal. In the prehistoric rock art of South Africa, for example, an unusual figure displays the same strategy as the deer head at Niaux. Here, an artist used the shadow made by a hole in the rock face to give the illusion of a rounded female belly (fig. 5.17).

Convex-concave ambiguity is also found in the tribal art of North America. A natural, circular depression in the rock at Tenabo, New Mexico, was made into a face by adding two eyes. A striking effect is that the face peers out of the rock and looks directly at the viewer. At Fisher's Landing, near Vancouver, Washington, an artist carved a deep concavity to represent a beaver in the Northwest Coast curvilinear style. A full-size human figure was carved as a concave reverse image, almost like one-half of a cast of a body, at Robertson Point, near Prince Rupert, British Columbia. Local legend refers to this carving as "the man who fell from heaven." It refers to the local raven god, Wegets, who is said to have fallen from heaven when in human form and to have left a concave impression. Mimbres pot painters used this type of illusion in virtuoso fashion. The artist Tony Berlant, describing their pots, wrote that "so adroitly do the images fit into the concave spaces that when approached frontally, the bowls sometimes create the illusion of being flat or even convex."[16]

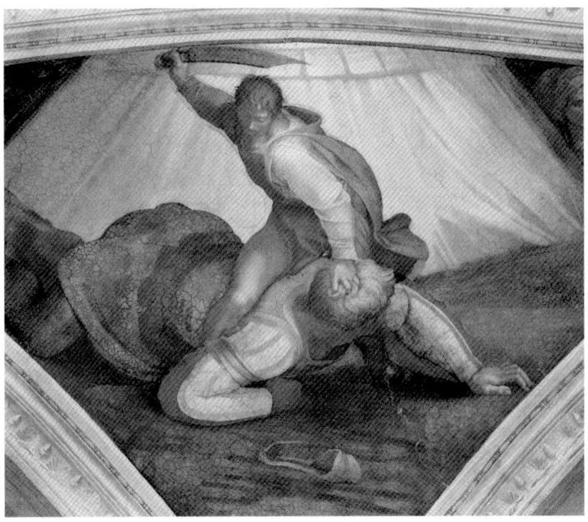

Figure 5.18. Michelangelo, *David and Goliath,* Sistine Chapel. The surface of the architectural vault is concave, but the head of Goliath appears to be convex and to protrude outward. Photo: E. Lessing / Art Resource, N.Y.

Perspective and Crater Ambiguity

Renaissance authors of the theory of perspective believed they had devised the means to make concavity appear convex. Leonardo da Vinci wrote in his notebook: "The art of perspective is of such nature as to make what is flat appear in relief and what is in relief flat."[17] In the huge vaulted ceiling of the Sistine Chapel, where the barrel-shaped vault meets the wall, twelve crests are formed that have even more accentuated curves. The most deeply concave surfaces of all are the four corner cloister vaults. In these most incurved of surfaces Michelangelo painted such Old Testament figures as David and Goliath (fig. 5.18). Goliath's about-to-be-decapitated head seems to project dramatically from the very point where the surface is farthest removed from the viewer.

But the artists of the Renaissance were not the first to achieve this feat of perspective. As we have seen, Ice Age artists knew how to do it even without the advantage of the mathematics of perspective. In caves, the artists often attempted to defy the actual irregularity of the surface and, as a serendipitous bonus, discovered they could make use of concavity to give the illusion of protruding, three-dimensional form.

Maurits Escher, in 1955, made a lithograph entitled *Concave and Convex*. In the dizzying space he created, a central ellipse on a dark, terracelike surface switches back and forth to the viewer's eye. At one moment it reads like a shell-shaped pool on a terrace and at the next like a sand dollar or sea urchin skeleton (fig. 5.19). At the same time, the staircases, which have been behaving more or less normally, flip into an inverted position, so that anyone on the staircase would fall off.

Escher was influenced by the writings of the Finnish psychologist Kai von Fieandt. In 1938 von Fieandt published some experimental patterns to demonstrate the change in depth perception from concave to convex and back again, depending on the direction of the illumination. He called this phenomenon the "Crater Illusion." Victor Vasarely and the Op artists later explored the ambiguity of the crater effect. In the 1960s, the California artist Robert Irwin made a series of sculptures that depended for their effect on the vagaries of perception. One mystical sphere floating in a shadowy space turned out to be a flat aluminum disc washed with light and shadow in such a way that the disc became a virtual globe. Artists relish ambiguity. In the preceding examples, as in the Ice Age, it is used as a source of wit. When the surface can be read first as concave and then as convex, the jester artist plays with our perception and creates the pleasurable little shock that comes from confounding mutually exclusive images.

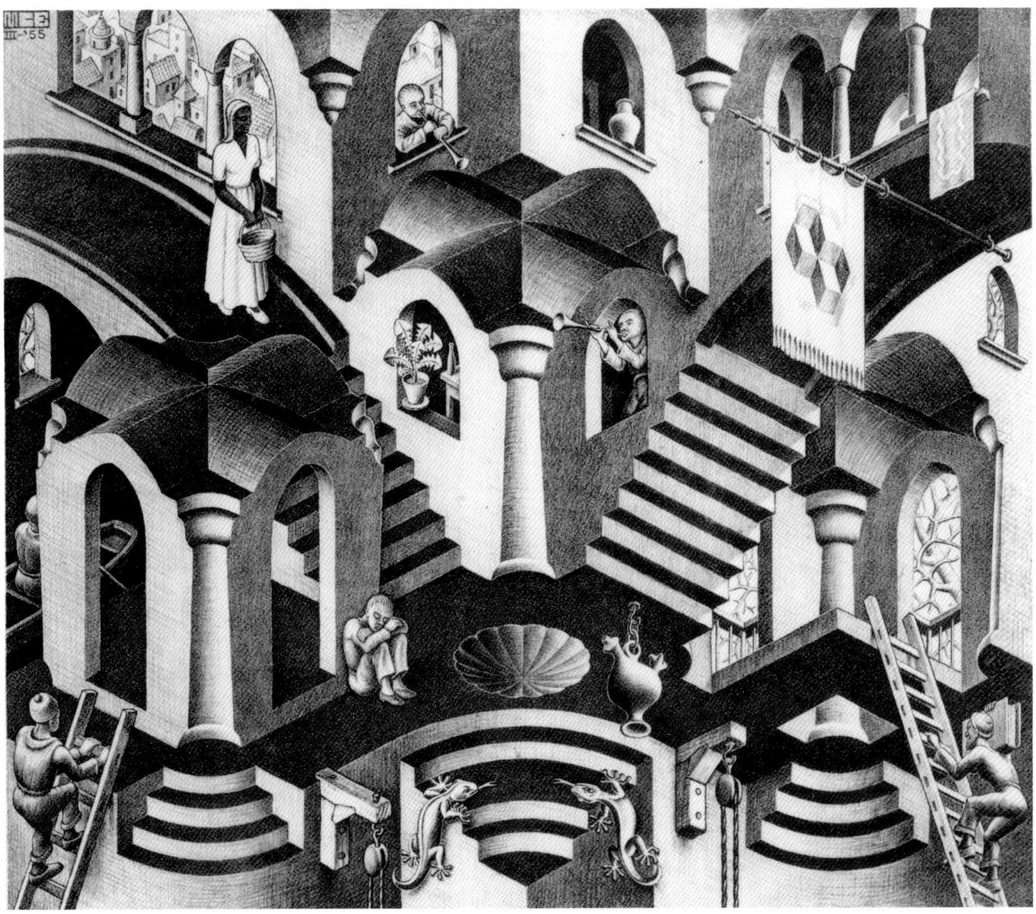

Figure 5.19. Maurits Escher, *Concave and Convex,* 1955. Lithograph, 275 by 335 cm. The shell formation in the center appears to flip back and forth from convex to concave, and the stairs flip as well. Photo credit: Art Resources, N.Y.

The shading produced by light is one of the clues our brains use for depth perception. Scientists Richard L. Gregory and V. S. Ramachandran performed experiments based on this illusion. Gregory made casts of faces and mounted some of them inside out so that they were actually concave replicas of the faces. In certain light they appeared to be as convex as the normally displayed casts. We humans have a powerful impetus to perceive such an illusion because we are preconditioned to read heads as normal and therefore as convex.[18]

The psychologists Terrence Sejnowski and Sidney Lehky devised a computer simulation modeled on the actual structure of the interconnected layers of neurons in the brain. They manipulated this simulation, called a "neural net," so that it would register depth as indicated by means of shading. Results from the computer model reinforced the conclusion that shading is a vital factor in enabling us to determine whether something is concave or convex.[19] If the form is ambiguous, then the interpretation depends on our understanding of the light source. Because the sun is our most common light source, we automatically assume that light comes from overhead. Light directed downward lightens the lower side of a concavity and the upper side of a convexity. Most people also automatically assume that light is coming from the left side. This is because the majority of people are right-handed, so artists usually place their illumination on the left side in order to avoid working in the shadow of the right hand. These unconscious assumptions about the source of light enable us to organize reality quickly. Artists use these assumptions but may take a different tack. They create convex and concave forms, and at times they deliberately startle us by causing us to confound the two.

SPATIAL AMBIGUITY

They weren't bound by the silly feeling that it is impossible for two figures to occupy the same space at the same time. . . . It happens all the time. One creature interlocks with another in a completely illogical way.

—Bill Reid, *Form and Freedom*

A stone plaquette from La Marche, dated to about 14,000 years ago, is engraved with a human profile, probably that of a woman (fig. 5.20). Human faces are uncommon in European Ice Age art, but they do exist, and many were found on a series of plaquettes at this particular site. Superimposed over the profile, and recognizable from a tangle of other lines, is the engraved torso of a nude woman. Superimposition is a commonplace, almost a hallmark, of Ice Age art and is frequently seen in rock art all over the world. Looking at this example, one is startled to see that the eye of the profile coincides precisely with the woman's nipple. It is difficult to believe that this was an accident. The juxtaposition must have been a deliberate choice by the artist who added the second figure and who may have planned for the eye and nipple to coincide from the start.

We all know instinctively that two solid objects cannot occupy the same place at the same time, something scientists call *cohabitation.* According to research done by the psychologist Renée Baillargeon, even infants understand this.[20] But artists, because they are exploring a different dimension of reality, can and often do defy the rule. The result is a complex kind of double meaning.

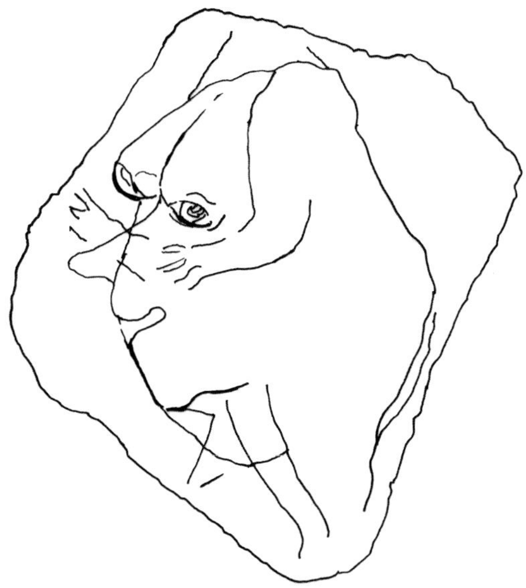

Figure 5.20. Human profile on a stone plaquette from La Marche. The face is also a body. After L. Pales

Body Sharing

In art from the European Ice Age, the sharing of body parts is frequent. Another Ice Age example of cohabitation is a complicated engraving on a piece of slate from Trois Frères (fig. 5.21). By rotating the slate, one can sort out and isolate five female figures from the entangled, superimposed lines. All of them share the same body, and each utilizes one or more of a selection of possible arms and legs. A similar graphic

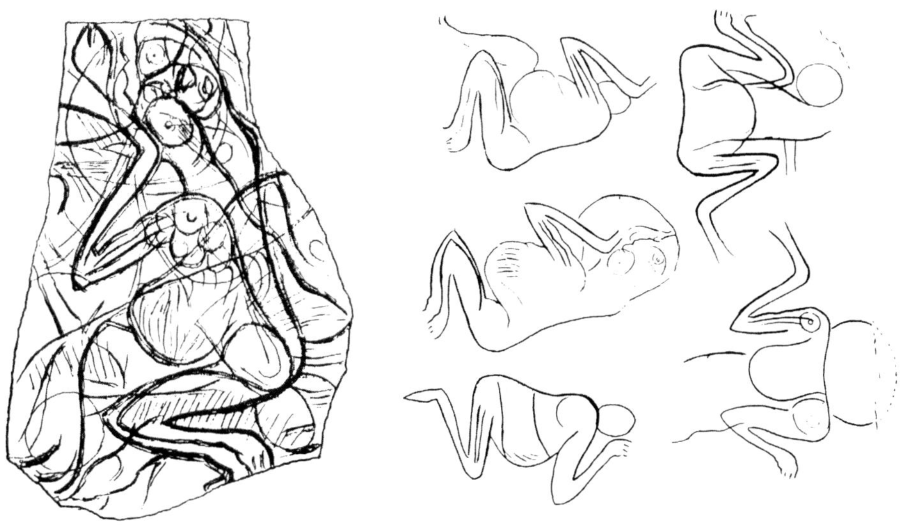

Figure 5.21. Left: Slate plaquette from Trois Frères showing five female figures superimposed. Right: The figures teased apart, with shared body parts separated. Drawing H. Brevil

puzzle device was used on a plaque from Gönnersdorf. In that case, seven figures were superimposed. An example from Les Combarelles has two horses sharing the same mane (fig. 5.22).

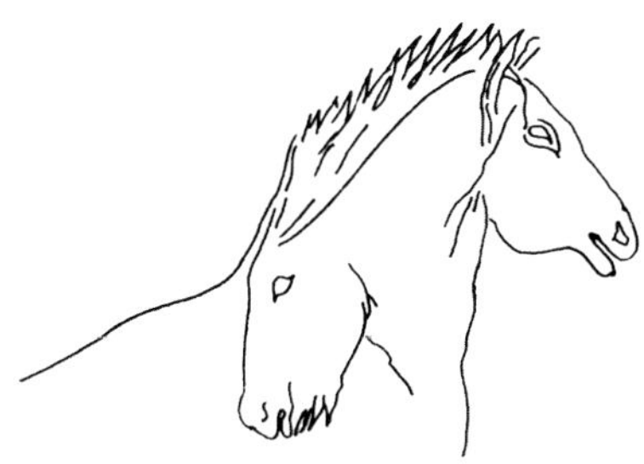

(left) Fig 5.22. Two horses sharing one mane, Les Combarelles.

Sometimes an entire body is shared. Again at Les Combarelles, a donkey and a cow cohabit one body. At Font de Gaume there is an amalgam of bison and reindeer. The bison head faces left and the reindeer head right, but they share one body. At the cave of La Pasiega we can make out a reindeer facing right sharing the body of a horse facing left. At Pair-non-Pair (Gironde), an ibex facing right shares a body with a deer facing left (fig. 5.23). In concept this is identical to the work of a sculptor at the amazing temple complex at Ellora,

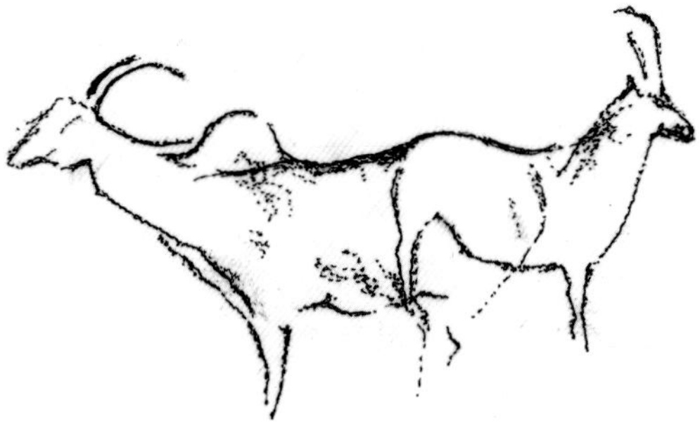

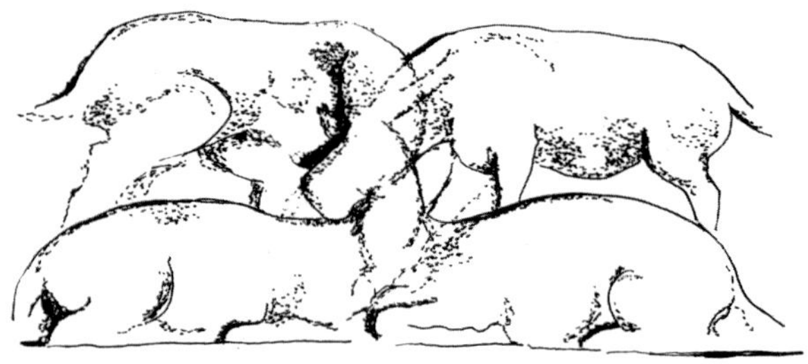

Left:Fig 5.23. An ibex sharing a body with a deer, Pair-non-Pair. (after photo M. Pillot)

Right: Figure 5.24. Four carved horses share one head on the lintel of a temple at Ellora, India.

India. From the fifth to the tenth century, 34 temples and monasteries for Hindu, Buddhist, and Jain worship were carved from the living stone of the Charanandra hills. On one unique lintel an inventive artist carved four horses that share a single head (fig. 5.24).

A surprising example of shared body parts is seen in an Australian Aboriginal rock art painting in Laura, west of Cairns, where a human male and a turtle are superimposed in such a way that the turtle shares its neck with the man's penis (fig. 5.25). An example of cohabitation like the Ice Age examples was made in the twentieth century by Salvador Dalí in a series of drawings and later in a series of paintings, all of which confound a horse and a lion. In one example, an image can be read as a lion facing left and as a horse facing right (fig. 5.26). This version is further complicated by cohabitation in the same figure of a sleeping nude woman.

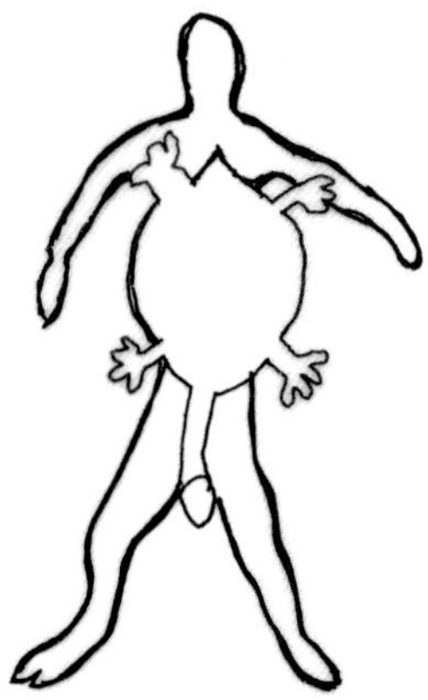

Figure 5.25. A turtle and a man share neck and penis, respectively, in an Aboriginal rock painting at Laura, Australia.

"Exquisite Corpse"

The Dalí drawings are similar to the results of a game called "exquisite corpse" that was popular among certain members of the Surrealist movement in the early twentieth century. In this game, each artist would draw a head of some sort and then fold the paper so that the head was invisible, but leaving tag lines that could be seen. Then the papers were passed around. The other artists would each begin at the lines they could see and extend them to create the next body part, in turn folding the paper until the new contribution was hidden except for tag lines with which the next artist would begin. The game continued until the feet had been drawn. When the papers were unfolded, the results not only were strange and amusing but were also held to stimulate creativity.

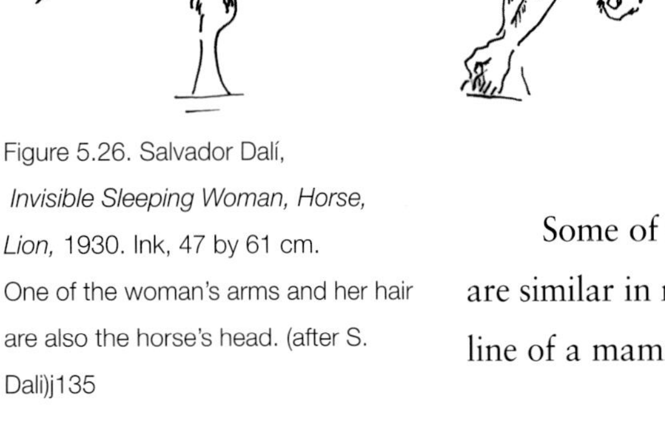

Figure 5.26. Salvador Dalí, *Invisible Sleeping Woman, Horse, Lion,* 1930. Ink, 47 by 61 cm. One of the woman's arms and her hair are also the horse's head. (after S. Dali)j135

Some of the figures created during the Ice Age consist of extended lines that are similar in result to the figures from this Surrealist game. At Gargas, the dorsal line of a mammoth continues to become the top of the head of a quadruped (fig.

5.27). In another example from that site, the jaw of a bear becomes the forehead of a mammoth. At El Castillo, in a painting of two bison, one following the other, the tail of the first is also the horn of the second. In a similar feat of economy at Font de Gaume, the tail of one bison is lengthened to become the tail of another (fig. 5.28). In another example there, the back of what looks like a reindeer becomes the jaw of a horse. At Hornos de la Peña, the line that describes the back of a bull is also the belly of a mare. At Lascaux, the horns of an ibex are extended and used to form the back of another, smaller ibex (fig. 5.29).

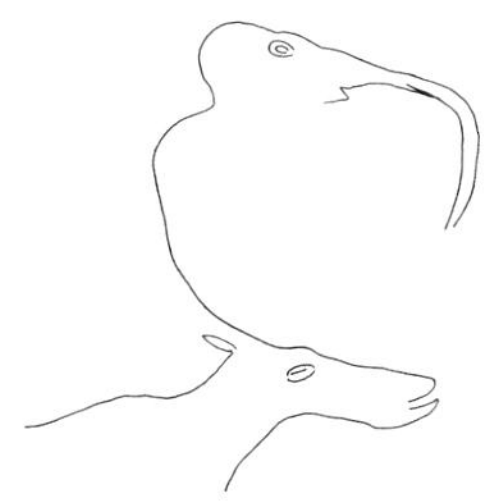

Figure 5.27. An extended line merges a mammoth with a horse at Gargas.

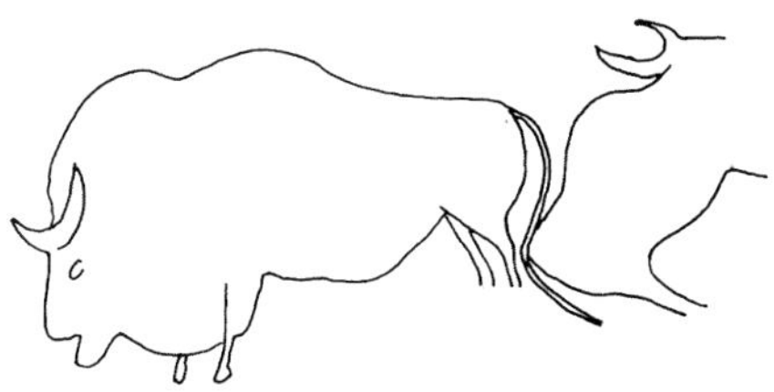

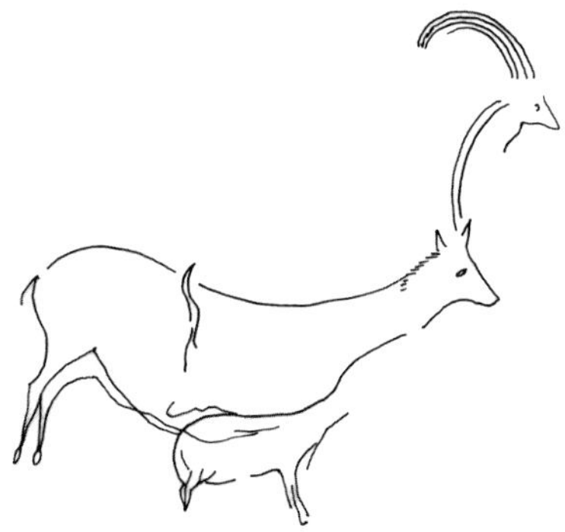

Left: Figure 5.28. At Font de Gaume, the tail of the larger bison on the left is shared by the smaller bison on the right.

Roght: Figure 5.29. The horns of an ibex at Lascaux continue to form the back of a smaller ibex.

The Duck-Rabbit Figure

Approximately 14,000 years after the Ice Age examples were made, a Mimbres pot painter in the American Southwest raised the punning concept of cohabitation to new heights. On a black-and-white figurative bowl is a design consisting of two stylized white rabbits on a black ground (fig. 5.30). The second rabbit is rotated 180 degree from the first, and the two are connected by a white band. At length we notice that the two rabbit heads can be reversed to become ducks. Each rabbit's ears become the beak of a duck, its nostril becomes a little topknot on the duck, and its front legs become the duck's wings. The information in the picture does not change, but the way we interpret it does. Further evidence that the artist intended the viewer to see both figures is that the eyes are in a position unusual for either rabbits or ducks in Mimbres painting; they are placed so that they can serve as eyes for either of the two animals. John Clegg found almost the same kind of figure reversal ambiguity in an Australian aboriginal engraving.

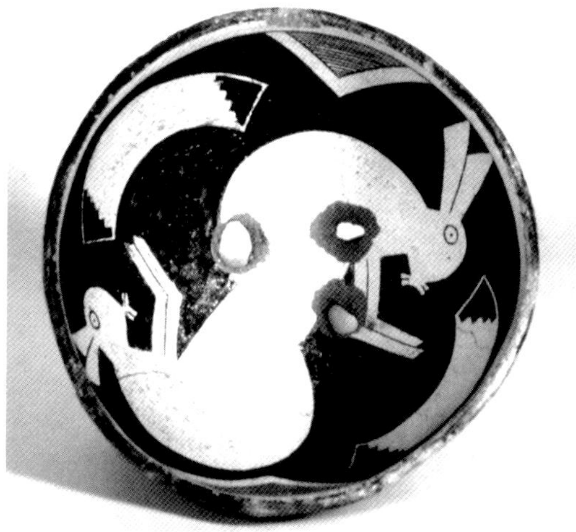

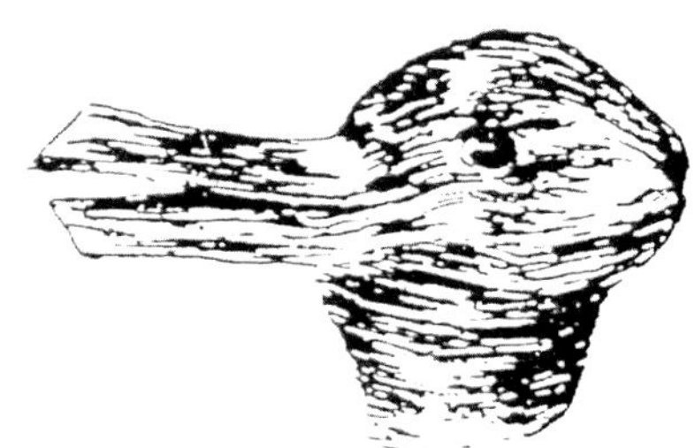

Figure 5.30. Mimbres pot on which two rabbits can be reversed to become ducks. © Maxwell Museum of Anthropology.

Figure 5.31. Duck-rabbit from a German joke book.

In some strangely coincidental thought process, a nineteenth-century German joke book made use of almost the same duck-rabbit reversal (fig. 5.31).[21] The artist who drew it did not know of the Mimbres duck-rabbit pot, which had not yet been unearthed. Perhaps influenced by this joke book, an artist at

Harpers Weekly made a very similar duck-rabbit cartoon.[22] The psychologist Joseph Jastrow, in a 1928 publication, used precisely the same duck-rabbit reversal as an example of perceptual ambiguity.[23] This ambiguous figure was not dismissed as an amusing or insignificant illustration. It was given serious consideration in intellectual circles and was singled out by the philosopher Ludwig Wittgenstein and later by the art historian Ernst Gombrich. Both of them found it of sufficient interest that they wrote about the phenomenon.

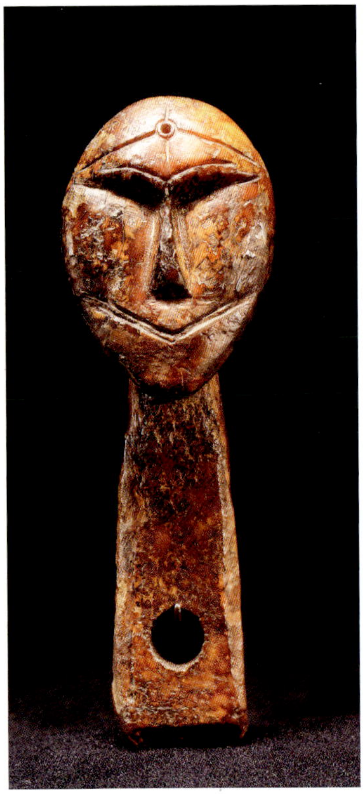

Figure 5.32. A carving on a walrus tusk from St. Lawrence Island, Alaska, can be read as both a human face and a whale's tail. The hole at the bottom may have served as an attachment to a staff or tool. 11.5 cm.

Alaskan and Northwest Coast Ambiguous Figures

Masters of the visual pun, both in antiquity and into the present, are the various Eskimo peoples. In a 2,000-year-old Okvik-style piece from the Gambell site on Saint Lawrence Island, Alaska, the eyes and nose of a human face carved on a handle or staff head can also be seen as the tail of a whale as it breaches the ocean surface (fig. 5.32). A Dorset Eskimo figure made about 700 years ago also makes use of ambiguity in such a way that it appears as a dog in some positions and as a man in others.[24]

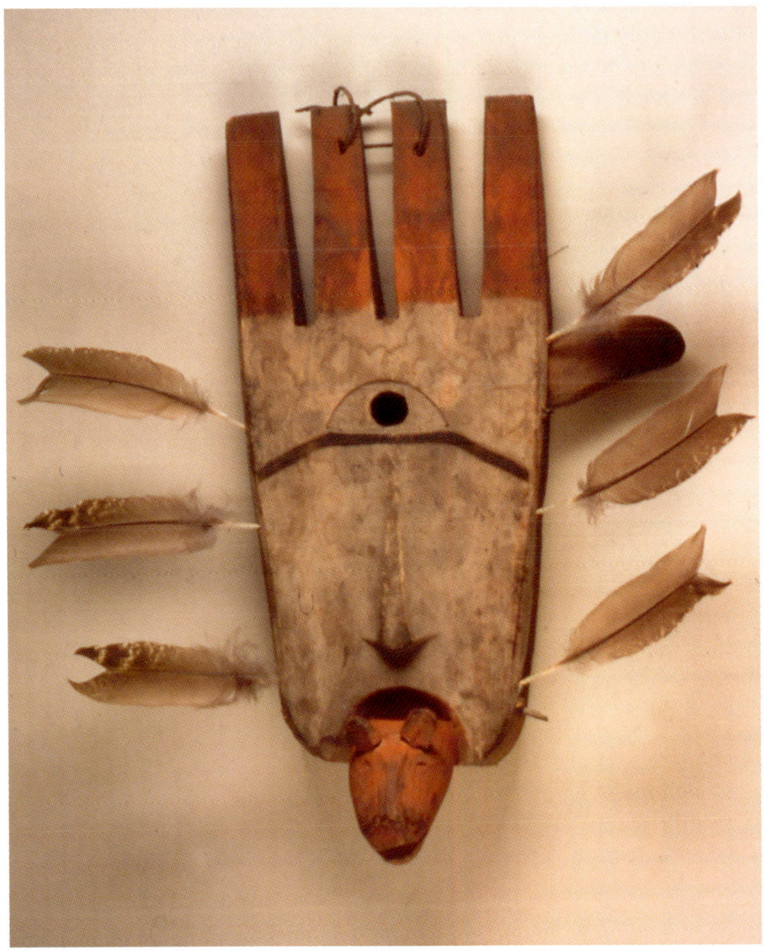

Figure 5.33. Yup'ik Kuskokwim mask portraying a mink or a muskrat, nineteenth century. The animal's tail is also the fingers of a hand, and one of the hind legs is also the thumb of the hand. The entire mask is also a face with a Cyclopean eye.

There are at least two figures in most Eskimo masks, because Eskimos traditionally believe that everything possesses an *inuit,* or soul, and this soul is interlocked with the figure in the mask. On a remarkable late-nineteenth-century Yup'ik mask, a mink or muskrat is shown swimming through the water. The animal's tail also forms the fingers of a hand, made complete by the addition of a thumb. The thumb serves also as one of the animal's hind legs (fig. 5.33). The ambiguity does not end there. The whole mask is also a Cyclopean face with one central eye. Its nose is simultaneously the animal's backbone, and its mouth is also the hole from which protrudes the animal's head—which doubles as the face's extended tongue. Multiple meanings and puns like these were ubiquitous in Eskimo culture and continue with unabated zest in their most recent art.

The native people of the Northwest Coast also reveled in spatial ambiguity leading to the cohabitation of figures. Often the body parts of one figure proliferate into smaller figures in an almost fractal fantasy. Tsimshian shamans used small bone charms and amulets to represent the animals that gave them power. In one example, a humanlike figure forms a bird's backbone. The human's head doubles as the bird's tail, and its moonlike face represents the wing joint. The Tlingit people made many examples of heads within heads. Spatial cohabitation is also commonly seen on the spindle whorls made by the Salish people. On one whorl, a female is flanked by two birds. The birds' wings contain human faces, and their feet also serve as the arms of a crouching figure.

Figure 5.34. Tlingit dagger hilt, walrus ivory or sperm-whale tooth decorated with abalone shell. Height 9.2 cm. The piece shows the cohabitation of animal and human figures.

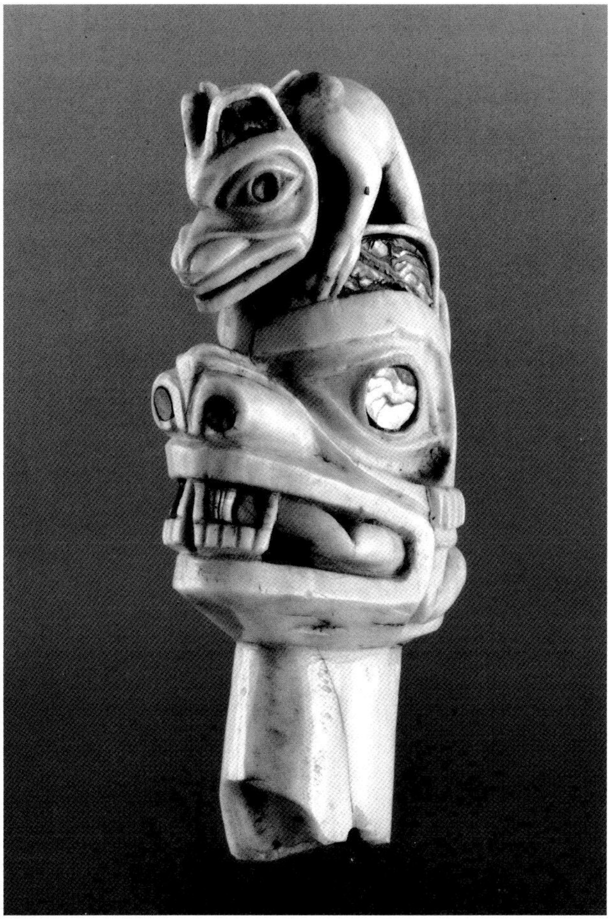

One of the most striking examples of the use of cohabitation in Northwest Coast art is a dagger hilt made of walrus ivory or sperm whale tooth (fig. 5.34). The carving is of an animal's head. Between its ears is a smaller, bearlike animal. A human figure extends through the animal's head, with its knees and legs sticking out of the animal's mouth. Its feet, made of abalone, double as the animal's teeth.

Bill Reid, the renowned Northwest Coast Indian sculptor, was quoted at the beginning of this section describing how native carvers from his region felt free to use interpenetrating forms. Bill Holm, another Northwest Coast artist working in the traditional art of his ancestors, is skilled as a carver, a dancer, and a singer. He has also analyzed the art of this region and attempted to explain aspects of both its narrative and its graphic art. In one revealing passage he discussed the much-favored use of multiple meaning in Northwest Coast Indian art:

> The Bella Coola seemed especially to enjoy this byplay. The joints of the two shoulders become the eyes of a face which fills the body area provided with ears, mouth and nose. . . . The famous "Rain Wall at Klukwan" is literally covered with over fifty such extraneous faces, many of them fitted out with little bodies, arms and legs. The tails of whales are often elaborated into faces because of the similarity of the fluke design to ears.[25]

Nested Figures

Sometimes the trick consists of constructing a whole figure out of smaller ones. Figures lie within figures like a series of Russian *matryoshka* dolls. In the celebrated panel from Pech-Merle, the spotted horses are extremely stylized, with small black "duckbill" heads (see fig. 1.1). The shape of the stone projection on which the right-hand horse is painted actually forms a natural horse's head better proportioned to the painted body. The result is a smaller horse's head within a larger one. Horse's heads that were small in proportion to the body may have been a stylistic convention seen again in the Chinese horses at Lascaux (see fig. 6.39). In the same cave, on a rock shaped like a mammoth, an artist painted a smaller mammoth. A spear thrower excavated from El Pendo in Ice Age Spain is decorated with the engraved heads of deer. A closer look reveals that the entire antler was shaped to appear like the head of a deer, so that the engraved deer heads lie within the head of the larger deer—another example of nested cohabitation.

An example at the cave of Cougnac strongly suggests the same intent. There, the dorsal line was the essential abbreviated statement understood to mean mammoth. That line, along with a second, smaller, but almost identical line below it, could have meant that a second mammoth stood in front of the first. But the ventral line of this mammoth repeats the shape of the mammoth once again. The artist seems to have played with the similarity of these outlines and made, in effect, three nested mammoths.

In a variation of nested forms, larger figures are composed of smaller, complete figures. The great master of this tour de force was the sixteenth-century artist Giuseppe Arcimboldo, a man much influenced by the work of Leonardo da Vinci. Arcimboldo devised his own fantastic style in which carefully rendered still-life objects or animals served as elements of portraits. Fortunately, his art was admired by the German Emperor Rudolf II, who became his patron and encouraged him to pursue his highly individual style. He composed faces out of fruit, vegetables, books, fish, other animals, and even people in a way that is not always immediately apparent. Sometimes the effect is metaphorical; often it is satirical. In Arcimboldo's *The Vegetable Gardener,* a face is made with vegetables (fig. 5.35). The face of the gardener is partially hidden, seen only when the bowl of vegetables is inverted. In the painting *Eve and the Apple* (fig. 5.36), Eve's face is composed entirely of intertwined nude figures.

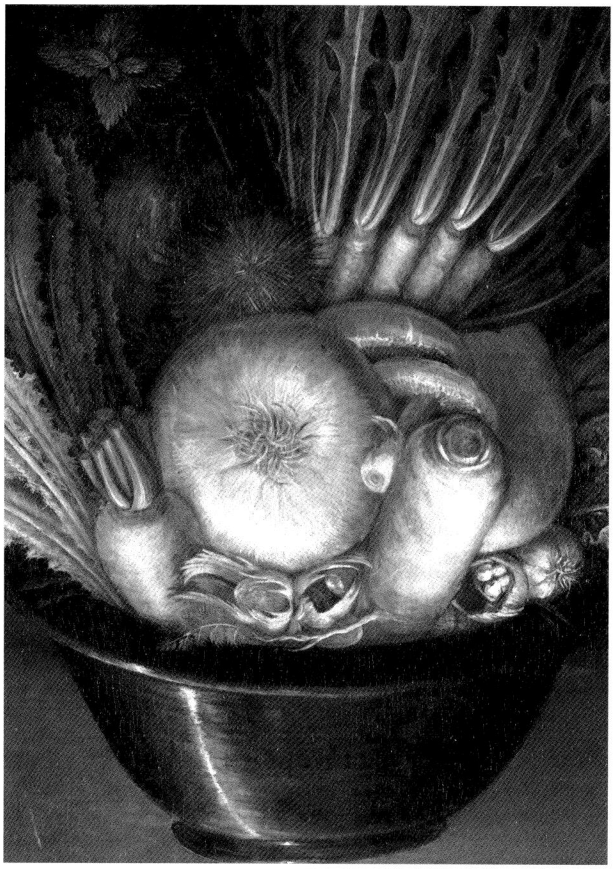

Figure 5.35. Giuseppe Arcimboldo, *The Vegetable Gardener,* 1590. Oil on panel, 35 by 24 cm. This painting is a double *tour de force* because the bowl of vegetables can also be inverted to show a face composed of vegetables. Collection of the Museo Civico, Cremona, Italy. Photograph by Erich Lessing. Art Resource, New York. Photo: E. Lessing/Art Resource, N.Y.

It is tantalizing to discover that at Orcha, in Madya Pradesh, central India, in the late sixteenth or early seventeenth century, an elephant painted on the walls of the palace of Raja Mahal was similarly composed of closely entwined women. We see the same concept used by an Indian painter in the eighteenth or nineteenth century in a painting on mica that shows Kama, the god of love, riding an elephant composed of women (fig. 5.37). In the late nineteenth century, in Edo-period Japan, the painter and printmaker Utagawa Kuniyoshi made woodcuts in the style of *yoko zu,* which means "portraits on several levels." His composite *Head of a Man,* made of entwined human figures (fig. 5.38), is surprisingly similar in concept to the earlier German and Indian examples.

Cohabitation has been used in works other than high official "art." Sometimes it is relished for its wit. It occurs in all periods and all over the world. Among the Etruscan sculptures in the Vatican collection is an unusual bronze dog whose body appears to be an erect penis. Hind legs and tail are attached to the body, as well as his own smaller genitals, the penis of the penis. The ribald and lubricious aspect of this sculpture is evident.

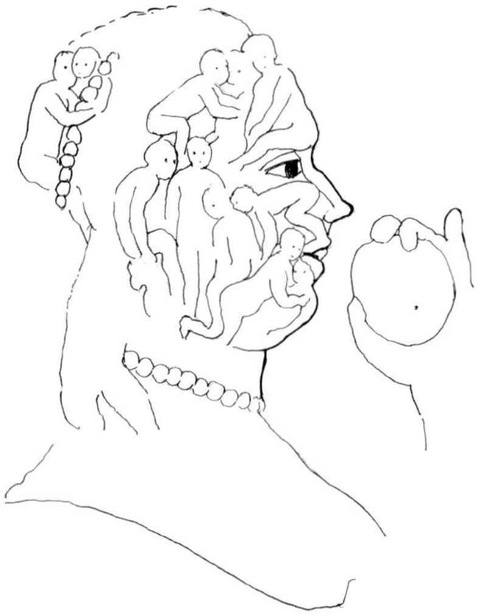

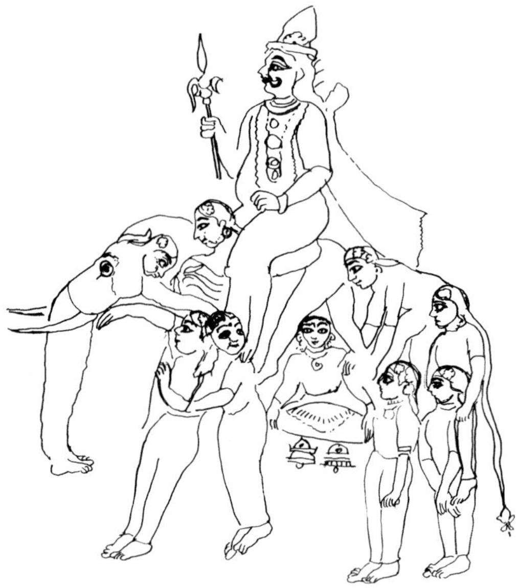

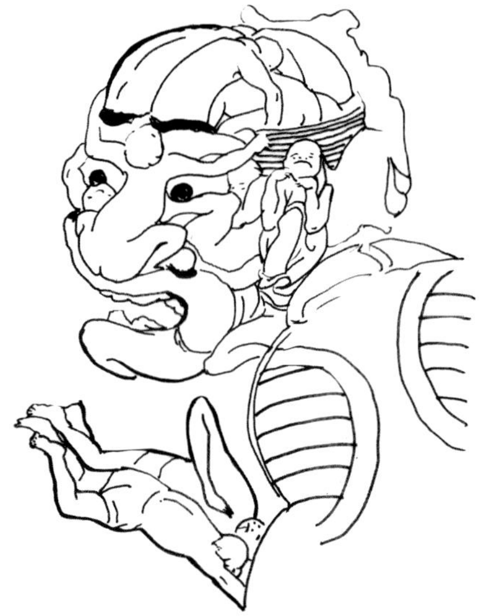

Left: Figure 5.36 Section of *Eve and the Apple,* by Giuseppe Arcimboldo, 1578.

Center: Figure 5.37. Indian painting on mica showing Kama, god of love, riding an elephant composed of female figures.

Right: Figure 5.38. *Head of a Man,* by Utagawa Kuniyoshi, Edo period, Japan.

In the nineteenth-century United States, the narrative aspect of such spatial confusion was frequently seen in cartoons. L. C. Gregg's cartoon *For President* (fig. 5.39) depicts the face of Teddy Roosevelt composed of war materiel. His nose and teeth are bullets, his eyes are cannons, and his chin is made of crossed swords. Sometimes spatial ambiguity seems to have been created purely to display graphic inventiveness. There are many modern examples. In Pavel Tcheletchew's famous landscape *Hide and Seek,* the central tree and the landscape itself are composed of people. A drawing for that painting shows a hand that is also a tree (fig. 5.40). In *Tatiana,* by René Magritte, the woman's figure is composed of faces. Salvador Dalí played with this particular visual pun, as he did with so many others, especially in the paintings *Invisible Man* (1929), *Portrait of Paul Eluard* (1929), *Invisible Sleeping Woman* (1930), and *Landscape of Woman* (1936–38). More recently, the cover of the *New Yorker* for March 1996 displayed a lamb cohabiting the body of a lion (fig. 5.41).

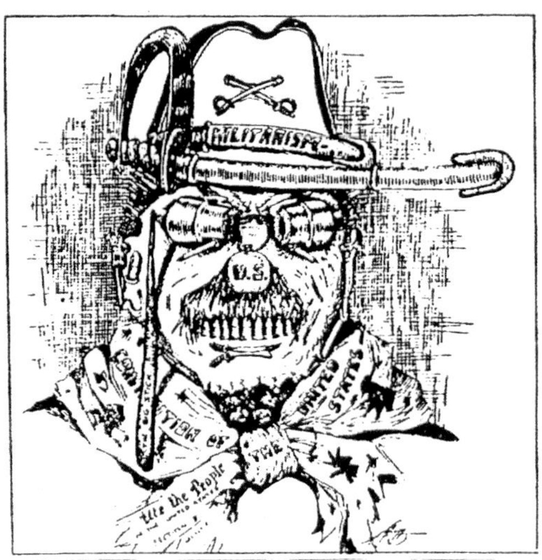

Figure 5.39. L. C. Gregg, *For President,* 1904.

In a category other than that of professional artists or professional cartoonists is the "outsider" art of the playwright Clif-

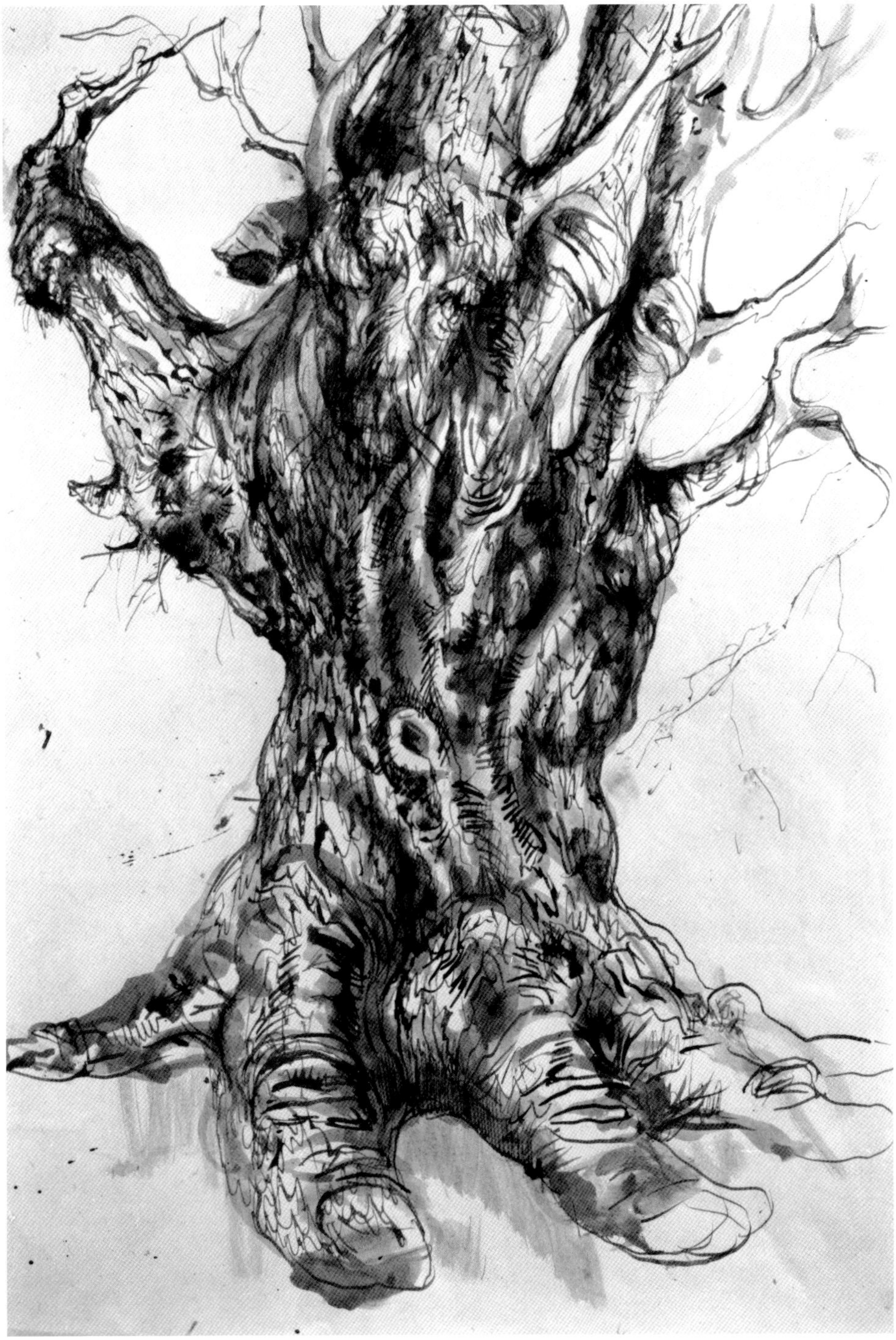

Figure 5.40. Pavel Tchelitchew, *Tree into Double Hand (Study for Hide and Seek),* 1938–39. Brush and pen and ink on paper, 35.5 by 24.7 cm. Photograh © 1998 the Museum of Modern Art, N.Y.

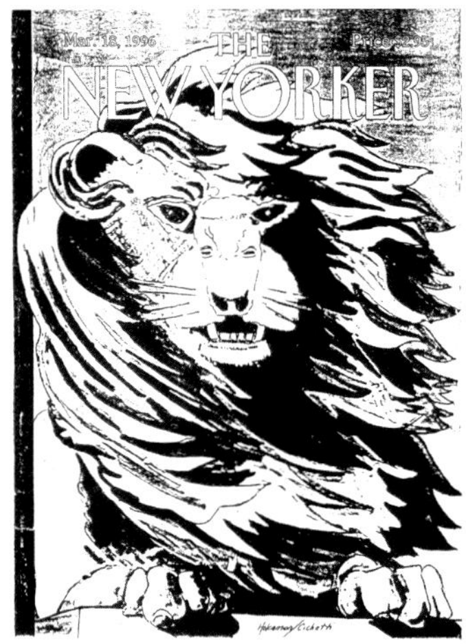

Figure 5.41. *New Yorker* cover, March 1996, by Hokanson/Cichetti, showing a lamb cohabiting within a lion. © New Yorker Magazine

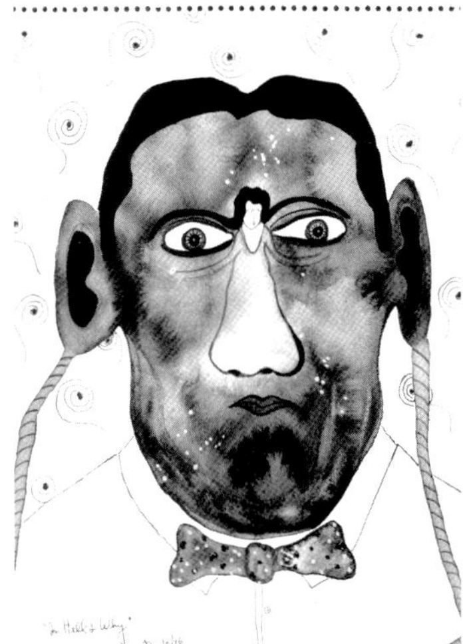

Figure 5.42. Clifford Odets, *To Hell + Why,* 1946. Watercolor, gouache, and ink on paper, 29.8 by 22.9 cm. The nose is also a hovering woman. There are spirals in the background and on the ears. © Clifford Odels Estate.43

ford Odets, who did a series of paintings beginning in the late 1940s. The work is highly emotional and personally revealing. In a self-portrait (fig. 5.42), a woman seems to pivot around the staring eyes, which may simultaneously be her insectlike wings. Double meaning is used here to reveal disturbing psychological depths.

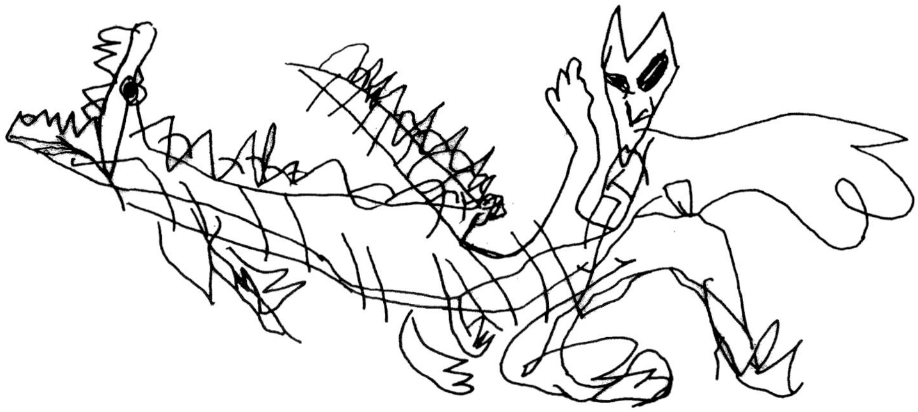

Figure 5.43. Nicholas's drawing.

Cohabitation also appears spontaneously in children's art. Nicholas, a six-year-old for whom drawing was a vital form of expression, drew so rapidly that the lines seemed to pour out unedited from his vivid imagination. In an elaborate example that conflated his interests in undersea creatures and in superheroes—including Superman and Batman—we see one section in which appears a monster with a fishtail (fig. 5.43). The tail is also a formidably toothed alligator head, and the alligator's own tail rises from the monster's back. Cohabitation appears to be a way of structuring images that are produced by the mind.

A painting by René Magritte establishes an astonishing parallel with the plaquette from La Marche, the example that began this section. It is called *The Rape* (fig. 5.44) and is one of a series of similar paintings by Magritte. Carl-August Ehrensvärd, a Swedish painter, used the identical device 135 years before Magritte in a drawing he called *Grotesque Portrait* (fig. 5.45). In a concept shared by artists separated by 15,000 years at the least, we see a visual pun based on the confounding of nipples and eyes. Pablo Picasso, following the same mental path, made a sketch of Marie Therese Walter in india ink on paper in which her eyes were at the same time her nipples. Neither Magritte, Picasso, nor Ehrensvärd knew of the Ice Age drawings. The plaquette from La Marche was not discovered until a generation after Magritte's 1934 painting or Picasso's 1936 sketch, and it was years later that the engravings were published by the archaeologist Léon Pales. These artists arrived independently at nearly identical images. Many examples suggest that humans, throughout history, have had similar perceptual abilities and limitations, causing them to arrive at similar pictorial creations.

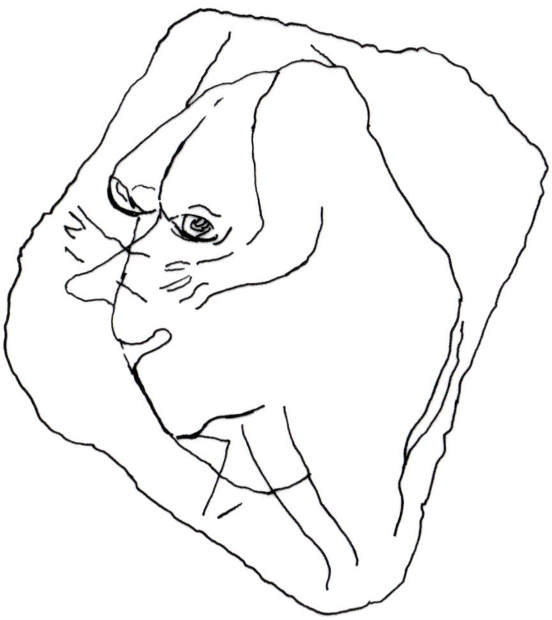

Figure 5.44 (same as 5.20). Human profile on a stone plaquette from La Marche. The face is also a body.

Below left: Figure 5.45. René Magritte, *The Rape,* 1934. The face is also a body.

Below right: Figure 5.46. Carl-August Ehrensvärd, *Grotesque Portrait,* 1882. The face is also a body. 32.0 by 20.5 cm.

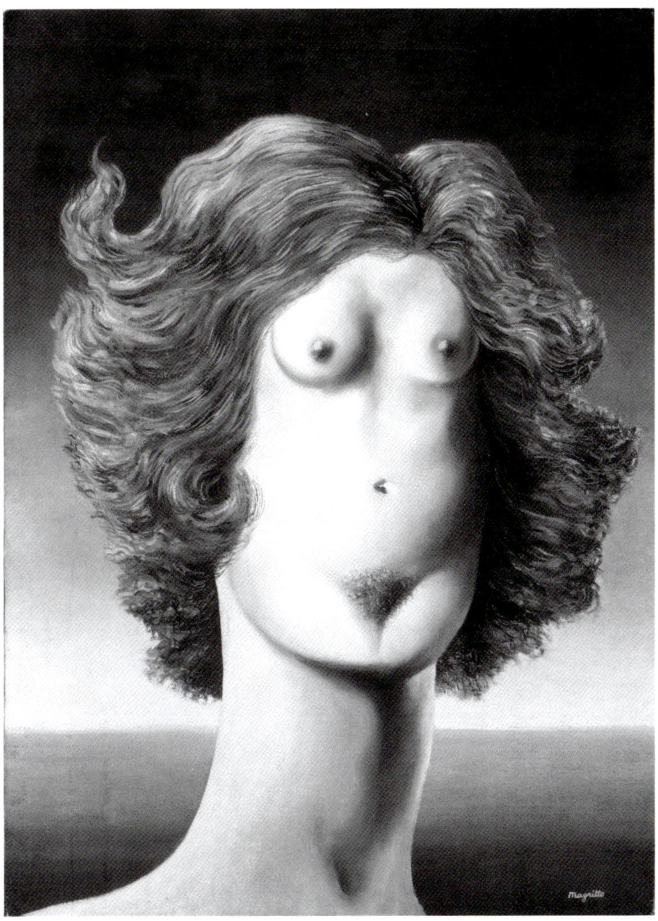

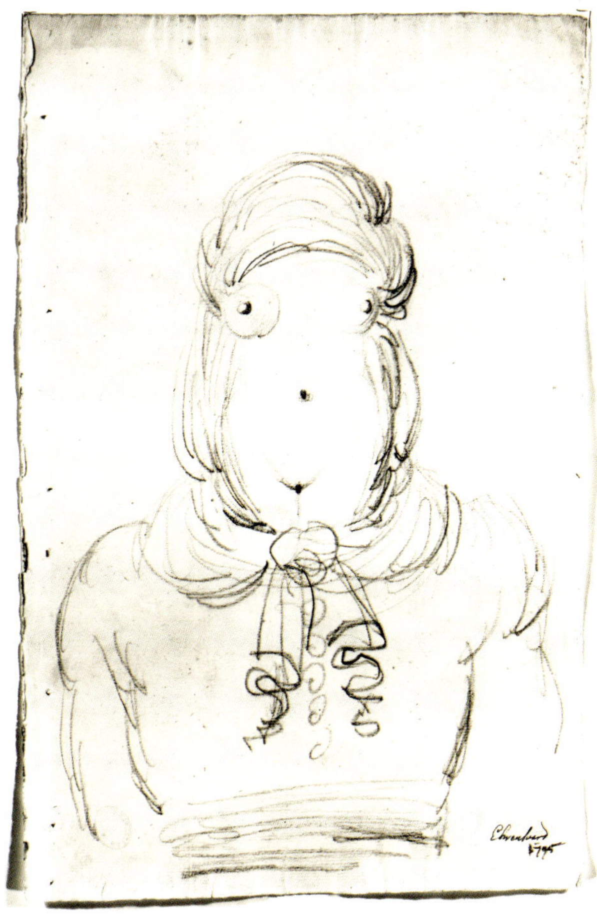

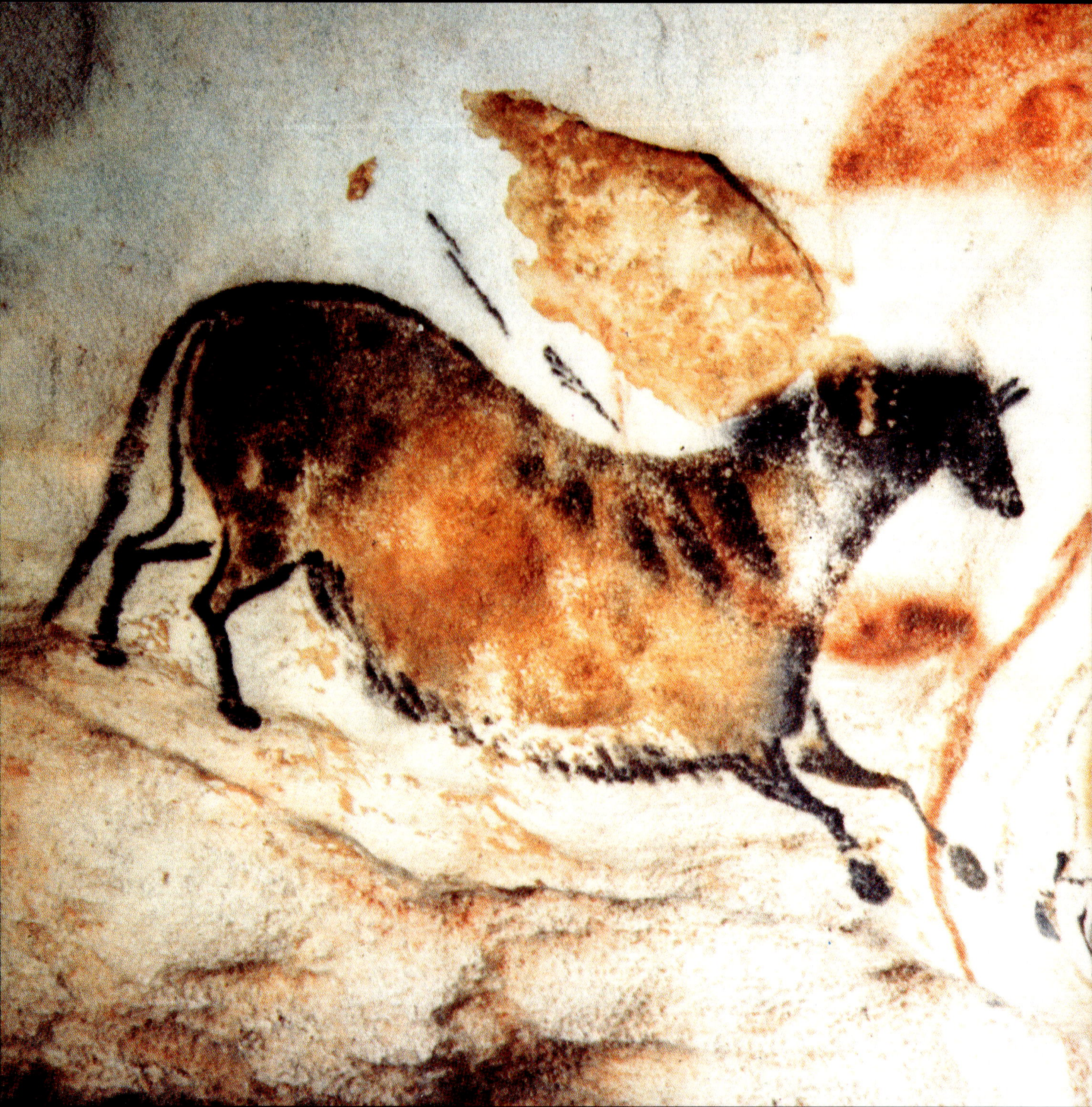

6

PARADOX

Reconciling the Irreconcilable

"A PARADOX, A PARADOX, a most ingenious paradox!" sings the chorus in Gilbert and Sullivan's *Pirates of Penzance.* The story's hero, Frederic, is a young man of 21, but as the plot unfolds we learn that because his birthdate was February 29, during a leap year, he has had only five birthdays. Depending on how his age is reckoned, he is simultaneously 21 and 5. In a paradox, two mutually contradictory statements may each be true, within its own context, but an attempt to reconcile the two will appear absurd.

We use our brains in order to understand the brain— a self referential paradox.
—RICHARD RESTAK, *Brainscapes*

One of the great paradoxes of modern science concerns the nature of light. Classical physics experiments showed that light traveled in packets of particles. Later, other experiments proved with equal authority that light moved in waves. The two descriptions were mutually exclusive, yet physicists now live with this paradox and view both models in a tenuous reconciliation within the overarching construct of quantum mechanics.

Riddles are a form of paradox. They play an important role in myths and stories throughout the world. The sphinx of Greek legend blocked a well-traveled road and, like a devastating toll booth, required all travelers to answer, on penalty of death, the most famous riddle of all time: "What walks on four legs in the morning, two at noon, and three at night?" Oedipus was the first traveler able to answer it: "Man, who crawls in infancy, walks upright in maturity, and uses a cane in old age." He resolved the conundrum, as is often the case, by shifting to a previously unexplored point of view. Paradox has creative potential because it forces us to cast off our accustomed ways of thinking in order to look for solutions in new and unusual approaches. In doing so, it sets free the imagination.

Opposite: One of three 'Chinese Horses' on the ceiling of the south wall of the Axial Gallery at Lascaux. The striped coat is typical of a Przewalski horse. The legs show a graphic device to indicate foreshortening. Photo by J. Vertut. CNP-MCC

We now know that our brains contain a built-in paradox. Each hemisphere processes information separately, and each sometimes arrives at its own model of reality. The two hemispheres communicate with each other along 800 million nerve fibers, and finally the incongruent messages are reconciled and experienced as a seamless unity.[1]

In this chapter I look at several examples of visual paradox that first appeared in European Ice Age art. The first is incongruity, which occurs when two or more seemingly incompatible qualities, such as an animal head and a human's body, are merged in one figure. Under the heading "Inversion and Reversion" I look at the visual paradox that occurs when a single image appears to be something different from each of two or more vantage points. The two-dimensional graphic description of space presents an unavoidable paradox, because three dimensions cannot truly be shown on a flat surface. The problem is exemplified by the dilemma of the cartographer: it is impossible to project our globe onto any flat surface map with accuracy. Each solution may solve one problem as it presents new ones. How this relates to art is seen in the third topic, "Space and Motion."

INCONGRUITY

If man had not encountered dragons and hippogriffs in dreams, he might not have conceived of the atom.

—LEWIS MUMFORD

Deep within the famous cave of Lascaux, a geological fault created a natural shaft 8m (26 feet) below the normal cave floor. Humans descended into the resulting pit with the aid of a rope. Near the bottom of the pit, a bison painted in black on the crystalline wall is shown pierced so deeply that its entrails appear to be spilling out. Facing this eviscerated, dying animal is a strange, sticklike, backward-falling figure with four fingers on each hand, an erect penis, and, incongruously, the head not of a man but of a bird (fig. 6.1). At the foot of the figure is what appears to be a spear thrower, an Ice Age tool used to greatly enhance the distance that a spear may be thrown. There is also a staff surmounted by a real or carved bird. On the other side of the falling figure, a rhinoceros appears to be leaving the scene.

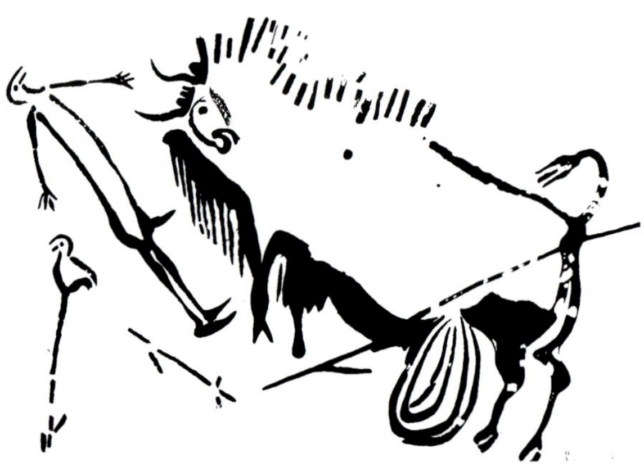

Figure 6.1. Scene in the pit at Lascaux, with a bird-headed man falling backward. Length of complete panel 185 cm.

This enigmatic painting has been dated to approximately 17,000 years ago. It is not only remarkable for its subject matter but also jarring because of its schematic style. The figures of the man and the bison are done in a manner unlike anything else in the cave and unlike any other figures of this culture. The bird-headed man is rare in Ice Age art but not unique. Another one appears in Spain, in the cave of Altamira (fig. 6.2). Others are found at Lascaux, Cougnac, and Pech-Merle. In the Hall of the Hieroglyphs at Pech-Merle is a bird-headed female figure, one of the figures discussed earlier as emerging from the cave meanders (see fig. 1.9). A curious and unusual cave engraving made on the island of Sicily at the end of the Ice age depicts a scene of men with bird heads (fig. 6.3).

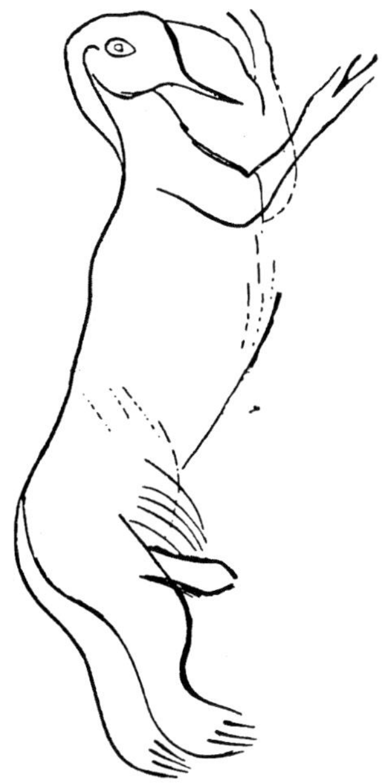

Figure 6.2. Bird-headed man in Altamira cave. Height 48.3 cm.

Subsequent Use of Bird Heads

Thousands of years after the Ice Age images were made, someone living in Siberia, some 4,000 miles from Lascaux, during the Asian Neolithic period made a petroglyph on a cliff above the Tom' River, one of several stick figures with, again, four fingers on each hand, an erect penis, and a bird head (fig. 6.4). Bird-headed humans are abundant in Neolithic art and the art of Mesopotamia and continue into the subsequent European Copper and Bronze Ages. Examples of bird-headed women have been found in Turkey at Çatal Hüyük, in Minoan Crete, throughout the Middle East, and in the area known as Indo-European. Looking back at a double-headed female figure we saw ear-

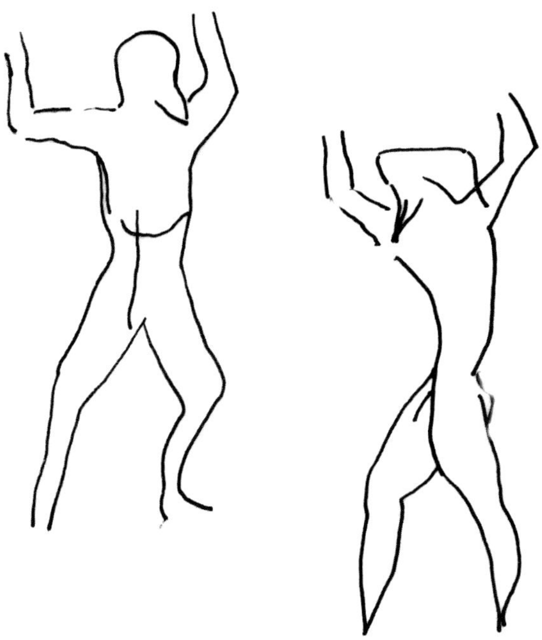

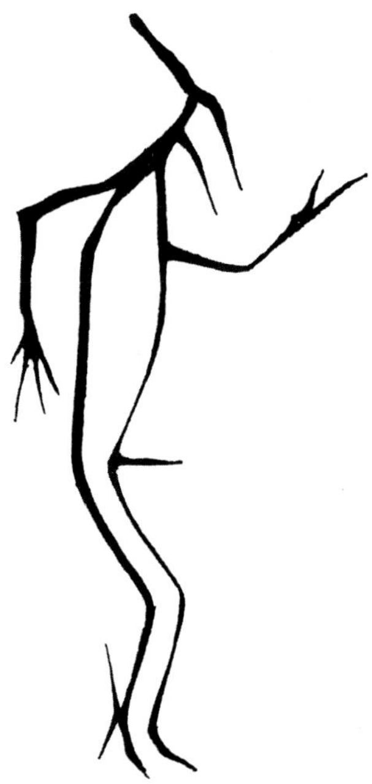

Left: Figure 6.3 Bird-headed men from late Ice Age cave of Addaura, Sicily.

Right: Figure 6.4. Bird-men from Tom' River, Siberia, early Neolithic period.

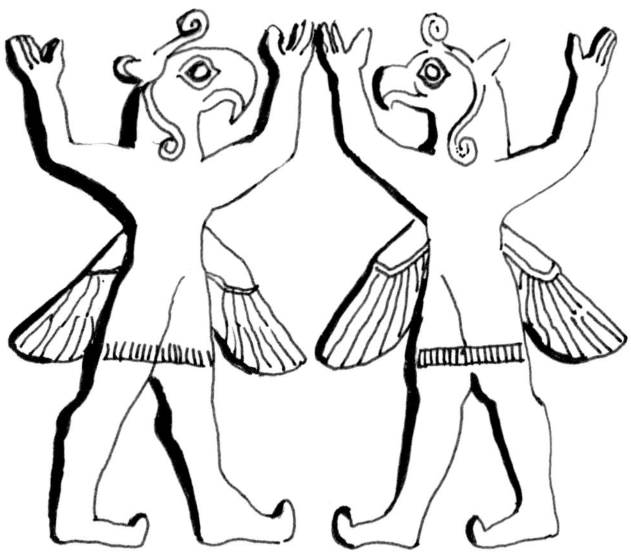

Figure 6.5 Bird-headed men on a carved stone relief from the ancient Hittite culture of Anatolia.

lier (fig. 2.13), note that the heads are beaked bird heads. An example from the Bronze Age is a carving of paired Hittite bird-men (fig. 6.5).

Halfway around the world from Lascaux and again thousands of years later, an American Indian artist made rock art that is curiously similar to the painting at Lascaux. At Three Rivers, New Mexico, an engraved human figure is being attacked by a lion or wildcat from the front and by another animal that looks like a bear from behind. As in the Ice Age painting from the pit at Lascaux, this figure has a bird head and holds a staff (fig. 6.6). Plentiful and often impressive examples of bird-man images are found in Barrier Canyon, Utah, and at the Dinwoody site, Wind River, Wyoming. Bird-headed men, particularly ones with ducklike heads, are common in parts of Utah and New Mexico, especially in association with the ancient Fremont culture. A spectacular example of a bird-headed figure from the early Basketmaker period is found in the San Juan River basin in Utah (fig. 6.7).

Bird-headed humans have been imagined all over the world. They are seen in Peru and Polynesia, New Zealand and the Hawaiian Islands (fig. 6.8). On Easter Island nearly 500 bird-man petroglyphs may relate to the creator

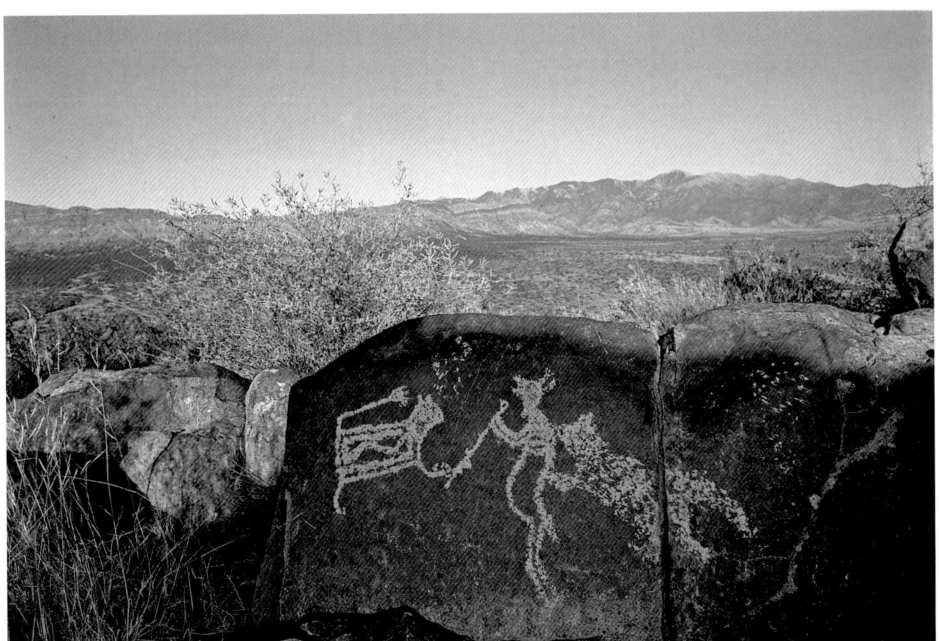

Figure 6.6. Bird-headed man attacked by two animals in a petroglyph at Three Rivers, New Mexico.
Photo by S. Mancini.

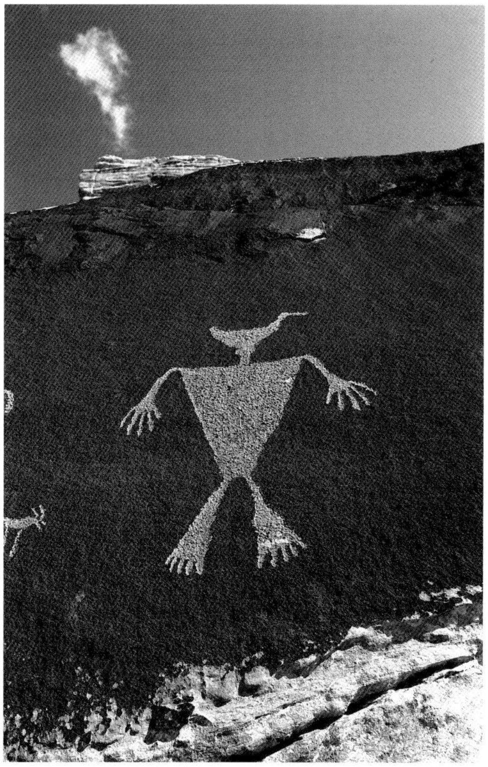

(left) Figure 6.7. Petroglyph of a bird-headed man from the San Juan River basin, Utah. Photo by S. Mancini.

(below) Figure 6.8. Bird-man image, Kaunolu, Hawaii.

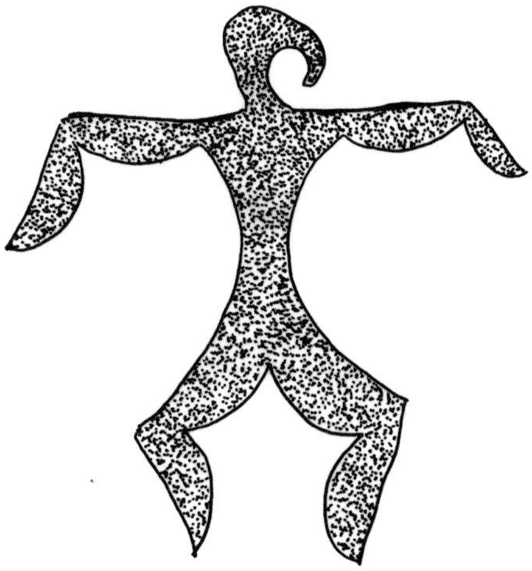

god Makemake, who is half man and half bird. A bird-man cult appears to have originated around the village of Orongo. Each year young men competed by swimming the shark-infested waters to a small atoll in an attempt to retrieve one of the first eggs of the speckled sooty tern. The one who succeeded was the bird-man and chief for the year. This practice continued into the nineteenth century.

Bird-headed humans were the sole characters in a fourteenth-century book from the upper Rhine area of what is now Germany. The book is a Haggadah, used specifically during the celebration of the Passover Seder. This time the purpose of the bird heads is known: they circumvented the Judaic stricture forbidding the representation of people.

How does one explain the appearance of all these bird-headed humans? Some were probably spread by cultural diffusion. Others seem to have arisen independently. Although bird heads have been said to be related to shamanism in some areas,[2] they seem to be a fundamentally human theme unlimited to any specific ritual or belief system. Perhaps birds have held a special meaning for humans at all times because they have the coveted power of flight. To earth-bound humans, this appears to be the ultimate freedom.

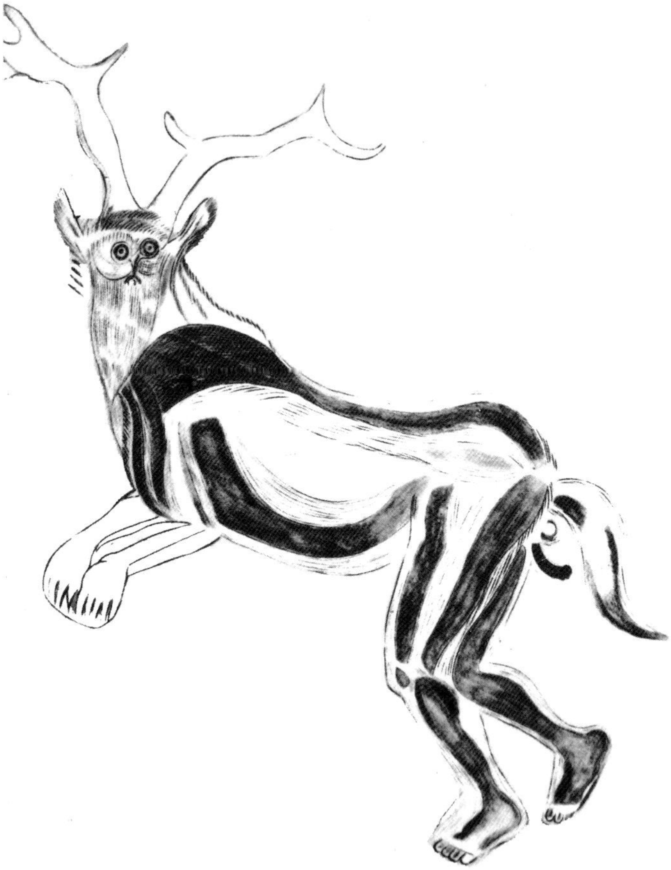

Figure 6.9. The "sorcerer" of Trois Frères. Height 75 cm.

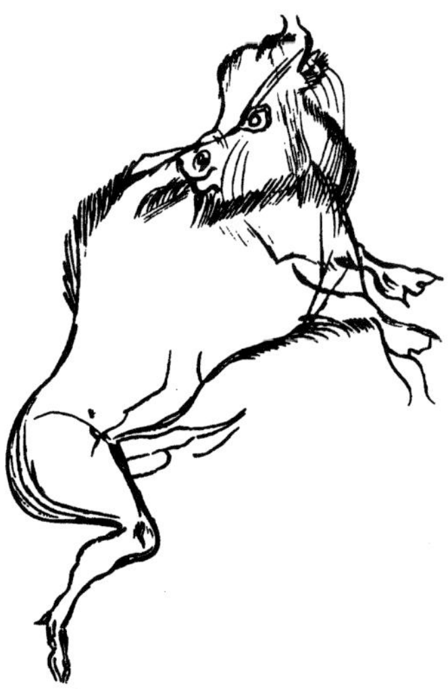

Figure 6.10. Bison-human figure, Trois Frères. Height 12 cm.

Other Human-Animal Hybrids

Birds were not the only animals that Ice Age artists combined with humans in ways that no doubt were meaningful to them but that seem incongruous to us now. Part human and part animal creations are called hybrids, anthropomorphs, or therianthropes. One of the most celebrated images in Ice Age art, dated to 15,000 years ago, is the "sorcerer" of Trois Frères. It is a painted creature with the antlers of a reindeer, the head or perhaps the mask of an owl, the arms of a human, the paws and claws of an unknown animal, the tail of a fox, the genitals of a feline, and the lower limbs of a human (fig. 6.9).[3] Below it is another, much smaller engraved figure with its head turned so that it is looking back over its shoulder (fig. 6.10). From the waist up it is a bison. Below the waist it is human, except that its genitals appear to be those of a bison. Not far from these is an engraved group with yet another figure that is bison above and human below (fig. 6.11). It appears to be holding an object that the scholar Abbé Breuil took to be a musical bow. More recently, others have seen these lines as an abstraction of speech and as a representation of nasal bleeding. The psychologist Noël Smith suggested that the lines are a graphic expression of the breath of life.[4]

At the cave of Gabillou, from about the same period as Lascaux, there are two anthropomorphic figures with bovine heads. A bison-headed creature from Chauvet is thought to be part human. It is far older than the figures at Lascaux, Trois Frères, and Gabillou—perhaps 15,000 years older. Painted on a hanging rock pendant, it follows the natural shape of the stone. The man-bison overlaps and appears to clasp the hips and legs of a woman. Its head is just over the woman's large, dark pubic triangle. This strange image is reminiscent of another image on a reindeer bone from Laugerie Basse, on which are engraved the hind legs and phallus of an animal apparently standing over a naked, possibly pregnant woman (fig. 6.12).

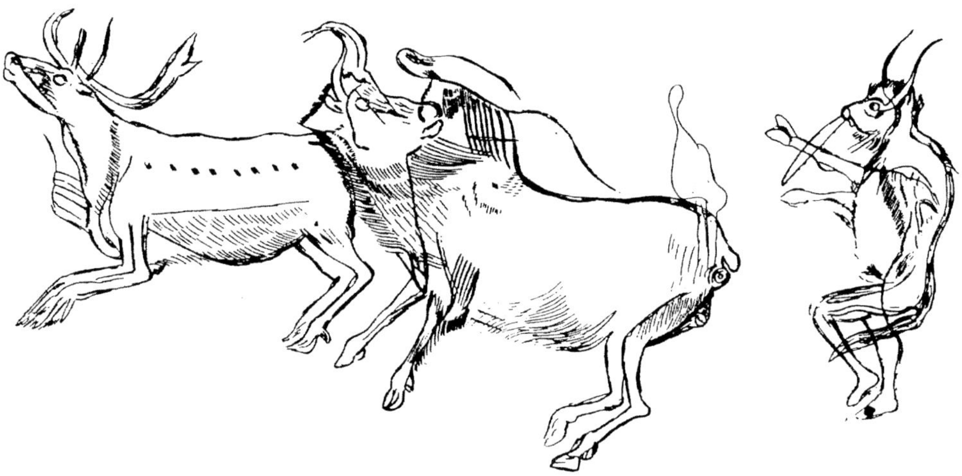

Figure 6.11. Left: Bison-human figure, Trois Frères, in context of the larger panel. Right: Figure in the same panel holding a bow-shaped object. Height 30 cm.

These Ice Age images, if we are interpreting them correctly, may be the first examples of an ancient and continuing theme of human-animal coition. In Greek legend, for example, Zeus raped Europa while he was in the form of a bull. Queen Pasiphae's lust led her to fornicate with the sacred bull from the sea. The result of this union was the Minotaur, part human and part bull. American Indian lore includes a number of stories of maidens who marry bison.

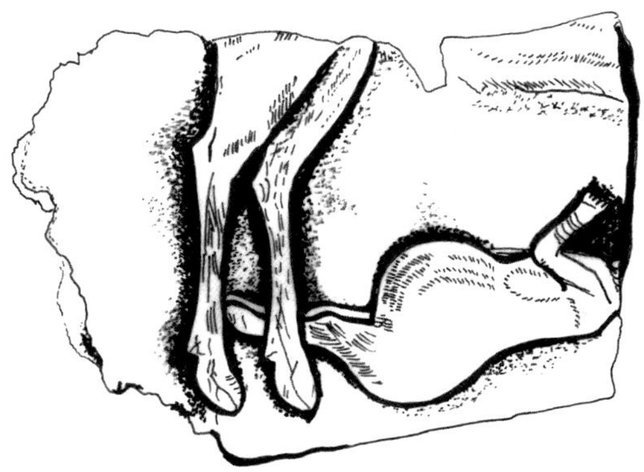

Figure 6.12. Engraved reindeer bone from Laugerie Basse showing the hind legs of an animal standing over a pregnant woman. Some interpreters have seen the animal as a reindeer, but too much of it is missing to identify it definitively.

The earliest known rock art in South Africa, dated to at least 27,000 years ago, was found at Apollo II cave, Namibia. Painted on one portable stone an animal figure appears to be a rhinosceros. On another stone, now broken is a figure that appears to be a feline with human hind legs. The native San frequently painted composite humans, called therianthropes, with eland heads and hooves in many respects similar to the sorcerer of Trois Frères.

One of the most peculiar examples of human-animal fusion is seen in a recently discovered face in Spain. At El Juyo (Cantabria), a face uncovered by archaeologists has been interpreted as half human and half lion.[5] An Ice Age statuette of a standing male human with the head of a cave lion, known as the *Löwenmensch* (lion-man), was carved from a mammoth's tusk about 32,000 years ago (fig. 6.13, see illus. p. ii). This approximately foot-high figure was found at Hohlenstein-Stadel cave near the Danube River valley in Germany. A tiny lion-headed human, less than an inch high and also of mammoth tusk, was found in Hohle Fels cave in southwestern Germany and is believed to be even

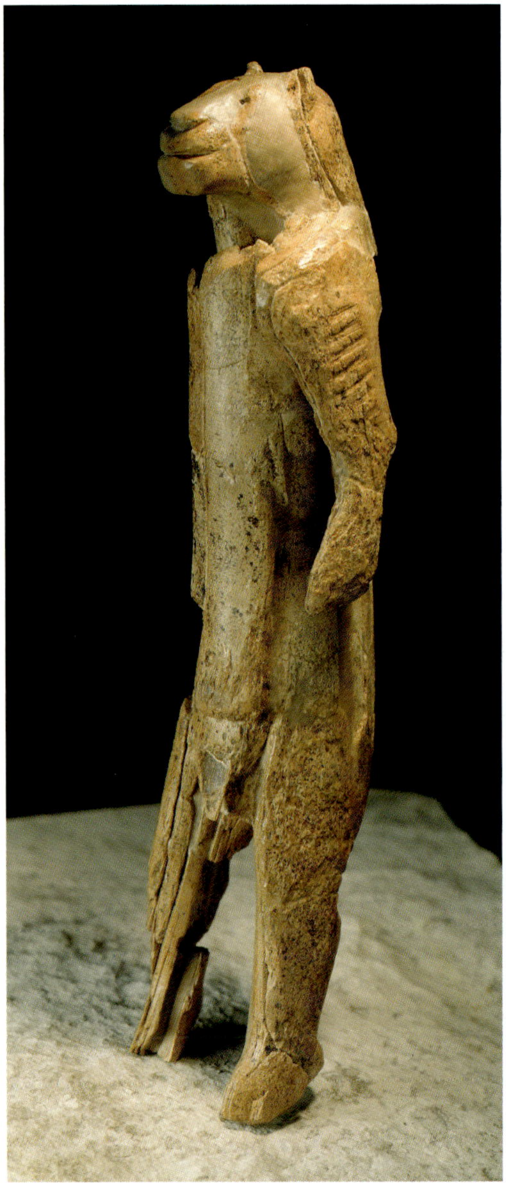

Figure 6.13. The *Löwenmensch* (lion-man) from Hohlenstein-Stadel cave, community Asselfingen, Baden-Württemberg, Germany. 296 mm, Aurignacian c. 32,000 B.P.

older. These dates tell us the surprising news that hybrid figures were being sculpted at the very beginning of known art making.[6]

And they continued to be made. An example paralleling the Ice Age lion man, done almost 30,000 years later, is a lion-headed man from the ancient Hittite culture of Anatolia (fig. 6.14). The Hittite artist may have been influenced by Egyptian art and its lion-headed goddess, Sekhmet. A parallel is found in Hindu mythology, in which Narasinha, an avatar of the god Vishnu, is half lion, half man. From the Mississippian culture of North America, only some 1,000 to 1,600 years ago, comes a woodcarving from Florida consisting of a kneeling human figure with a leonine head (fig. 6.15). On the Northwest Coast of North America, in the Prince of Wales archipelago, similar hybrids have been found: two carved figures with panthers' heads and claws on the forefeet but human legs and feet attached to the lower torso.[7]

Ancient Egyptians portrayed many kinds of animal-headed gods and goddesses in sculpture at least 2,500 years ago. Anubis, for example, had the head of a jackal. The sphinx, in both Egyptian and Greek mythology, had the body of a lion, the wings of an eagle, and the torso and head of a woman. Later, the human-headed sphinx was said to be composed of four animals, with the body of a bull, the feet of a lion, and the wings of an eagle. Ancient Greek mythology told of the centaurs, with their horse bodies, and of Pan, whose nether regions were entirely goat. About 4,600 years ago at Ur, in southern Mesopotamia, an artist used a sophisticated technique of gold, lapis lazuli, and shell inlay to construct a scorpion-man on the sound box of a lyre. The creature is human except for its ominously coiled tail. The Assyro-Babylonian legend of Gilgamesh, said to be the oldest written story in the world, mentions a scorpion-man. Hybrid creatures were portrayed in sculpture as well. A statue from Tel Halaf in Syria portrays a scorpion-man with coiled tail and splayed pincers.

In the North American Southwest, hybrid humans and animals are found in the rockshelter paintings of the lower Pecos River, some of which are believed to date back a minimum of 4,000 years. One particular example of a composite figure is found in Seminole Canyon, Texas, under a rocky overhang known as Fate Bell shelter. At this now almost inaccessible site, a large, mysterious painted figure has been interpreted as having the wings of an eagle, the claws of a bat, the head of a bear, and the antlers of a deer (fig. 6.16).[8]

Why Human-Animal Hybrids?

As in the case of the bird-men, we must ask why people across the centuries have so persistently merged humans with animals in their art. A plethora of theories has been offered to explain such amalgams. Early viewers claimed that part-human, part-animal composites were sorcerers—hence the appellation that has clung to them in reference to Ice Age art. It is now popular to call such figures shamans or animal spirit helpers, because shamans are said to be completely or partially transformed into animals in order to make dangerous voyages to the spirit world. Other interpreters have viewed them as hunters in animal disguise and as spirits taking the form of animals. In some instances—in certain parts of Africa, for example, where each clan is believed to descend from an ancestor that is part human and part animal—hybrids are viewed as ancestor figures. Another possibility, as we saw in the interpretation of San art, is that they are images derived from oral myths. There is no single accepted meaning. Possibly, as in so many other instances in art, the images had multiple or layered meanings.

One explanation has been offered by the archaeologist David Lewis-Williams and his followers, who believe that San artists entered trance states during which they envisioned composite figures. At such times, according to these proponents of "shamanic representation theory," a psychological state called "participation" was induced. The trancer felt dissociated from his body and became part of his own imagery. According to this theory, composite animal-humans were images dredged up from the deepest states of trance.[9] I use the past tense here because the once art-making San are now almost extinct, and the few who remain no longer make art. As a result, it is impossible to submit the shamanic representation theory to scientific inquiry. Not all archaeologists, even in South Africa, accept the theory. Anne Solomon, for example, went back to the ethnographic material on which the theory was largely based. Analyzing it in depth, she found an important source for San visual art in myth. Solomon believes the hybrid images in San art "are not well explained solely by reference to trance and shamanism."[10]

Although it seems possible that images seen in visions and dreams influenced the beliefs and myths of this culture, it is even more likely that the

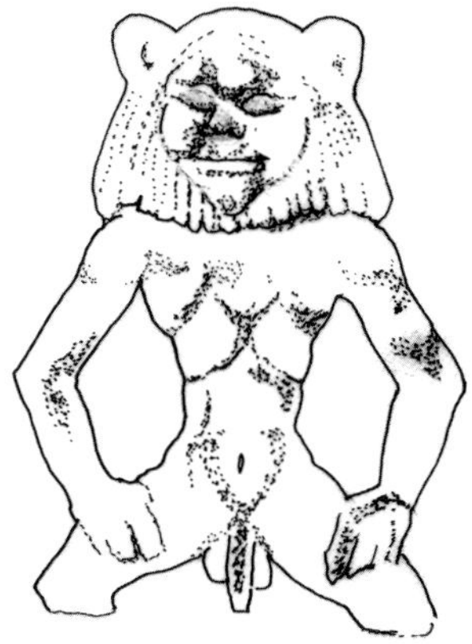

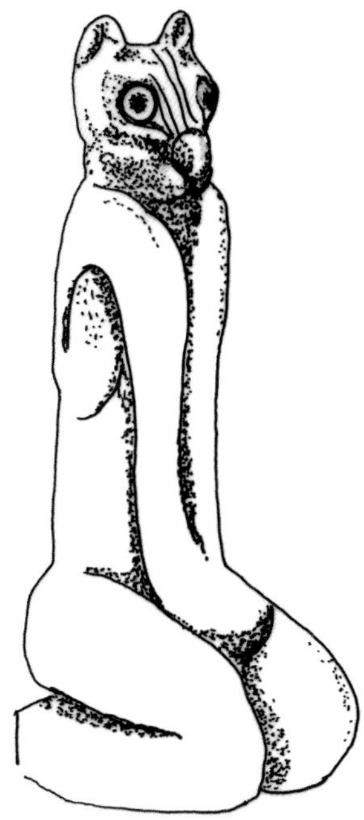

Top: Figure 6.14. Lion-headed man thought to be the god Bes, from Alacahoyuk, Turkey, Old Hittite period, 3500–3400 B.P. Bone, height 4.9 cm.

Bottom: Figure 6.15. A puma- or cougar-headed human figure from the Mississippian culture in Florida.

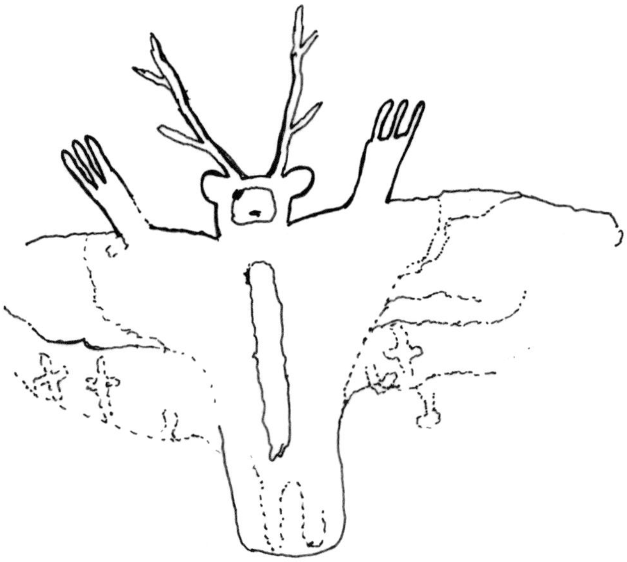

Figure 6.16. Composite figure at Fate Bell shelter, Texas.

reverse is true—that the myths influenced what people subsequently saw in their dreams. Such a view is reinforced by the beliefs of the psychologist and cognitive neuroscientist Merlin Donald, who states that pictorial representation first appeared in the context of an older, oral mythic culture and can best be understood in terms of the preservation of myths.[11] This view of the importance of myth was reinforced by the neuroscientist and polymath Francis Crick when he discussed what happens in the brain at the level of neuron function: "Human gray matter is 90% interpretation equipment—(that is) 90% storyteller."[12]

Even if it could be shown that some animal-human hybrids were related to shamanism, this explanation could not account for all hybrid creatures in early art. Nor can it account for the subsequent use of almost identical forms in art up to the present. Compound figures are found in societies with very different religious and spiritual concepts. What they all have in common is a belief in a life force that can be transformed into a variety of life forms.

We do know that hunting people everywhere strongly identified with prey animals and often depicted them bound together with humans. It may be that the merging of humans and animals expresses a primal worldview in which people and animals are seen as closely related. Hybrid images may express an underlying intuition of kinship with other animals that humans experienced even before that kinship could be proved scientifically. Many American Indian tribes express in their stories a sort of reverse evolution, with animals having once been people.

We now know that some animals are phylogenetically very close to us—that chimpanzees have DNA more than 99 percent identical to that of humans. We humans feel the need to be in some way connected with other animal life, sensing that if the web of nature were broken, our relationship to the planetary matrix would be lost. By means of their art, early humans invoked a world in which animals and humans were indissolubly connected with one another. Artists are still doing that. The contemporary artist Daniel Lee works in that vein, producing haunting animal-human images (fig. 6.17) that have a strong resonance with the Ice Age sorcerer (see fig. 6.9).

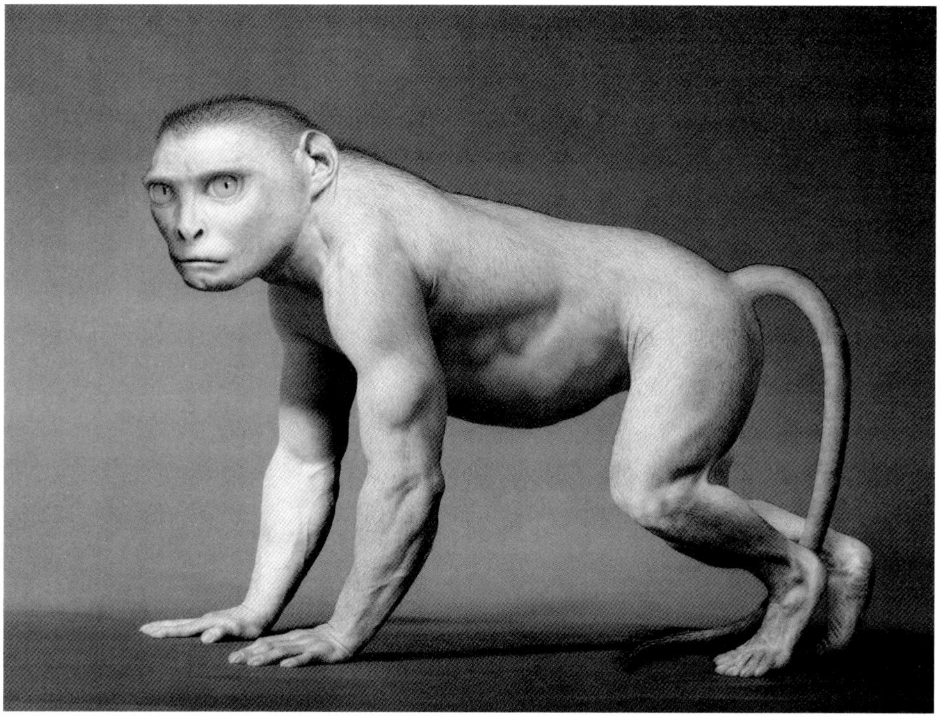

Figure 6.17. Computer-generated image by the contemporary artist Daniel Lee.

Animal-on-Animal Incongruities

Animal-human combinations are not the only instances of the incongruous mixing of species in Ice Age art. Many other hybrids are known in which attributes of different species were melded in startling ways. One example, from Mas d'Azil, is a quadruped, perhaps a horse, carved from reindeer antler, that clearly has wings (fig. 6.18). In an example we have already seen from Trois Frères (fig. 6.11), one reindeer has the head of a bison, and another appears to have webbed front feet. Incongruously webbed feet are seen on rear legs at Les Espélugues (Hautes-Pyrénées). Also in Trois Frères are hybrids of deer and bird, wolf and bear, and bear and bison. A panel of composite animals, half feline and half bull, is found at nearby Tuc d'Audoubert. A bison with deer antlers appears in Le Portel. Three fantastic animals at Pech-Merle have huge bodies and disproportionately small heads. One appears to have a bird head, and another, the head of an antelope; the third has a megaceros hump. A curious animal at La Baume-Latrone, made by drawing with fingers dipped in pigment, has the body of a reptile and the head of a feline.

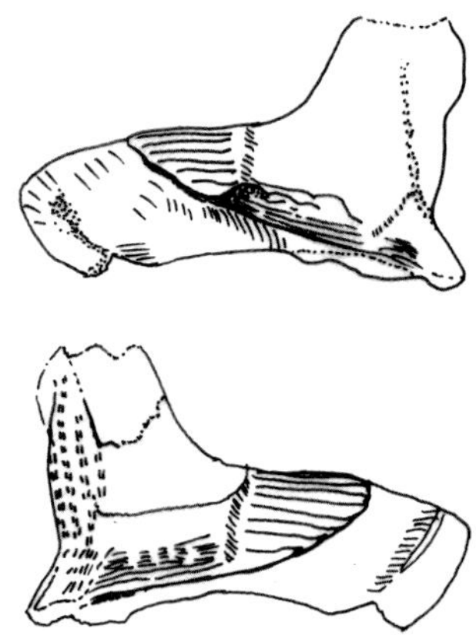

Figure 6.18. Winged quadruped, Mas d'Azil.

Ice Age artists invented a variety of preposterous images in a good number of caves. Two fanciful creatures from Tuc d'Audoubert each have a moose-like head and a hunched, striped upper body. On a stone from La Cauna, the engraved bird, thought to be a crane, that we saw in figure 4.14 seems normal until we note that it has four legs. A composite man-mammoth is seen at Les Combarelles. As a mammoth, it has long curved tusks, but these can also be interpreted as arms because at their terminations appear human hands. In the entry of what is known as the Chapel of the Lion at Trois Frères, a lion is engraved with two tails and two heads. And then one of the two tails appears not to be a tail at all but an arm, complete with elbow and hand (fig. 6.19). Discordant or disparate parts have been intermeshed to yield ever more absurd forms.

We do not know the meaning of these strange Ice Age creatures. The prehistorian Jean Clottes, remarking on the placement of some fantasy animals, noted that some were positioned in places where the underground passages were especially difficult to traverse.[13] That may have been one usage in a particular group of caves at a particular time. The impetus for creating fantastic creatures, however, still needs an explanation—perhaps more than one.

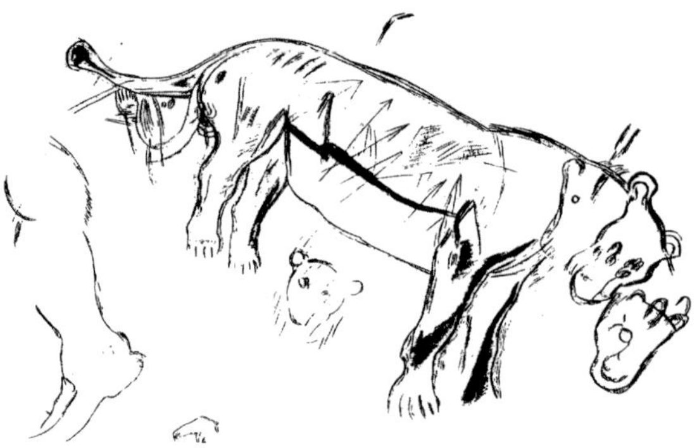

Figure 6.19. Two-headed lion, Chapel of the Lion, Trois Frères. Lower tail is also an arm with a hand.

Ice Age artists were not alone in using such incongruity. Paleolithic artists in Africa at a much later date produced surprisingly similar graphic inventions. In Namibia there is a striking petroglyph in which a lion's tail terminates in a pawprint, an image reminiscent of the lion at Trois Frères (fig. 6.20). The San of South Africa created imaginary rock art animals such as the pictograph surrounded by realistic elands at Horatio rockshelter in Orange Free State (fig. 6.21). San artists imagined felines with tusks on the rocky walls at Clanwilliam and Fouriesburg and a hippopotamus with two horns like those of a rhinoceros at Bosworth, Klerksdorp. On the wall of a South African rockshelter, another San artist depicted an ostrich with two arms extending from its neck. Similar incongruity revealed itself in the Americas. For example, a figure in gold repoussé with reptiles serving as hands was found in South America. On a Toltec relief from Pyramid B at Tula, Mexico, is a creature with a frog's body and a human head.

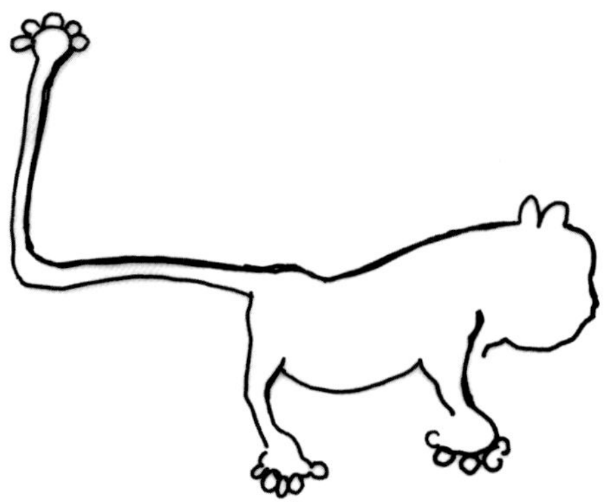

Figure 6.20. San petroglyph of a lion with a pawprint at the end of its tail, Twylfelfontein, Namibia.

The Native people of North America were also impelled to make seemingly absurd images. Colonel Garrick Mallery, one of the earliest ethnologists in North America, mentioned seeing many petroglyph hybrid figures such as eagle and elk, eagle and horse, and eagle and bear.[14] Even earlier, during the Jolliet-Marquette expedition of 1673, Jacques

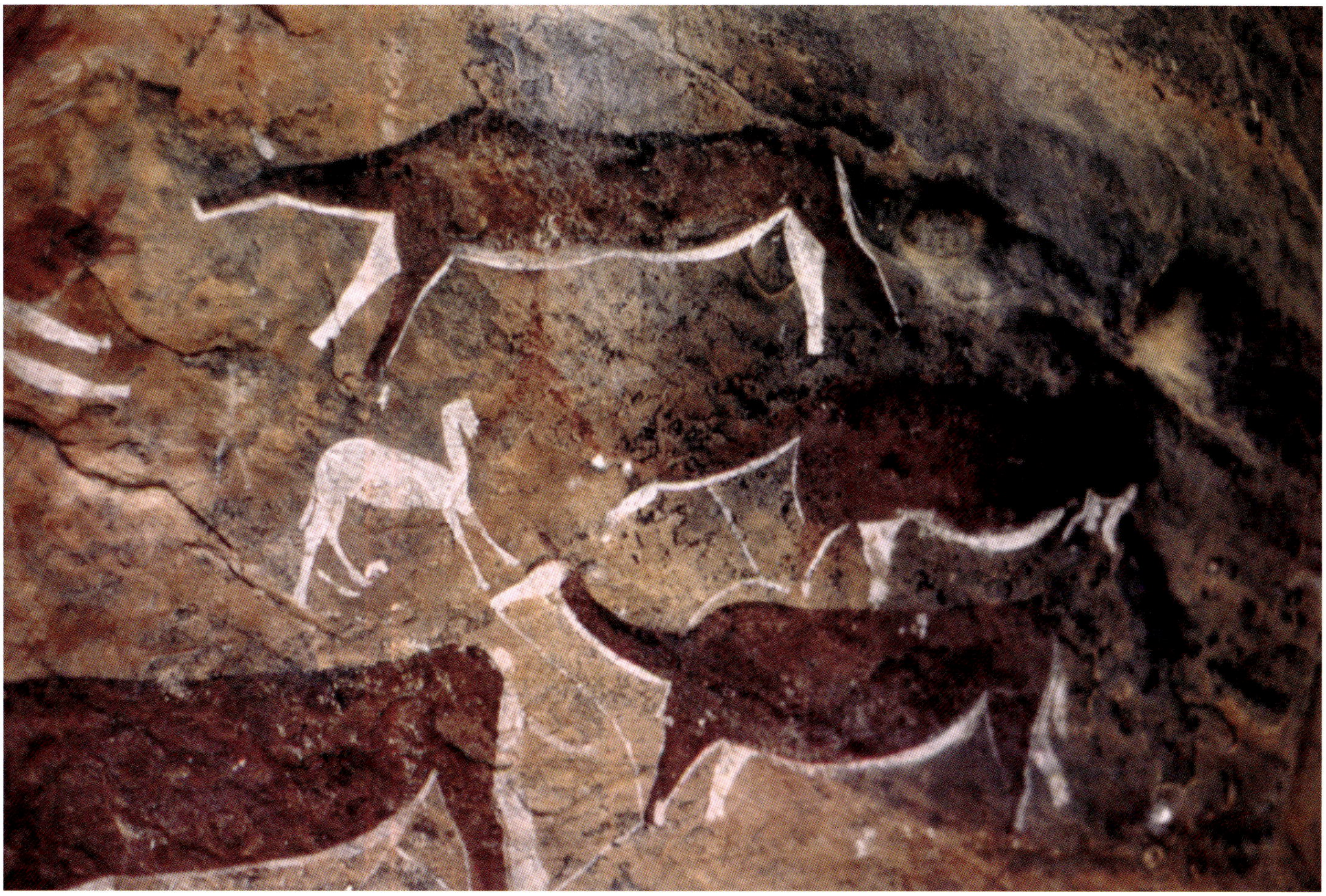

Figure 6.21. San pictograph of an imaginary creature surrounded by elands, Orange Free State, South Africa. Photo by B. D. Alpert.

Marquette described a rock painting he saw in what is now Illinois. It consisted of "two painted monsters which at first made us afraid. . . . they have horns on their heads like those of a deer, a horrible look, red eyes, a beard like a tiger's, a face somewhat like a man's, a body covered in scales, and so long a tail that it winds all around the body, passing above the head and going back between the legs, ending in a fish's tail."[15] In the American Southwest, Mimbres pot painters were masters of incongruous figures. They portrayed a fantasy world that included, among myriad other images, fish, bighorn sheep and a curious animal with the forepart of a bird, the hindpart of a fish, and a horned, deer-like head. A pictograph at Tenabo, New Mexico, shows a head with feathered headdress. Ultimately one is aware that the figure's open, semi-smiling mouth is also a bird.

Imaginary cross-species hybrids were not the exclusive fabrications of prehistoric people. The Sumerians, recording in cuneiform about 5,000 years ago, devised a demon called Pazuzu who was a composite of lion and eagle. The

Hittites of Central Asia, also users of a type of cuneiform, concocted the gryphon with the body of a lion, the head and wings of an eagle, and a back covered with feathers. The early Greeks wrote of the monster Chimaera, which had the forepart of a lion, a goat in the middle, and the hindpart of a dragon. The Hippalectryon was part horse and part rooster. The Celts may have borrowed this image in their own horse-rooster, which had the added fillip of a tail ending in a bird's head. The Manticore had the head of a man, the body of a lion, the tail of a scorpion, three rows of teeth, and the voice of a flute. Other mythic hybrids were the part dog, part bird *simurgh* from Persia, the part fox and part cat *gulon* from Sweden, Pegasus, the winged horse of Greece, and the *catoblepas,* a winged buffalo from the lower Nile. Better known, because it appeared in stories and was depicted in tapestries, is the mythical Unicorn. The oldest unicorn pictures seem to have been those carved on seals at ancient Harappa, part of the Indus River civilization, about 50,000 years ago. A one-horned creature is mentioned in the Bible. The Roman naturalist Pliny the Elder described the unicorn as having the body of a horse, the head of a deer, the feet of an elephant, the tail of a boar, and a single black horn. By the Middle Ages it had been embellished to have the body of a white horse, a goat's beard, and the tail of a lion.

At Sarna, India, several stupas dating from the first to the third century are famous for their carvings. Stupa II, less famous than Stupa I, has carvings that are equally skillful but much more fanciful. One is an image of an elephant with antlers and hooves, and another is an elephant with the tail of a fish (fig. 6.22).

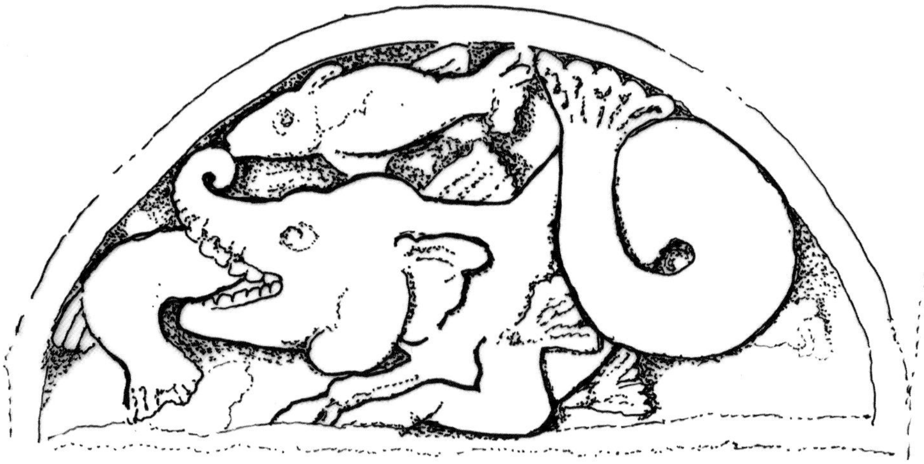

Figure 6.22. Elephant with fish tail, Stupa II, Sarna, India.

In the Western belief system, hybrid animals and animals fused with humans have been used in art based on Christian belief as manifestations of evil, especially as denizens of hell. Hieronymus Bosch, Joachim Patinir, and other artists of the late Middle Ages in Europe depicted these hybrids with much greater relish than they did the treacly inhabitants of heaven. Even Michelangelo, the consummate Renaissance man who looked to nature for truth, allowed that artists might "convert a griffin or deer downward into a dolphin . . . [or put] wings in place of arms . . . since sometimes they desire to see what they have never seen."[16]

Surrealism

The self-conscious use of incongruity reached new heights in the early-twentieth-century artistic movement known as Surrealism. To be effective, surrealist art must provide both familiarity and surprise. Joan Miró, a celebrated painter of the incongruous, produced many objects and creatures that metamorphose: feet become paws, limbs take on the shapes of insects' wing cases or else melt into stumps, mouths change into razor-edged beaks, teeth turn into fangs. René Magritte, another practitioner of such strange transformations, made paintings titled, for example, *Rhino Climbing a Greek Column* and *Giraffe in a Wine Glass*. One subject that fascinated him enough to make several versions of it was a pair of shoes transforming into feet. Magritte wrote: "I believe I've made an altogether startling discovery in painting. . . . I have found a new possibility things have: that of gradually becoming something else—an object melts into an object other than itself. . . . Using this means I get pictures in which the eye 'must think' in a way entirely different from the usual."[17] Magritte discovered this for himself, but it has been well known, as we have seen, at other times and in other parts of the world.

Paradox and the Human Imagination

We humans have conceived of incongruous images in our most ancient legends and in our earliest art. There is some indication that children's minds, unbidden, do the same thing. In one bit of anecdotal evidence, a three-and-a-half year-old girl named Madeleine reported to her mother that she had dreamed of a "scary animal" with the head of a cat and the body of a rooster. She had visited a farm and seen chickens the week before, and she had lived with cats from infancy, but it is unclear what made her merge them in her dream.

It has been estimated by neuroscientists that the human brain has more than 10 trillion synaptic connections. This astronomical number, resulting in overwhelming complexity, is likely to protect the mystery of the human response. Some brain researchers believe that it is this very unpredictability and randomness that allows for what we call inventiveness. In this view, incongruity is the result of the rich interconnectedness of the brain, which can result in seemingly aleatory connections. All humans have the potential to make unique associations. J. Allan Hobson, who studies the dream state of the mind, has written: "Each of us is a surrealist at night. . . . At night everyone is a Picasso, a Fellini."[18] Assembling things in new and surprising ways is one of the definitions of human creative thought.

INVERSION AND REVERSION

Figure inversion was something which was in some way especially appealing to these [Ice Age] artists.

—ANN SIEVEKING, *Engraved Magdalenian Plaquettes*

In Ice Age art, inversion was sometimes a deliberate choice. It was not, as has been suggested, the inevitable result of awkward positions assumed for working in the constricted spaces of the caves. At Niaux, an artist had ample space to stand upright when drawing an inverted horse's head. The same was true at Ebbou, where an engraved figure is turned a full 180 degrees. In sculptural examples as well, inversion was a deliberate choice. On portable objects inversion consisted of overlapping two images, one of which was upside-down in relation to the other. These images have been thoroughly studied by the prehistorian Ann Sieveking, who wrote that although inversion appeared on only a minority of found plaquettes, a sufficient number existed for her to conclude that it held special appeal for certain individuals.[19] Examples have been found in Isturitz, Bruniquel, La Colombière, Lourdes (Hautes-Pyrénées), Mas d'Azil, La Vache (Ariège), and El Castillo.

Symmetrical Inversion

MOM
WOW

An Ice Age bas-relief carved at Laussel has been called a "playing card" image because its two nearly identical women are inverted in relation to each other (fig. 6.23). A similar image was found at Tursac (Dordogne). Both of these might be interpreted as childbirth scenes, although if so, the child is nearly the same size as the mother. Or they might have been intended to show copulation. In either interpretation they would be the only known examples of the use such a theme in European Ice Age art, with one possible exception. These are puzzling images. We do not understand what they represent, but we do know that they are paradoxical. A single image that can be viewed in two inverted orientations, each of which presents something different, is an example of visual paradox. Sometimes the images may appear almost the same either way they are turned, which is a further level of refinement and difficulty in the *tour de force* of inversion.

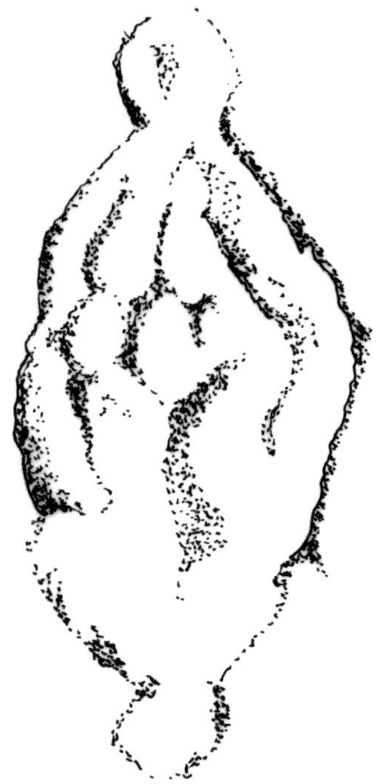

Figure 6.23. "Playing card Venus," bas-relief in limestone at Laussel. 20 cm.

Other examples of the paradox of inverted symmetry are seen in the Ice Age statuettes of females called "Venus figures" because of their generous female endowments. Unearthed all over Europe since the early nineteenth century, they generally adhere to a formula in which the breasts and belly are included within a large central sphere that contains the reproductive organs. In many of these small figures the breasts are so pendulous that they fall into the central sphere formed by the abdomen and vulva. In some cases, such as the figures from the Czech site of Dolní Vestonice and Russia's Kostienki, the breasts hang down to cover at least half of that implied sphere. The head and lower legs taper off from this sphere and are often so unrealistically attenuated that they become mere appendages.

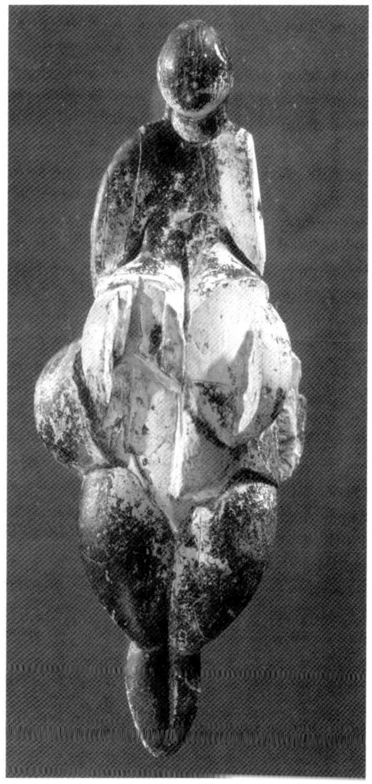

Figure 6.24. The Venus of Lespugue, carved in mammoth tusk ivory, now broken. Height 14.7 cm. Photo: Scala/Art Resource, N.Y.

The Female figure from Lespugue is an example. Carved in mammoth ivory and believed to date from more than 20,000 years ago, it is larger than most—about 15 cm high (fig. 6.24). The distortion of the figure's body is extreme; her breasts cover about three-quarters of the abdominal sphere. Her legs taper to a single oval knob, very like the small oval knob of the highly abstracted head. When seen from the rear, the steatopygous buttocks are roughly in the center of the figure. A series of vertical lines descends from under the buttocks to behind the bulge of the legs. These have been interpreted as depicting a grass skirt, but it would be unusual to place a skirt below the buttocks and the vulva. Rather, these lines appear to mimic the vertical lines of the woman's hair, which falls from the back of her head, in the same way that the swelling thighs mirror the pendulous breasts. Apparently the sculptors who produced these figures felt it was important to make them vertically symmetrical, even at the sacrifice of realism. With such a premise, the distortions make sense, because they achieve for these figures a symmetry of inversion. We see images that suggest a desire for this kind of inversion in the depiction of

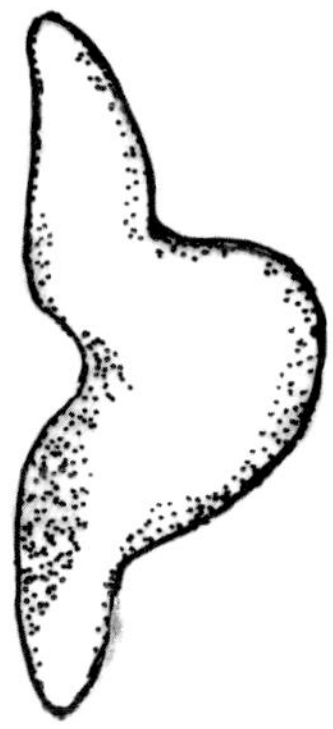

Figure 6.25. Female figure from Peterfels, Germany. It looks roughly the same when inverted. 4.5 cm.

females from Tursac, Sireuil, La Gare de Couze, and Peterfels (fig. 6.25). The small stone female figure from Peterfels, Germany, appears, in its abstraction and simplicity, to be have been crafted by the French sculptor Arp. It seems to be almost completely invertible.

Inversion as Description or as Paradox

In Ice Age art one finds figures unexpectedly turned 90 to 180 degrees from their normal orientation. The most famous is the "upside-down" horse painted on a false pier at the entrance to a passage known as the Meander in Lascaux. It falls hind-feet-first, with forelegs flailing the air, and seems all the more in jeopardy because there is a space between the pier on which it is painted and the ground on which it will presumably land. Also at Lascaux is a smaller, less well known, engraved falling horse. This one is shown falling headfirst. A vertical and upside-down bison was engraved at Le Portel, and an upside-down bison appears at Ebbou (Ardèche). Two falling bison and an inverted horse are found at Santamamiñe in Spain's Vizcaya province. Perhaps the artists were giving a literal description of Stone Age hunting practices, in which horses were sometimes forced to flee toward cliffs, where they fell to their deaths. Solutré in France is a site that confirms that animals were killed in this way over a long period. The same kind of hunting took place in North America at bison drops. It occurred in Africa as well. In Orange Free State, South Africa, at Pelendaba, Herschel, stampeding elands are portrayed as they plunge over the edge of a steep *krantz*. The descriptive meaning usually given to an inverted figure, whatever the culture, is death.

But another aspect of inversion is relevant here. Inversion may be used to present two figures both of which cannot be fully perceived at the same time—and that is a paradox. A figure may be cleverly constructed so that when rotated 180 degrees, the same lines form another image that had gone unnoticed in the original orientation. Sometimes the second image is entirely different from the first. At other times the second image presents the same subject but a different example of that subject. Playing with inverted images was not unknown in the Ice Age. Edouard Piette, an early French prehistorian, described an engraved piece in his collection of Ice Age artifacts that had three heads for one body. He wrote, "It appears as a swan whichever way one holds it. Sometimes the belly becomes the back, sometimes the back becomes the belly."[20] He also noted that sometimes the figure appeared to have outspread

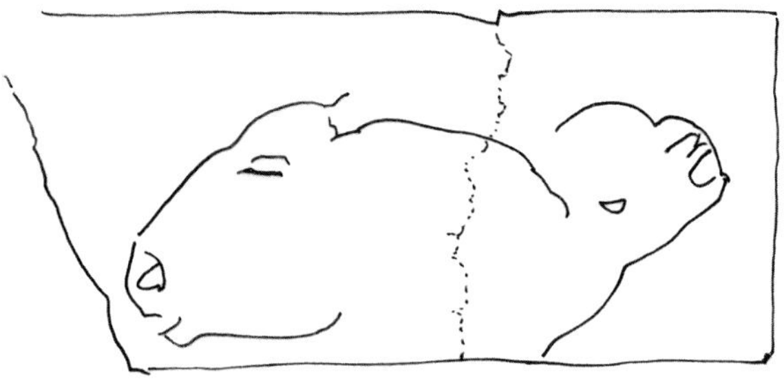

Figure 6.26. Bone from Gourdan with inverted engraved horse heads.

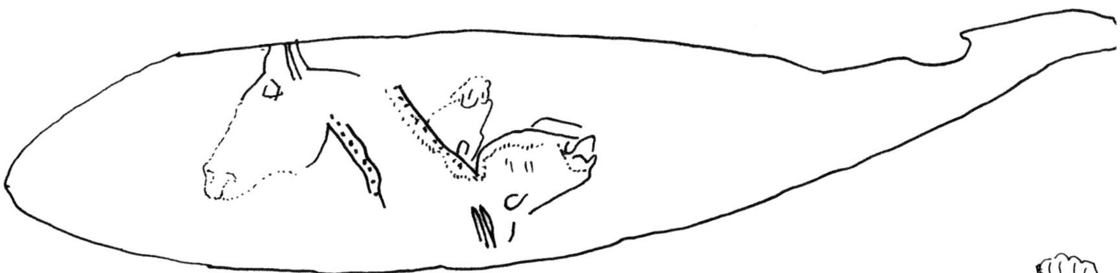

Figure 6.27. Bone from Pekarna with inverted engraved horse heads. Probably a knife.

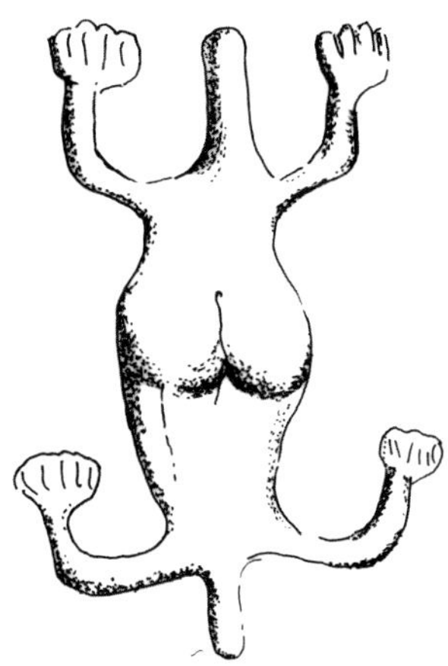

Figure 6.28. Inverted anthropomorphic figures sharing one buttock, a relief on a large vase from northeastern Romania dated to about 6500 B.P. Height 9.5 cm.

wings, and in other positions it appeared to be at rest. Ice Age portable art offers other examples of play with inversion. A bone from Gourdan (Haute-Garonne) is engraved with a horse's head. If the bone is inverted, one sees a different, smaller horse's head (fig. 6.26). Another bone from Pekarna, Czech Republic, shows a similar inversion (fig. 6.27).

Use of inversion to reveal hidden figures can be seen in examples from Isturitz, Bruniquel, Mas d'Azil, Les Espélugues, La Colombière, Lourdes, La Vache, and El Castillo. The device seems to have been most favored in certain geographical areas, particularly western France, the Pyrénées, and northern Spain. Only occasionally is it seen elsewhere.

Inversion has captured the imaginations of some artists in many other cultures throughout the years. By way of a few examples, in Neolithic Europe two anthropomorphic figures were made to share one buttock and appear almost the same upside-down or rightside-up (fig. 6.28). On the island of New Guinea and throughout Melanesia, shields and masks made by native people may contain double images. Iatmul shields from Papua New Guinea often present two different, frightening, open-mouthed faces whether seen rightside-up or inverted to reveal an alternative, equally terrifying face (fig. 6.29).

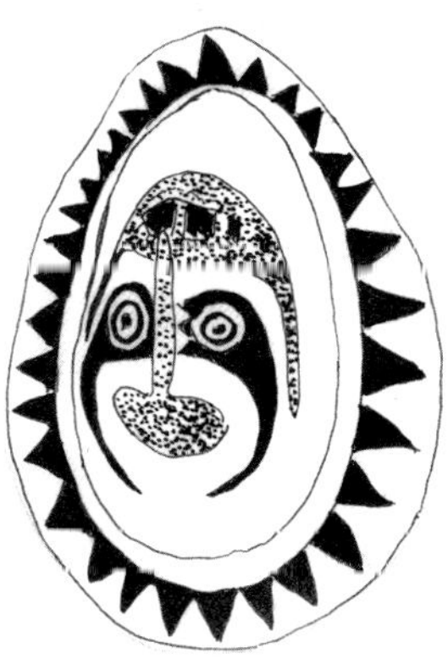

Figure 6.29. Iatmul invertible shield. The Iatmul people live along the Sepik River in Papua New Guinea and are best known by Westerners for having been the subjects of studies by Margaret Mead.

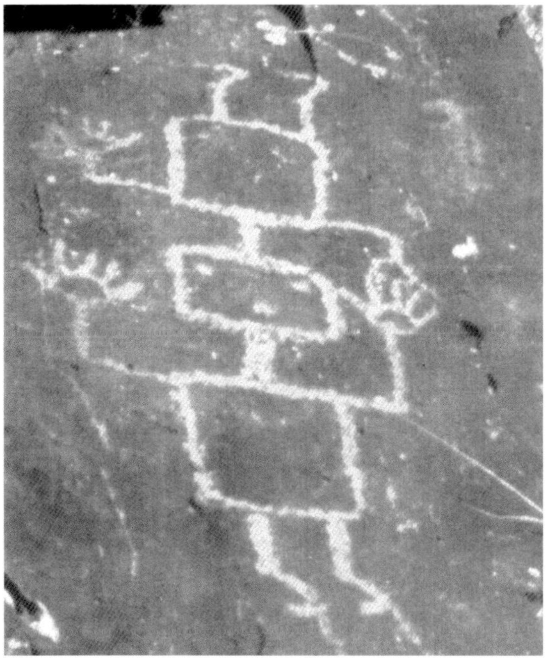

Figure 6.30. Inverted figures share one head in a petroglyph at La Bajada, New Mexico.

On the American continents, inversion is found over a wide geographic range. A puzzling but seemingly witty petroglyph at La Bajada, New Mexico, presents two figures who share one head and are upside-down in relation to each other (fig. 6.30). A common image in Pueblo Indian iconography is the flute-playing fertility figure. He is often depicted with a sack of seeds on his back and with a large erection; infrequently hc is shown copulating. An unknown Pueblo artist cleverly devised a unique invertible image that portrays a flute player both rightside-up and upside-down in the same petroglyph, which delights by its droll ingeniousness (fig. 6.31). Impressively, it was made using the inflexible medium of stone pounding on stone, in which it is difficult to sketch out an idea or to present a fine definition.

On occasion an artist appears to have chosen certain subject matter primarily because it allowed for the use of inversion—for example, in the Eskimo theme of a bear standing on ice looking at its own reflection. This theme was carved by at least two Alaskan sculptors, Manno and Eviluanjuk. Another example from a very different culture is a sculpture of two inverted wrestlers from the Bembe tribe in the Congo (fig. 6.32).

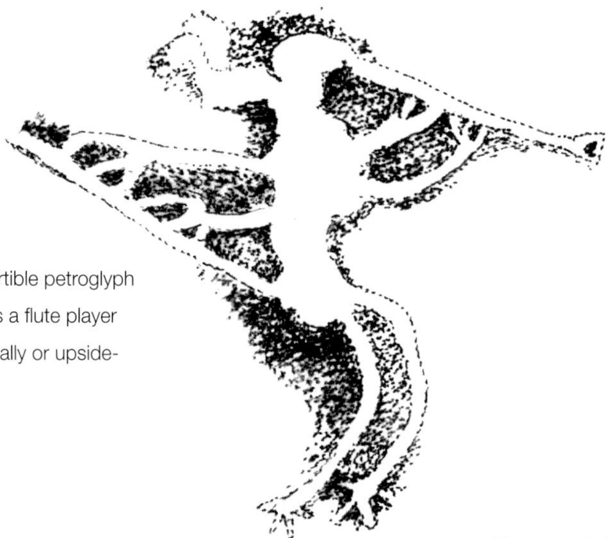

Figure 6.31. This invertible petroglyph image can be seen as a flute player whether viewed normally or upside-down.

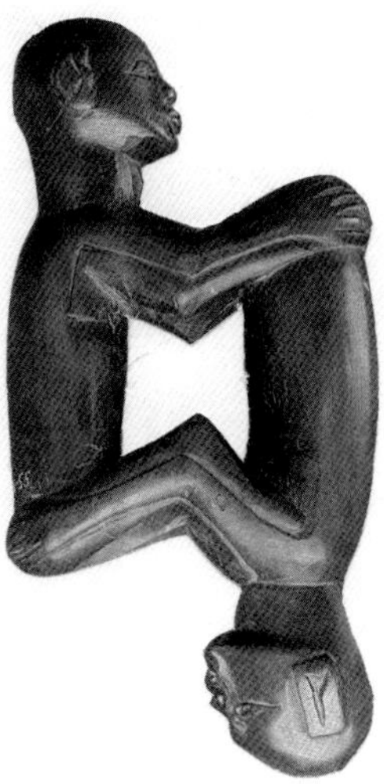

Figure 6.32. A pair of wrestlers in wood by an artist of the Bembe tribe, a seminomadic group that migrated from the area surrounding the Congo River to the border of Zaire in the Democratic Republic of Congo.

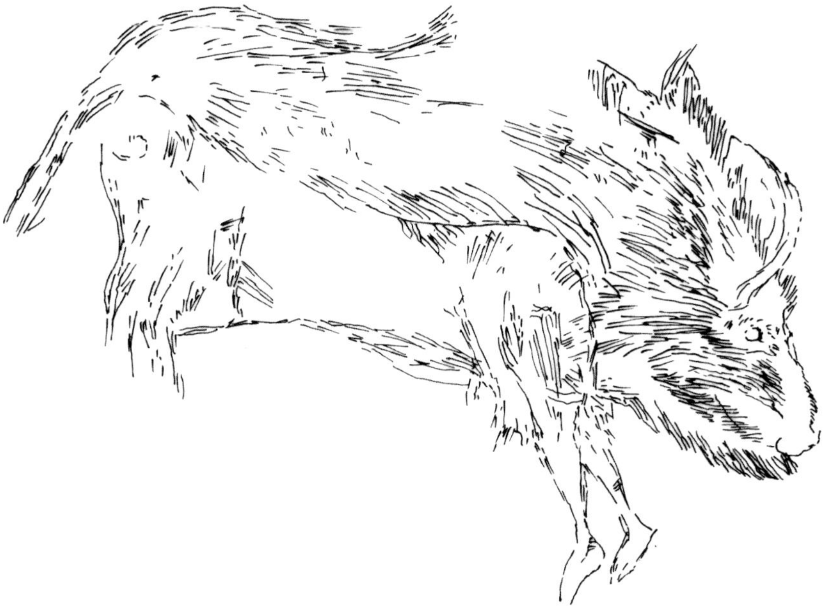

Figure 6.33. Bison sharing legs and feet with a part-human creature, Fontanet. (After D. Vialou)

Bizarre Use of Reversion in Feet

In the Spanish cave of El Castillo, an artist saw a bison in the natural formation of a stalactite and completed the image with strokes of paint (see fig. 3.10). As we examine this sculpture more closely, we are startled to find, in place of one of the rear hooves, the engraving of a human foot. At Fontanet (Ariège) a panel is covered with two highly realistic engraved bison roughly facing one another across a crack in the wall. One of them appears to share legs and feet with a creature that is human from the waist down (fig. 6.33). Because of their placement, one cannot rid oneself of the feeling that the human legs are meant to serve simultaneously as legs for the bison. Then one notices, with some surprise, that not only do the legs and feet belong simultaneously to man and bison but they are attached so that on the bison they are backward.

Backward legs or feet have, curiously, had widespread appeal, as can be seen by their appearance in far-flung places over a vast range of time. The Inuit believe in humanoid demons called Tuurnigait who have their legs turned backwards. Eskimos in the Baffin Bay area believe in a mythical giant who is always shown with his feet reversed. In Africa the Nuloi are mythical creatures with backward-turned legs. The Greek God Hephaestos, known in Roman mythology as Vulcan, was a blacksmith and an artist. Unlike the other, physically perfect Greek gods, he was born with a club foot and is also sometimes described as having his feet facing backward.

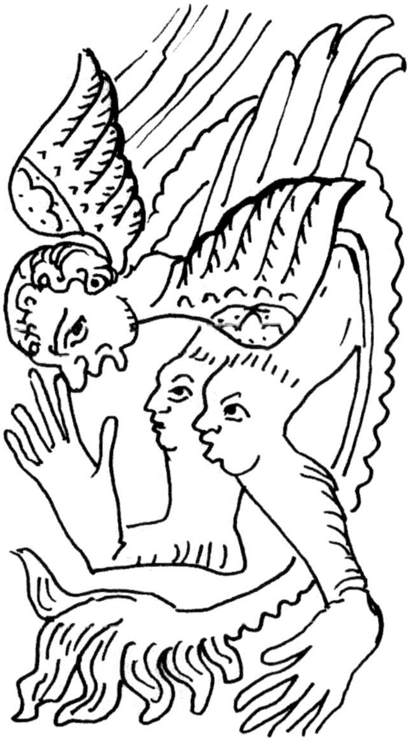

Figure 6.34. Foot reversal is seen in a page from the book of Numbers in a thirteenth-century German Jewish Bible.

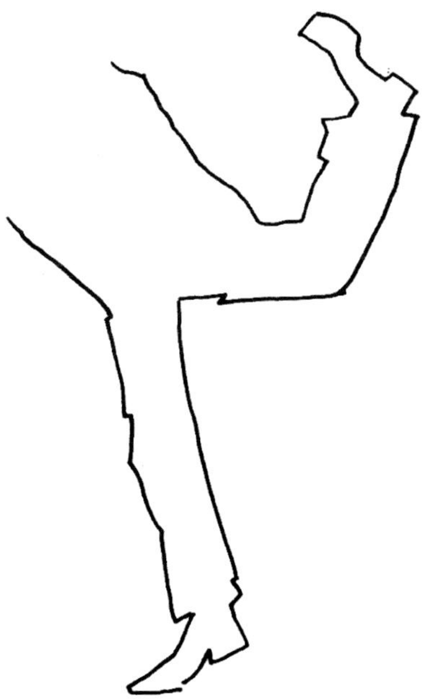

Figure 6.35. Drawing of a section of a theater curtain painted by M. Chagall. in his *Homage to Gogol.*

In listing some of the creatures who possess this abnormality, one feels one has stumbled upon a universal image in mythology and folk belief. The leg twisted or bent backward is a dominant motif in the animal style of Central Asia. In Europe, a legend circulated during the Middle Ages about a group of people called Abanmon, all of whom had their feet turned backward. There are many others with backward feet: the yeti from Tibet and ghosts in India. In Africa, on the Ivory Coast, there are mythic dwarfs. In the Amazon, especially Brazil, there are strange red-haired creatures. Belize has goblins with feet reversed. Indications of similar stories appear in the rock art of North America. A petroglyph at La Cienega, New Mexico, shows a quadruped with backward feet. Quadrupeds with backward feet are also found at Indian Creek, Utah. The Ice Age engraving from Fontanet that began this listing of backward feet appears to have been intended to portray the greatest possible naturalism, and in this context the appearance of backward feet strikes the viewer as all the more incongruous.

Occasionally, a different sort of foot inversion appears. At Velarde, New Mexico, two sets of large, carefully pecked hands reach up in two adjacent petroglyphs. Upon closer examination one finds that these overlarge hands belong to two upside-down figures. The hands are where the feet should be, and the actual hands are schematic feet. The same perverse foot-hand reversal is found on an angel in a thirteenth-century illustrated German Jewish Bible (fig. 6.34).[21]

We find puzzling foot reversal in more recent times in a painting by Marc Chagall called *Homage to Gogol* (fig. 6.35). Showing a man flying through the air with one foot reversed, it evokes a mood of dreamlike fantasy. The foot reversal here may have some deeper meaning, but it might also serve as the artist's conspiratorial wink to the viewer.

Inversion in Recent Art

Artists have always been fascinated by inversion. Salvador Dalí was one of its most devoted practitioners, owing in part to an incident that occurred early in his career. He was searching for an address

Figure 6.36. Image on a postcard that, because of its changed orientation, Dalí mistook for a picture of a head by Picasso.

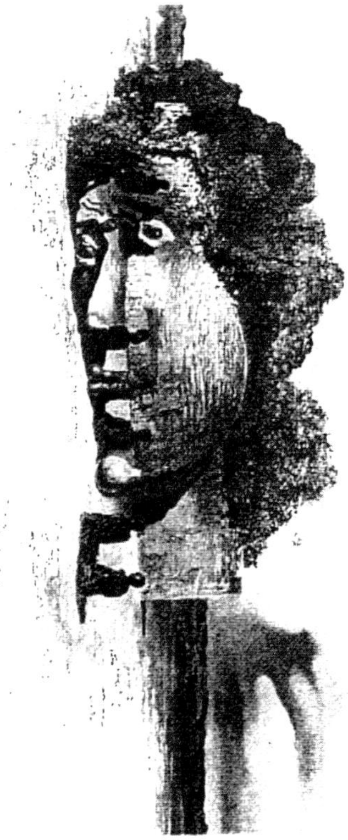

amid a clutter of papers on his desk when, unexpectedly, he found a reproduction of a face by Picasso that he did not know he possessed and could not recall ever having seen before (fig. 6.36). A moment later he realized that it was an ethnographic photograph showing a group of natives seated before a stone hut. Inadvertently giving it a 90-degree turn had made it into a likeness of a Picasso drawing. "All at once," he wrote, "I was aware of the illusion."[22]

A fascination with the power of that illusion haunted Dalí. In 1923 he did a portrait of his sister that can be inverted 180 degrees to become a different portrait of his sister. Again in 1967 he produced a double image in a sculpture called *Swan/Elephant.* When inverted, the wings of the swan change into the elephant's ears, and the swan's neck becomes the elephant's trunk. Dalí wrote about this illusion: "It is by a specifically paranoiac procedure that it has been possible to obtain a double image: that is the image of an object which, without the least figurative or anatomical modification, can at the same time represent another, absolutely different object."[23] In this sense "paranoia" means self-delusion, and Dalí was talking about the artist's ability to manipulate perception for himself as well as for others in order to achieve an exhilarating moment of discovery.

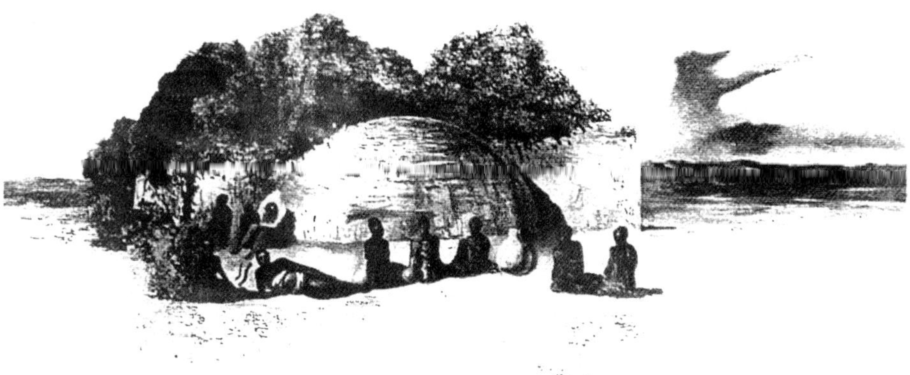

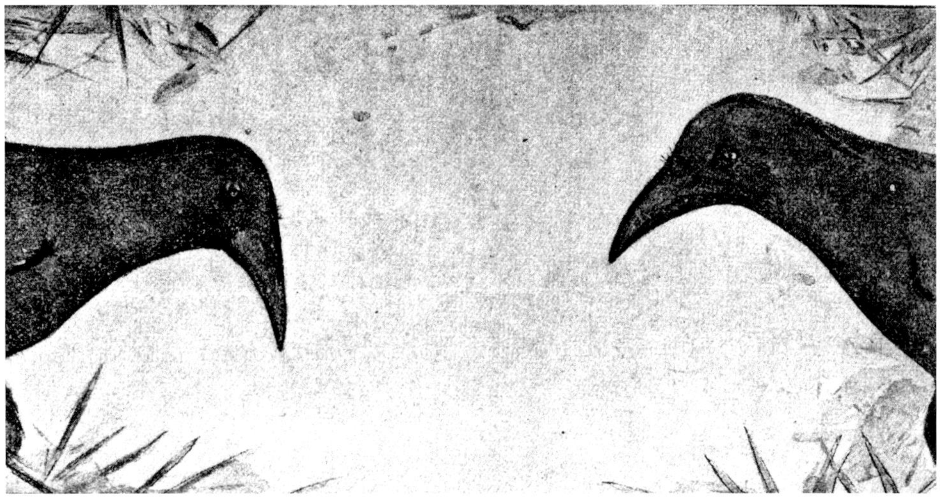

Figure 6.37. Illustration from Peter Newell's *Topsys and Turvys*. When iin-verted crows become rhinos.

It was this aspect of inversion that made for the popularity of "transformation cards" in early-nineteenth-century England. These could be rotated to show differing images depending on how they were held. A century later, in 1903 and 1904, Gustave Verbeek created a similar series of cartoons for the *New York Herald* that made sense (but a different sense) both rightside-up and upside-down. Peter Newell drew what he called *Topsys and Turvys,* published first in 1894 and followed by further examples in 1902 (fig. 6.37). These were a series of cartoons when viewed in one orientation and a different but equally comprehensible series when inverted. Such games have an ongoing fascination. An extravagant example of the genre is a book written in English that reveals another story, this time in French, when turned upside-down. The book is not strong on plot, but it exerts a peculiar pleasure for other reasons.[24] Douglas Hofstadter playfully devised an altered alphabet in which letters appeared identical whether seen normally or rotated 180 degrees. He called it a "whirly alphabet" and displayed it in a book called *Ambigrammi,* published in 1993.

It is said that the painter Wassily Kandinsky entered his studio one day to find an exciting painting that he had never seen before propped against the wall. In a few moments he realized that it was one of his own paintings placed carelessly upside-down. Perhaps the story is apocryphal, but it is true that he abandoned figurative work to devote himself entirely to what was then revolutionary non-objective art. The painter George Baselitz has for the last 30 years inverted all the figures in his paintings. He says he does this in order to force the viewer to be aware of his color, his brushwork, and other purely painterly qualities. By inverting the image, comprehension of it is deliberately delayed.

In the popular instruction book *Drawing on the Right Side of the Brain,* Betty Edwards has her students copy pictures that are upside-down. Again the purpose is to hide the figure, this time so that the beginning artist can concentrate on the lines without being distracted by the meaning of the image. Artists and art students routinely invert their canvases so that after hours of working on them they can see them with fresh eyes and, as in the Kandinsky example, better critique them in terms of abstract elements.

Inversion (and Reversion) in Music

Inversion is not only a common device in Western graphic art but is also basic to Western music. In harmonically structured music, triads and other chords are taken through a continuous series of inversions to achieve the desired chord progressions. Melodic inversion can also be used when successive intervals of a melody are inverted, as in a mirrored exchange of upward and downward movements. Bach used both reversion and inversion in his canons. For example, a section of *The Musical Offering,* containing both, is called a "crab canon" because it can be played backward and upside-down. In the gigue movement of his *French Suite Number 5* and in other compositions as well, Bach used inversion to explore compositional possibilities. Then, in an even greater tour de force, he wrote *Tafelmusic,* in which two players sit at opposite sides of a table playing from one sheet of music. The music is played rightside-up and upside-down simultaneously.

Mozart played the same game in pieces such as *Serenade Number 12 K. 388 in C Minor,* in which parts of the trio are upside-down in relation to the music's original statement. Anton Webern also wrote music meant to be played either normally or upside-down. Handel's *Concerto Number 13 in F Major,* called "The Cuckoo and the Nightingale," first musically represents the cuckoo's call and later inverts it. Beethoven used inversion in the scherzo movement of his *Symphony Number 4*. Darius Milhaud used inverted themes in the slow movement of a suite for two pianos called *Scaramouche.* Camille Saint-Saëns, in *Carnival of the Animals,* quoted folk tunes upside-down. Melodic inversion formed an essential ingredient of Arnold Schönberg's twelve-tone music.

Neurological Explanation

Because the appeal of inversion is so ubiquitous, we look for some neurological explanation. One answer is that it opens up new and unforeseen possibilities. It disorients and thereby provides a feeling of surprise. Such momentary revelation startles us. Cognitively explained, the brain stem has sent out acetylcholine to induce a chemical and ultimately an electrical stimulation in the affected brain cells to respond to the challenging new image. We seek this stimulation just as we crave the experience of the novelty that can set the process in motion. The scientist J. Allan Hobson wrote that the "startle reflex," in some rare instances, can be powerful enough to initiate a trancelike state in susceptible persons. The rush of acetylcholine, he says, acts as a chemical exclamation point.[25] It reinforces and intensifies experience, serving in turn as further stimulus for artistic exploration.

SPACE AND MOTION

The structures of space begin in structures of the mind which are utilized to construct representations of objects, patterns and events including the self.

—DAVID R. OLSON AND ELLEN BIALYSTOK, *Spatial Cognition*

Ice Age humans probably experienced space in a way similar to that of other hunting and gathering people. Perhaps their perception of the world was comparable to that of Eskimos, of whom the anthropologist Edmund Carpenter said: "I know of no example of an Eskimo describing space primarily in visual terms. They don't regard space as static, and therefore measurable; hence they have no formal units of spatial measurement, just as they have no uniform divisions of time."[26]

There might also be parallels with the concept of space held by Australian Aboriginals, who described space in terms of spoken or sung information rather than in terms of visual maps. These "songlines" served as mnemonic devices enabling people to remember great expanses of land in minute detail. Ability to recall the exact location of a waterhole could mean the difference between life and death for people walking about in the vast arid spaces of central Australia.[27] We can hypothesize that Ice Age people's sense of space was different from ours, but certain problems in depicting space were the same for Ice Age people as they are for us.

Three Dimensions on a Flat Surface

There is an essential paradox in portraying a three-dimensional world on a two-dimensional surface. Ice Age artists devised a variety of means to attempt to resolve this paradox. As we saw in chapter 1, contour lines are more successful than outlines in suggesting three-dimensional form, and cross-contour lines are most successful. Artists during the Ice Age experimented with shading to mimic the look of real objects. We see shading used expertly in the oldest known cave art, that at Chauvet, in bear and horse heads (fig. 6.38, see illus. p. 62).

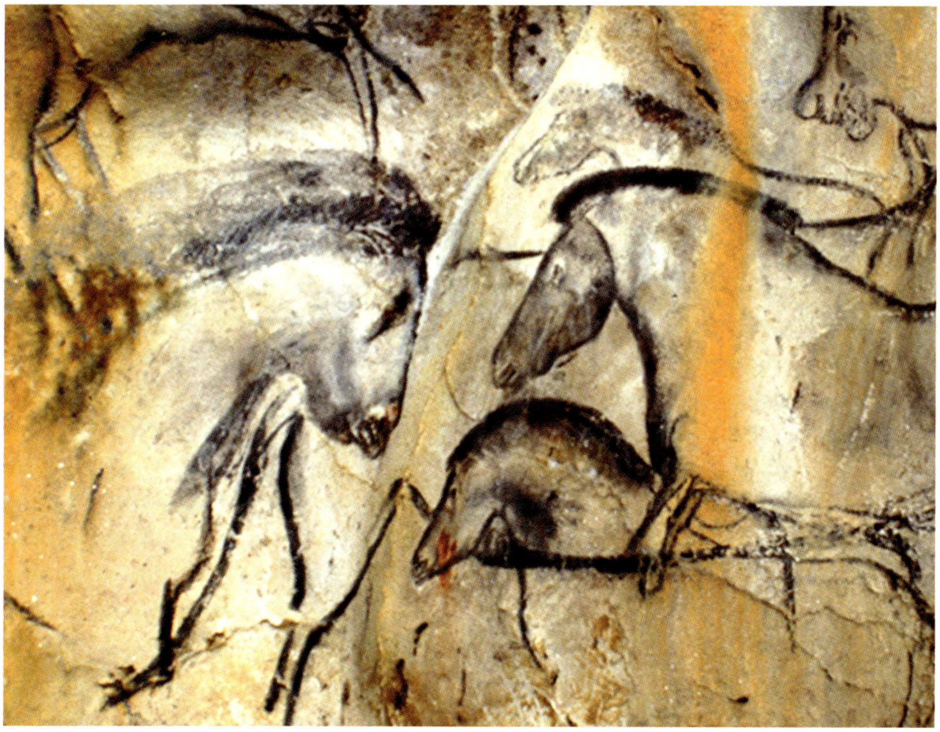

Figure. 6.38. Detail of the horse panel from the Third Chamber at Chauvet. The artist used shading to model the horses' heads and give the illusion of relief. Sections that seem highlighted in white appear to be the underneath surface of the limestone where the yellow ocher outer surface has been scraped away. Three red ocher finger marks have been placed on the head of the lowest horse.

Figure 6.39. One of the "Chinese" horses in the Axial Gallery, Lascaux, so-called because they resemble images of horses from the Han Dynasty. Empty space between leg and body indicates the distance between the near and far legs, a graphic device suggesting foreshortening. Note the striped back, which affirms the relationship of the Ice Age horse to the still extant Przewalski horse.

Although the real world can never be reproduced on a flat surface, the illusion of reality can be created by following certain optical guidelines. It can be observed that things that are closer appear larger and more distinct. To be visually accurate, the two legs on the far side of a quadruped in profile should be made to appear more distant than the two that are nearer to the viewer. An ingenious solution to this problem was devised by one or more Ice Age artists. One clear example of this solution is seen in the depiction of a horse in the Axial Gallery at Lascaux (fig. 6.39, see illus. p. 144). Stencils were used to give a distinct and clean line, especially on the underside of the neck and on the near leg. This line contrasts with the paint on the far leg, which fades gradually and disappears before the far limb joins the body, leaving a bit of empty space between leg and body. The same graphic device was used in the much earlier cave paintings of Chauvet and appears in other sites throughout the Ice Age. It was reinvented tens of thousands of years later by Chinese landscape painters,

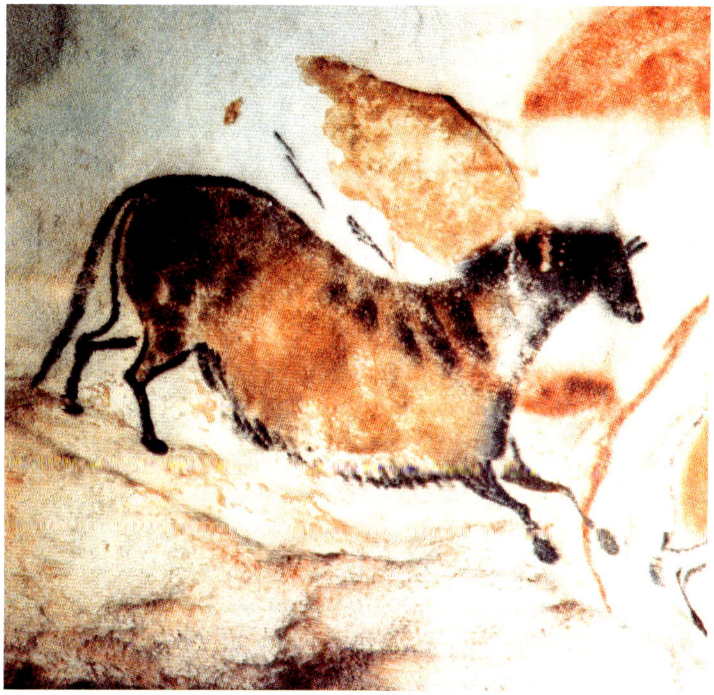

who used what we now call "plane-and-void" to show distance in mountain scenes by leaving white space between one peak and another, more distant one.

Body parts that are farther away appear smaller, a visual illusion called *recession*. This did not present a problem for Ice Age artists in the usual practice of showing quadrupeds in profile, but if an artist wanted to give a figure a look of natural movement, then recession had to be acknowledged. In that case the artist had to deal with foreshortening, which is difficult to do accurately because it is counterintuitive. The first Greek artist to use foreshortening, called *catographia,* was Cimon of Cleonae, around 500 B.C.E. (2,500 B.P.).[28] Paleolithic artists attempted foreshortening 10,000 years earlier. Very occasionally they employed three-quarter views, but a more common solution was what I call the "foldback view." It gives the impression of natural movement while avoiding many of the anatomical problems of true foreshortening. In the foldback view, the artist takes a profile drawing of an animal and folds the head backward. Both head and body are still shown in profile, but they face in opposite directions. This graphic device suggests movement and makes the animal seem more alive, but it does so without the artist's having to undertake the more difficult task of showing the stretched and turned neck with anatomical accuracy.

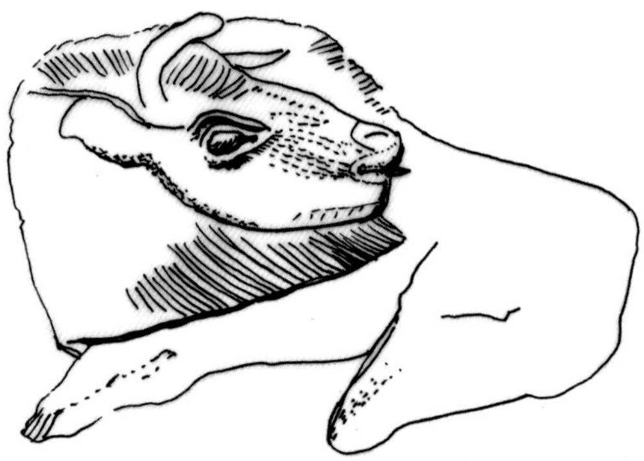

Figure 6.40. Bison from La Madeleine in which use of the "foldback view" conveys motion. 10,5 cm.

The foldback view was used in a sculpture of a bison found at La Madeleine. The head was turned backward, and the animal was further enlivened by showing the tongue extended, licking its flank (fig. 6.40). The foldback view also appears in the half-bison, half-reindeer creature in the panel at Trois Frères (fig. 6.11) and in a stag engraved on an antler baton from Lortet (fig. 6.44). Other examples are a fawn from Bédeilhac (Ariège), a deer from Tito Bustillo, an animal from Covalanas, and another from Abri Murat (Lot). Farther afield, the same device was used on an engraved horse or wild ass in a late Ice Age cave in Levanzo, Italy.

One of the most fascinating drawings in all of Paleolithic art is a boy engraved on a plaquette from La Marche. He may be throwing something, juggling, or, more probably, dancing. His head is in profile, his body close to full frontal (fig. 6.41). His raised left hand has been foreshortened. Hands present one of the greatest difficulties to artists of all periods. Greek artists finally succeeded in foreshortening hands and feet to much acclaim in the fifth century B.C.E. (2,400 B.P.) Yet this Ice Age hand from La Marche, more than 14,000 years old, is shown skillfully foreshortened.

In geographical space, parallel lines appear to converge and to vanish in the distance. It was the emphasis on lines and vanishing points that gave the name *linear perspective* to the set of rules that was to dominate the Western art world for almost 500 years. More frequently known as Renaissance perspective, these rules consist of a scientific, mathematical formulation of optical laws. Although there had been precursors in Greece and Italy, the discovery of the rules of perspective was credited to the artist-engineer Filippo di Ser Brunelleschi, who articulated and demonstrated them in Florence in 1452. By means of sheer observation, Ice Age artists had been able to achieve many of the same results more than 25,000 years earlier.

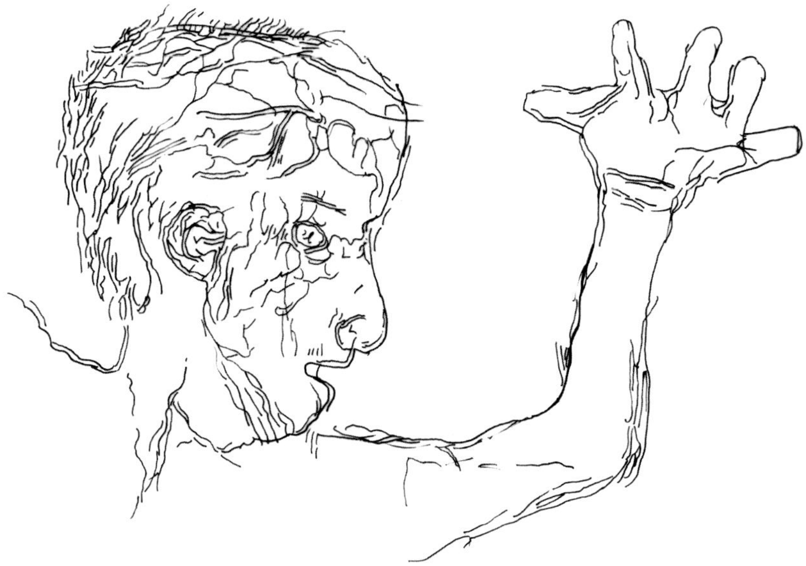

Figure 6.41. Part of drawing from a stone from La Marche, discovered by H. Breuil and analyzed by Léon Pales. Whereas most hands in Ice Age art are schematic, the left hand of this figure is brilliantly foreshortened. (After L. Pales)

Overlap

In order to give the illusion of space when depicting more than one figure, Ice Age artists discovered and used depth cues. One such cue is overlap, which signifies spatial depth because something is occluded by and therefore behind something else. The rearmost figure is partially hidden. It is now so familiar a convention that we forget how disturbing it might once have been to truncate a figure in this way. Overlap was used during the Ice Age, but rarely and with apparent reluctance. On a wall at Lascaux, two bison are painted surging toward the viewer, their hindquarters overlapping. There are also examples on portable pieces. On a baton from El Pendo, two deer heads are overlapped, and on a bone from Mas d'Azil, two bulls are overlapped. Other examples appear on pieces from Teyjat, Isturitz, and Chaffaud (Vienne). But these are exceptions. Almost uniformly, early artists avoided overlap, perhaps seeing in it a kind of amputation.[79]

Ice age artists generally preferred to use transparency, which allowed each of two or more figures to exist, as in a double exposure. An example of the use of transparency by Paleolithic artists is seen in the now familiar spotted horses from Pech-Merle. The composition can be read alternatively with

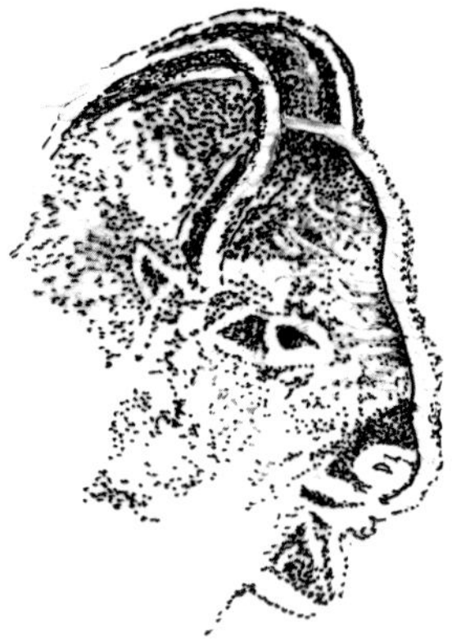

Figure 6.42. Painted and engraved bison head from Trois Frères.

either horse in front. Another example is the bird-headed woman drawn with fingers in clay in the Hall of the Hieroglyphs at Pech-Merle (see fig. 1.8). Transparency enabled both breasts to be shown complete, even though one is behind the other.

Another way to avoid overlap was to use a convention called "twisted perspective," in which horns or antlers were shown frontally even though the animal's head was shown in profile. We see this at La Mouthe (fig. 1.13). The convention is better known in its use by ancient Egyptian artists, but some 12,000 years before Egyptian artists used twisted perspective, Ice Age artists had discovered how to show perspective in a more visually realistic way. At Teyjat, a cow and a bull that we looked at earlier (fig. 1.14) each have the near horn as an *S* shape and the far horn as a *C* shape, a commonly used solution to the problem of horn perspective. This usage is also seen in a magnificent painted and engraved bison head from Trois Frères. Note that the head has been just barely turned toward the viewer to make the positioning of the horns appear more realistic (fig. 6.42).

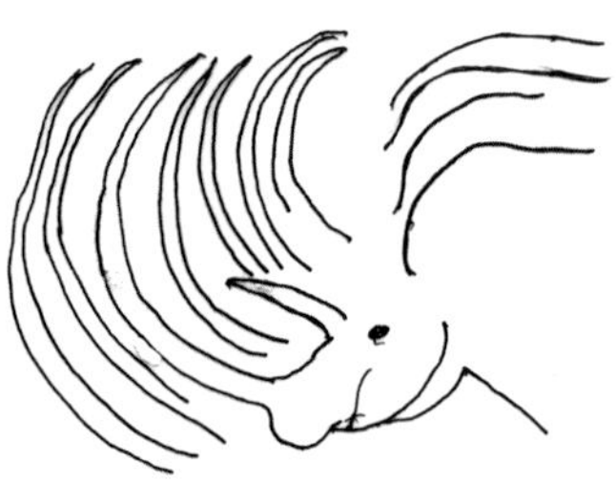

Figure 6.43. Rhinoceroses shown in perspective at Chauvet.

Sometimes artists used conventionalized distortion of the horns. At other times they placed the horns parallel, one above the other. On rare occasions Ice Age artists did use overlap in a limited way. A phalanx of rhinoceroses at Chauvet is placed one behind the other (fig. 6.43). The bodies are overlapped, but their horns are shown one above the other and demonstrate the painter's understanding of perspective, which causes objects to diminish in perceived size as they recede in space. At Lortet, however, an artist with enormous skill and sophistication allowed the near tine of a reindeer's antler to overlap the far one, giving an accurate recording of what was actually perceived from that viewpoint (fig. 6.44).

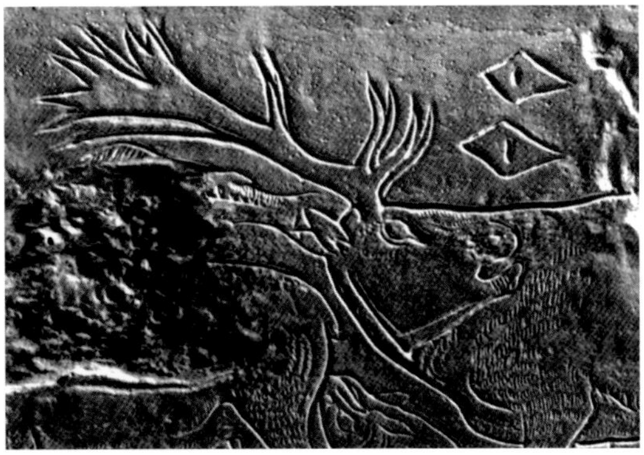

Figure 6.44. Visual realism in a reindeer engraved on a baton from Lortet. The antlers are shown overlapped as they appear to the eye.

Occasionally, strange images arose from the attempt to avoid overlap. An artist at Chauvet painted a large lion over a group of three horses. Superpositioning of this sort was the normal practice in Ice Age art and in much of the rest of the world's rock art as well. But the lion painter seems to have wished to spare the exceptionally beautiful horses and reached a curious compromise with one of them. The line of the feline's stomach crosses behind the head of the horse but over its neck, making it appear that the horse's head is peering out from inside the lion's belly (see fig. 6.38, see illus. p. 62).

The Frieze

One system for organizing figures to suggest their three-dimensional existence in two-dimensional space is by means of processional rows, or friezes. At Lascaux, a frieze extends around the natural rotunda called the Hall of the Bulls. Animal friezes are also found on the rock walls at Chauvet, Cap Blanc, Rouffignac, and many other Ice Age sites, as well as on many pieces of engraved bone or antler. The art historian Charles Bouleau wrote that

> sometimes [the figures] run the whole length of a wall or of several walls, inviting us to follow them; we march beside them, their suggested movement becomes our movement, and the figures succeed one another in time as well as in space. A similar processional format can be seen in the Egyptian frieze, the Panathenaic frieze of the Parthenon, the mosaics in the nave of Apollinare Nuovo. . . . the Bayeux Tapestry, danses macabres, [and] frescoes of Giotto all echo this sequential view of space.[30]

In a frieze, each figure is viewed separately. The earliest artists apparently viewed rows of animals from many individual viewpoints. Probably the artist moved from figure to figure as the work progressed, creating a perspective called "moving focus," in which aspects of a scene are shown sequentially and then assembled in the mind. The modern equivalent is a comic strip. If the artwork is large, like the aurochs at Lascaux or the carvings on the Parthenon, then the viewer, moving from one section to another, re-creates the original movement of the artist. A variation of such spatial organization is seen in the scroll, a form particularly developed in China.[31] In the scroll, as in the frieze, a scene is viewed little by little over time as it is unrolled. Revelations over time involve a thought process different from the compacting of visual experience into a single moment that is the great feat accomplished by what we call Renaissance perspective.

Working in the caves made a necessity of this kind of spatial organization, in which each figure in a group is viewed separately, for in the dark interiors the artists could not have seen the entire grouping all at once, even if they had desired to do so.[32] In Font de Gaume, a 3.5m composition of two reindeer facing each other was placed in a corridor so narrow that it would have been impossible for the artist to step back far enough to see both animals at once.

Abbé Breuil knew the art as intimately as anyone because he spent long days in the caves making sense of the often enigmatic art and then meticulously tracing the images he found. He wrote that in some cases the areas decorated were so inaccessible that he had to draw the art reflected in a mirror and then reverse it to correct for the mirror's reversal. At Altamira an artist had to kneel or squat close to the ceiling in order to paint many of the figures in the Polychrome Chamber. The original floor was so close to the ceiling that it would have been impossible to see clearly more than one animal at a time. Each figure had, of necessity, to exist in its own separate space.

Anamorphism

Anamorphism, from the Greek roots *ana* (again) and *morphoun* (to form), is the process of making an image systematically incorrect so that under specific circumstances it will appear correct. Because of the inaccessibility of some of their selected surfaces, Ice Age artists often worked in such awkward positions that the images had to appear distorted to them in order, paradoxically, to appear correct from the anticipated viewing point. In addition, the surfaces themselves were often so irregular that the artists had to compensate by distorting the figures so that they might appear normal. It is almost impossible to show photographs of anamorphic examples because, depending on the camera position, the images will appear normal or distorted but will give no sense of how moving in one or another direction magically changes them.

For example, the bulls on the right side of the Rotunda at Lascaux are larger than those on the left, probably because they are farther away from the place where the viewer was expected to stand. By making them larger, the artist gave them the appearance of being the same size as the nearer bulls on the left. In another example at Lascaux, the legs and tail of the "red cow with a black collar" are unusually long in comparison with those of the animals surrounding it. The legs and tail were painted on a receding surface, so they are actually farther back than the body of the cow and, if not effectively enlarged, might have appeared to be too small for the body.[33] An aurochs in the Rotunda at Lascaux has one unusually elongated front leg, which appears to be of normal size when viewed from the entrance of the hall.[34] The use of anamorphism in a bison at Bédeilhac was mentioned by both Abbé Breuil and the archaeologist Annette Leroi-Gourhan. Another bison example at Pech-Merle was brought to my attention by Norbert Aujoulat. Also at Pech-Merle, Eric Teyssedou pointed out a bear that, viewed from another angle, becomes a horse. A horse at Ebbou is another likely example.

The science writer John Pfeiffer described an experience he had at the cave of Tito Bustillo in Spain, where a large red horse outlined in black appeared distorted because its head and neck were severely elongated. When he commented on this to Mouré Romanillo, the archaeologist excavating the cave, he was told to lie on his back beneath an overhanging ledge. When viewed from this position, Pfeiffer said, the image was transformed into a correctly proportioned horse (fig. 6.45).[35]

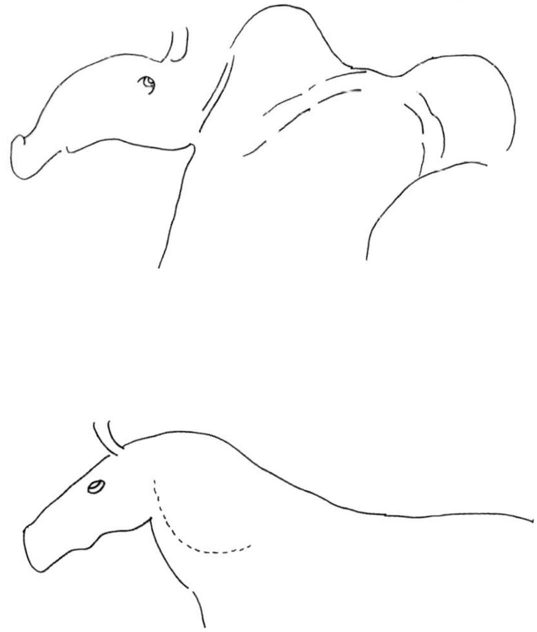

Figure 6.45. Anamorphic horse at Tito Bustillo. Above viewed from where artist probably stood, below viewed from special specified position.

Anamorphism has been known in Western art at least since the Renaissance. Artists of that time played with the newly articulated rules of optical perspective to achieve deliberate distortions that could be resolved only by viewing a painting from a certain angle. Leonardo da Vinci made the earliest known Western anamorphic drawings—a child's face and an eye. For his patron, François I of France, he made an anamorphic painting, now lost, of a dragon battling a lion.

In the sixteenth century, anamorphism in paintings became more frequent in northern Europe. One of the most famous is the painting by Hans Holbein the Younger called *The Ambassadors*. In the foreground a strange shape like some space-age disc seems to intrude into the picture. When viewed from the upper right at a specified angle, this shape is discovered to be a human skull. Chinese artists also toyed with anamorphic perspective; they achieved it with the use of distorting mirrors to create and then decode the picture. We can deduce a certain levity on the part of these artists, because virtually all their pictures are pornographic.

Perspective boxes were developed in the seventeenth century. Images examined from the open end of the box appeared incomprehensible, but they became normal when viewed through a specially placed peephole. A similar anamorphic device has been used by the contemporary Swiss sculptor Markus Raetz. In at least two of his pieces, twigs are suspended on strings, producing what appears to be an unmoving mobile, but the point of the sculpture is actually its shadow. When the light source is positioned correctly, the shadow duplicates a famous Matisse drawing of a reclining nude. Raetz made a similar piece whose shadow gives the illusion of a drawing of the head of Mickey Mouse.

Because Ice Age artists had long experience painting on irregular surfaces and adjusting their images accordingly, it seems reasonable that they were able to discover and produce anamorphic effects even without the knowledge of optical rules or the assistance of mirrors. All these examples and many others suggest that the earliest artists struggled to create on bone and stone illusions of their visual experiences. Perhaps not again until Classical Greece and, most significantly, the European Renaissance were artists so concerned with producing a construct to parallel the perceived appearance of visual sensation.

As people moved from a migratory hunter-gatherer existence into more settled Neolithic communities, it appears that their sense of space changed. An attempt to deal with surrounding space—what we now call landscape—dates as far back as 8,000 years ago. On a wall at Çatal Hüyük in Anatolia is a unique landscape painting, a bird's-eye view of a group of rectilinear houses with an erupting volcano in profile behind them. By 3,000 years later, in Egypt, depiction of fields and marshes was common. Instead of the unspecified space of the Ice Age, the space Egyptian artists were concerned with was specific and contained. The ultimate containment was achieved with linear perspective in the Italian Renaissance. It may be no coincidence that it was devised by architects such as Bramante and Alberti, who were trained to contain people in circumscribed spaces. That containment is not unlike the solution of linear perspective, in which the viewer's eye is directed into an implied space framed like a window.[36] Objects and figures, previously scattered, could now be coordinated and located in the virtual space extending on the other side of the picture frame. The seemingly unruly space of the Ice Age artists had been controlled and confined, perhaps paralleling what people were doing to control and contain the land itself.

Motion

Everything moves, everything runs. . . . Owing to the persistence of images on the retina, objects in motion are multiplied and distorted. . . . Thus a galloping horse has not four legs: it has twenty.

—UMBERTO BOCCIONI, "Futurist Manifesto"

Motion is another aspect of space. It is a paradox that movement and shape cannot be seen at the same time. This is because the eye uses larger sweeps to see movement and smaller scans to analyze the details of shape. Each kind of information uses different receptors.[37] It is a further paradox that artists attempt to show motion by means of fixed lines on a stationary surface. In the Ice Age caves, the flickering light of the lamps might have helped to give an illusion of motion. When a lamp is carried, the angle of viewing changes, and lines visible at one moment disappear as new lines appear. Moreover, the irregularity of the stone surface causes endless distortions and corrections. Figures emerge from the multitude of engraved lines; in a moment they disappear, and new figures emerge and recede.

In Ice Age Europe, artists depicted many figures with multiple legs, heads, and tails. For example, a wild boar painted in polychrome on a wall at Altamira has eight legs (fig. 6.46). Other examples can be seen at Les Combarelles, Lascaux, Trois Frères, Limeuil and Chauvet. One explanation relates these multiple limbs to shamanism. Another finds them to be an accepted convention for suggesting motion. By lambent torchlight, viewers see first one set of legs and then another, or one head and then another, in quick succession, receiving the impression that the legs, heads, and tails are moving.

Aboriginal artists in the Americas may have used the same means to show motion. The Kwakiutl of the Northwest Coast depicted a wolf with two tails. At Zuñi there is a petroglyph of a mountain lion with five legs. A Ute petroglyph of a horse and rider shows a horse with nine legs (fig. 6.47). In prehistoric African art, the aboriginal San, especially in the southeastern mountains of what is now South Africa, often portrayed figures with extra limbs.[38]

Another convention invented during the Paleolithic and more commonly used by later cultures was an exaggeration of spread legs to give a sense of frantic motion. At Lascaux, both the "fleeing horse" and, opposite it, the "leaping cow" display this graphic convention, which has been called the "flying leap." A horse at Altamira is another good example (fig. 6.48). San artists used the same device much later, calling it *run-run* (fig. 6.49).

Ice Age artists also devised a way to show prancing motion. One sees it at El Portel and El Buxú, where animals' back legs are extended and their front legs are bent forward. An even more sophisticated analysis of a galloping horse is seen on a schist plaque from Paloma, Asturias. There appear to be two horses on it, one behind or within the other. The front legs are bent backward and the hind legs are bent forward—an accurate depiction of a running horse. Ann Sieveking has pointed out that the movement of the horse was misunderstood in subsequent Western art and not rediscovered until the work of the photographer Eadweard Muybridge in the nineteenth century.

Efforts to animate figures are evident in prehistoric art all over the world. During the Ice Age, an artist at Trois Frères engraved a little reindeer with one leg raised in an animated position that suggests the animal is preparing to lie down or perhaps to burst forward (fig. 6.50). Appearance of motion has been attempted not only in two-dimensional work but also in sculpted pieces. The

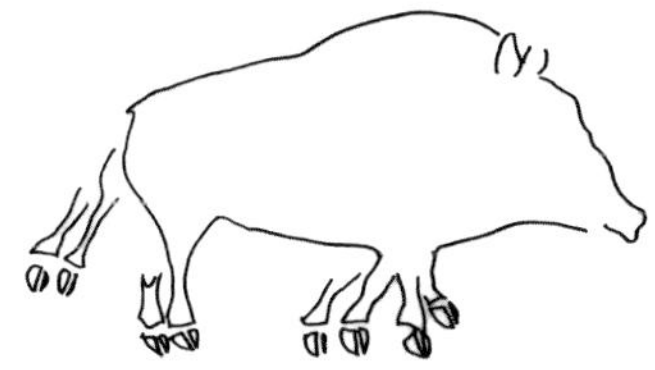

Figure 6.46. Painted boar with eight legs on the ceiling of Altamira.

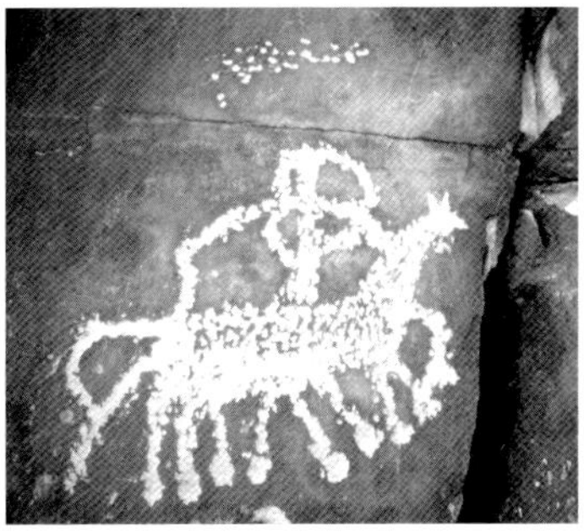

Figure 6.47. Ute petroglyph of a horse with nine legs, Shivano Valley, Colorado.

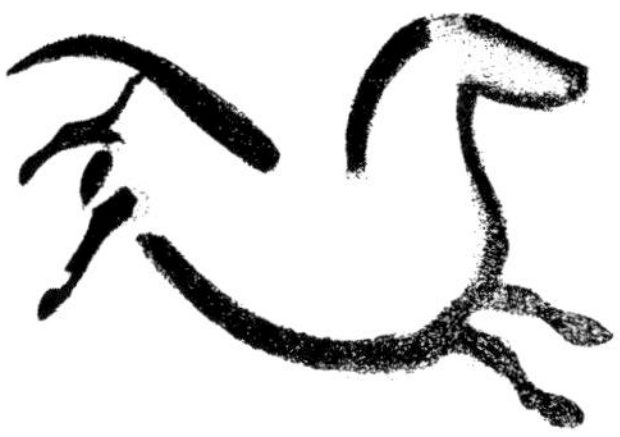

Figure 6.48. Horse in "flying leap," Altamira. 1.8 m.

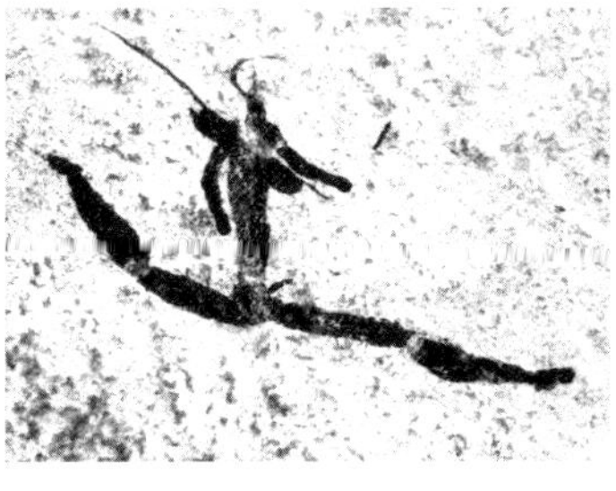

Figure 6.49. San pictograph depicting the *run-run* graphic device.

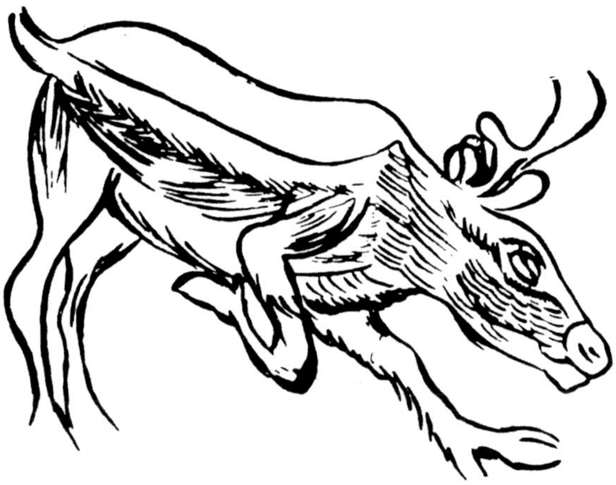

Figure 6.50. Reindeer with one leg raised in an animated position, Trois Frères.

Kwakiutl made puppets that were moved by pulling a string. On the other side of the world, at sites of the Indus Valley civilization, dated to about 4,000 years ago, archaeologists have unearthed one of the earliest known toys, a small clay animal whose head had been attached to its body by means of a string. When a child pulled the string, the head nodded. Similar toys are still used in the area. Motion or the appearance of motion makes a figure come to life.

At various times in the subsequent history of art, the depiction of motion assumed paramount importance. Artists such as Muybridge in his photography and Marcel Duchamp in paintings such as *Nude Descending a Staircase* devoted much of their effort to this goal, and for artists such as Boccioni and Balla in the Italian futurist group, it was a near obsession.

The Eye, the Brain, and the Movies

The art of the Ice Age caves, seen by the light of small lamps, did not reveal itself all at once. The viewer moved past sections of the cave wall, around protuberances, and into recesses and culs-de-sac. Some of the images in cave art can be seen in their entirety only if the viewer is in motion. One example is the falling horse in the Axial Gallery at Lascaux The upper part of the horse is on one side of a stone outcrop. The body then wraps around this rocky projection so that the lower half ends up on the other side of the outcrop almost exactly 180 degrees from the upper half. It is as if the image were on a canvas and that canvas were twisted like a towel. The viewer holds the partial image in mind while moving around it to complete the image. We do this naturally and effortlessly because in our minds a visual stimulus can remain clearly visible for 10 seconds after we have first seen it.

The falling horse of Lascaux cannot be captured on film except by a motion picture camera, because to see it whole one has to move around the column on which it is painted, as only a motion picture camera can do. When movie film is projected, individual frames are separated by spaces of between half a second and a tenth of a second. At this speed, we are unaware of seeing discrete images. We have the illusion of continuous vision. If the frames are slightly different from one another, we have the illusion of motion. In modern movies, 24 frames per second are presented to the viewer, and in television, 30 frames per second.[39]

The process of movie making may be more like our actual visual process than is still photography. It is part of the nature of our perception that our eyes are in continuous movement. They make rapid motions, almost tremors, known as saccades, and larger, slower motions known as sweeps. At only one tiny spot on the retina, called the fovea, can we resolve an image with clarity, and that is because of the density of receptor cells there—200,000 for each square millimeter. Our eyes must move continuously across the field of vision so that the foveal point receives information from every part of that field. Although we are unaware of it, our restless eyes focus on no one thing for long. And in the same way that movie film consists of a sequence of still shots, we assemble our multiple views to form what is essentially a collage of images viewed over time. The profusion of visual data that has been processed in bits and pieces in many different sites in the brain comes together and is assembled to form an informational map. All this information gives the viewer the feeling of viewing a picture even though no picture is involved. Seeing is an externally and internally active process. The movie picture, like the process of seeing itself, is a collage composed of many bits.[40]

Cubism

The problem is now to pass, to go around the object, and give a plastic expression to the result. . . . All of this is my struggle to break with the two dimensional aspect.

—PABLO PICASSO

A paradoxical limitation of visual realism on a two-dimensional surface is that the more artists limit themselves to what is seen from one position at one moment, the less can be shown about the other side, the unseen part of the figure. Sometimes artists have attempted to resolve this dilemma. A number of Ice Age examples appear to show two views of one animal's head in the same engraving. A particularly enigmatic example, a drawing in charcoal, was made in the Salon Noir at Niaux (fig. 6.51). The archaeologist Denis Vialou said that it "evokes cubist drawings."[41] The head of a bison with a barely suggested mane is superimposed on another, fully realized bison. The effect is that of one animal with its head in two positions. The artist may not originally have intended the two heads to appear to belong to one animal, but the final effect would have been as apparent to the Ice Age artist as it is to us and the artist chose not to change that effect, which could have been easily accomplished by drawing the body of the right-facing animal. An American Indian from the ancestral Pueblo period attempted to deal with this limitation by creating an

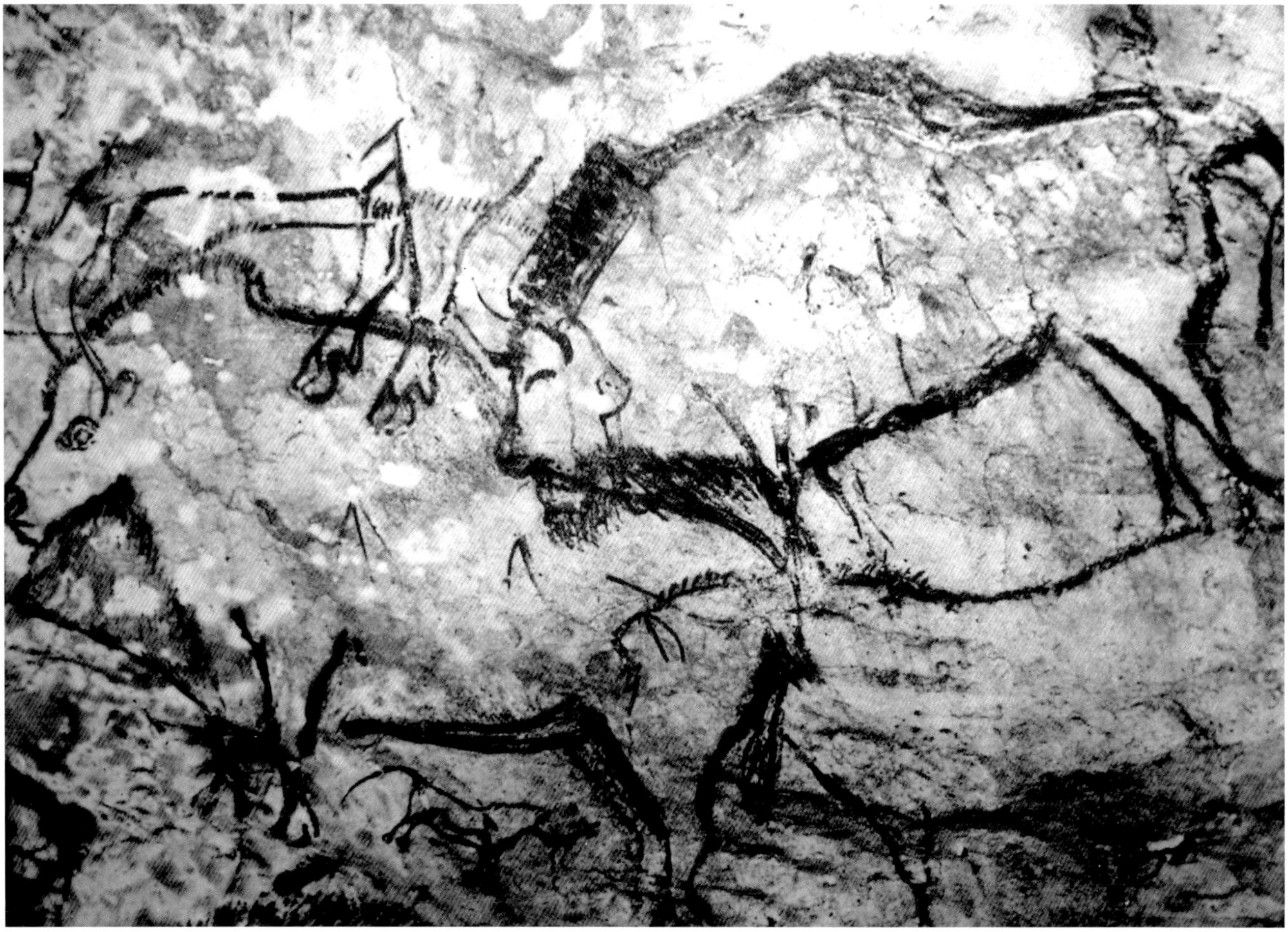

Figure 6.51. Bison with folded or overlapped heads drawn in black charcoal in the Salon Noir, Niaux 1.27 m. CNP-MCC

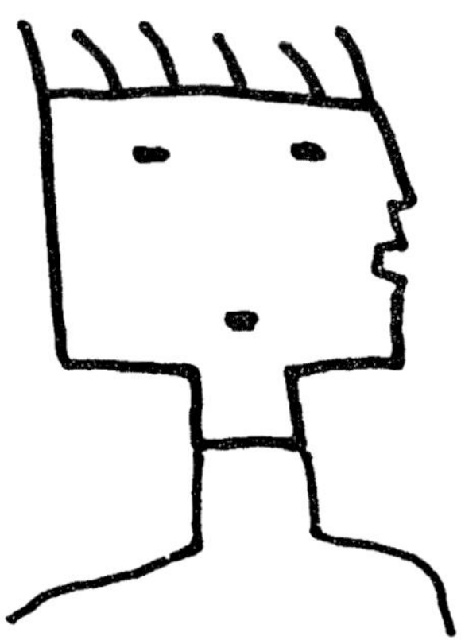

Figure 6.52. Ancestral Pueblo face, front and side views, La Bajada, New Mexico.

unusual face or mask with frontal and profile views shown simultaneously (fig. 6.52). So the solution adopted by Braque and Picasso in the cubist movement was deliberate but not unique. An example from Picasso's notebook of 1946 shows this graphic device, which was later used in many of his cubist portraits (fig. 6.53).

When we speak of portraits, we have seen that there are individual cells in the brain's fusiform gyrus, called face neurons, that respond to individual faces. Some of them are so specific that they fire only to particular views of particular faces—for example, only to a full face or to a profile. But that poses the question of how we recognize the same person in differing views. Fortunately, there are other neurons that respond to all the possible views of an individual face. One of the achievements of Cubism was to give graphic expression to this cognitive capability.[42]

The Cubists were concerned with an overarching conceptual problem: the representation of three-dimensional reality on a flat surface. Picasso would walk around the favored subject, generally a seated figure or a still life, and then collate a number of views.[43] Recently, the painter David Hockney, who has been obsessed with problems of depicting space in photo collages, discussed the way he dealt with space in his painted landscapes, particularly one called *The Road across the Wolds*. He spoke of using another form of perambulation: “The space is utterly impossible, but it is possible through time—you are moving through time driving in an open car.”[44] Walking has been superseded by the automobile, but in this new possibility of locomotion, artists are still dealing with the same problems the earliest artists first recognized and puzzled over.

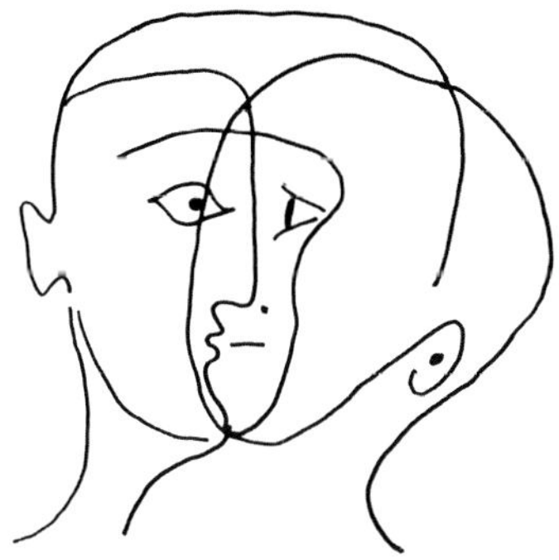

Figure 6.53 After early Cubist sketch by Picasso.

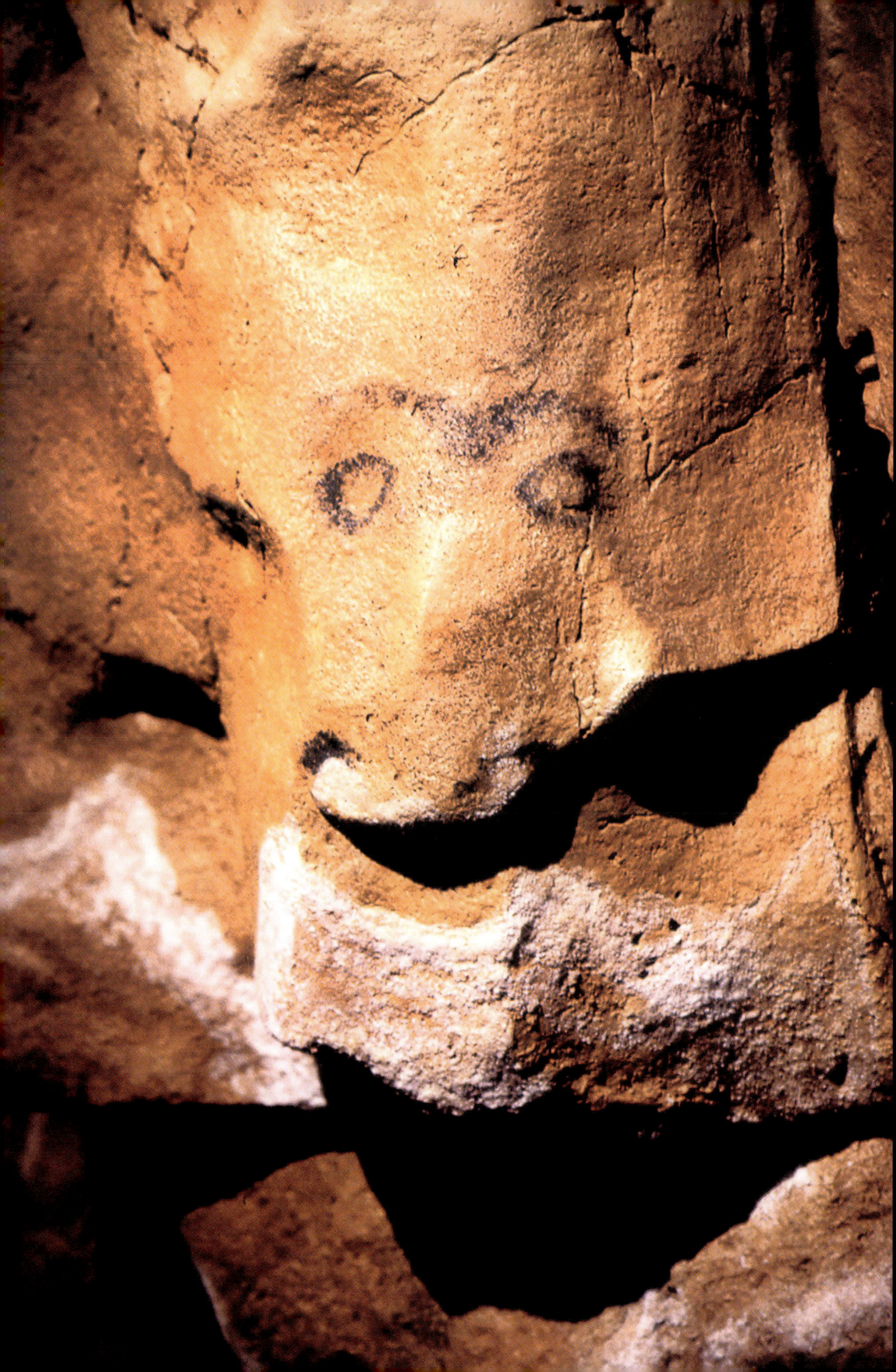

After the difficult entry into the cave of Tuc d'Audoubert, one traverses a long passage to reach the chamber with the clay bison described in chapter 3. When I visited the cave, I saw along the way bones and skulls of cave bears, which were probably already extinct by the time the Ice Age explorers found them. The bones appeared to have been rearranged, and most of the canine teeth were removed from the skulls to be used for jewelry. Stalactites had been broken off and set down. On the muddy floor I saw human footprints preserved exactly as they had been originally found. On a small ledge were the little footprints of a child about three or four years old, toes clenched in preparation for a jump.

Count Robert Bégouën, the owner of the cave, believes that some of the marks left on the clay floor may be indications of game playing. Near the end of the cave, in a small side chamber with a very low ceiling—three to five feet high—are some 50 heel prints made apparently by children or adolescents. Bégouën has speculated that these unusual prints were made as part of a ceremony or game.[1] Nearby is a large hole from which someone took the clay used to make the sculpture of the two clay bison. To the left of the hole, lying within a heel print and therefore made after the ceremony or game, are two coils of clay that some prehistorians have called phalluses. But they could as likely be rejected beginnings of the bison's horns. It seems to me even more likely that these coils represent nothing more than someone's having prepared the clay by rolling it into workable pieces, just as a contemporary artist working with clay would do today.

Next to the coils is a small arrangement of shards of delicate stalactite or stalagmite spikes. Although this construction has not been much discussed in

Opposite: Face or Mask from the 'Horse's Tail' at Altamira makes use of the natural formation of limestone. Eyes and brows and parts of nostrils are drawn in red ocher. Photo by P.A. Saura Ramos. ©Museo de Altamira

the description of the caves, I find it of enormous interest. It is hard not to surmise that it represents an example of creative play devised by some child, adolescent, or adult. This crystallized construction, made of debris found in the area, is very likely the first example of the thought process involved in making sculptural constructions from found objects. It is an example of the activity of *Homo ludens.*

HOMO LUDENS

La peinture est un jeu d'esprit.
—PABLO PICASSO

The Latin word *ludens* has no adequate translation in English, involving as it does not so much play as a sense of playfulness. The ludic sense was described by John Dewey as a state of mind. Johan Huizinga's book *Homo Ludens* is an early important work devoted entirely to this subject.[2] The ludic sense may be thought of as a freewheeling, pleasurable, exploratory state of mind that manifests itself in game playing, inventiveness, humor, and creative activity in general.[3]

For the archetypal artist Picasso, art was a serious, even subversive play. Françoise Gilot, who lived with him and viewed him as closely as anyone, wrote analytically about his creative powers: "There was something special about his creative spirit which could remain ablaze only with playful attitudes and gratuitous games."[4] Max Beckmann, the dour and bitter twentieth-century German painter, unexpectedly described a game-playing element in his own work. Art, he said, "is a game and a good game at least for me; one of the few games which make life, difficult and depressing as it is sometimes, a little more interesting."[5] Maurits Escher played an almost Mephistophelian game with the laws of nature to create his highly cerebral art: "My subjects are often also playful. I can't keep from fooling around with our irrefutable certainties. It is, for example, a pleasure to knowingly mix up two- and three-dimensionality, flat and spatial, and to make fun of gravity."[6]

The ludic spirit unleashes creativity not only in the arts but also in science. This state of mind has been an important catalyst for the release of insights in scientific research and has enabled scientists to reach solutions to previously insoluble problems. Albert Einstein mentioned the link between playfulness and creative scientific thought: "But taken from a psychological viewpoint, this combinatory play [using signs and images] appears to be the essential feature in productive thought."[7] A most ludic contemporary physicist, Richard Feynman, wrote about a malaise he experienced at a certain time of his life, a sort of scientist's block: "Physics disgusts me a little bit now, but I used to enjoy doing physics. Why did I enjoy it? I used to play with it. . . . So I got this new attitude. Now that I am burned out and I'll never accomplish anything . . . I'm going to play with physics, whenever I want to, without worrying about any importance whatsoever."[8]

One day in the cafeteria at Cornell University, Feynman saw someone throw a plate into the air. The plate's trajectory interested him. His lighthearted response was nevertheless that of a physicist. He worked out an equation to explain the wobbles of the plate as it flew through the air. Then he realized that the equation could relate as well to the movement of the orbits of electrons. The equation ultimately made an important contribution to the study of particle physics. Feynman later explained how his playful attitude freed him and turned on a veritable stream of creativity: "It was effortless. It was easy to play with these things . . . everything flowed out effortlessly. I almost tried to resist it! There was no importance to what I was doing, but ultimately there was. The diagrams and the whole business that I got the Nobel Prize from came from that piddling around with the wobbling plate."[9]

Playfulness and curiosity seem to be associated primarily with the higher mammals. Some birds such as corvids and parrots appear to play, but that is exceptional. For young mammals such as dogs, cats, wolves, and lions, play seems to serve some vital function in social development relating to future adult activities such as mating and hunting. Young chimps are as curious and playful as human children. We may be surprised to learn that mother gorillas play peek-a-boo with their babies much the way human mothers do. But play, even in these animals who are so like us in many ways, diminishes or stops as they age. Occasionally adult mammals demonstrate such behaviors, but by and large *Homo sapiens sapiens* is the only animal that continues to be playful throughout adulthood. This is another example of our neoteny, the process by which childlike mammalian attributes are prolonged into maturity.

Play is energy costly. Therefore it must be valuable. Nature, though seemingly profligate in some areas, in reality seems to be frugal with energy and material. Many researchers, including the animal behaviorist John Byers, believe that games and play stimulate brain fiber formation.[10] If so, play and games would encourage neurons to sprout large numbers of axons and dendrites. Such growth is vital in the early years of development for many animals and is more important in large-brained species, for which development goes on over a much longer period.

The ludic state of mind induces creativity. Robert Fagen, an authority on cognitive play, acknowledges this relationship: "By some unspecified mechanism the cognitive processes of transformation, abstraction and innovation involved in . . . animal play are hypothesized to propel human artistic activity, paradoxically recombining experience and creating novel forms of expression."[11]

Thoughts occur with the reception and transmission of electrical charges in the brain. Chemically induced electrical charges travel from one cell to another by means of changes in the electrical potential of individual nerve cells. The nerve impulses are carried from one nerve cell to another over the minute space between them—the synaptic cleft—and ferried over the gap by chemicals called neurotransmitters. Neuroscientists tell us that when we learn we are forging new synaptic pathways and that each time we use these connections they become more accessible, which explains why learning requires repetition. It may be that in a ludic mode we ignore the old pathways, causing our neurons to flail about for new connections. Exploration of this kind takes us to unexpected regions, yielding surprising results and, often, creative discoveries.

With these new discoveries we may sense the mental jolts that accompany them, and we may experience the consummate thrill of inspiration. Ludic-inspired activity seems to be related to one of the oldest parts of our brain, the limbic lobes, which are associated with our emotions. The involvement of ludic play and creativity with our limbic system may help to explain why the process itself can be so intensely pleasurable. The most recently evolved part of the limbic system is the cingulate gyrus; scientists have found that when it is destroyed, an animal is no longer playful.[12]

The archaeologists B. Spencer and F. J. Gillen reported that Aborigines in central Australia called their secular art "play-work."[13] This is a cogent description of the art-making process. To say that making art is exhilarating does not mean that art comes without effort. Long periods of study may be required to become sufficiently skilled. In some Ice Age caves, such as Niaux, it appears that an apprentice worked side by side with a master. Apprentices or other assistants would have had to learn to make tools as well as to use them. They would have had to learn to prepare pigments, some of which appear to have required complex formulas. Entering caves was difficult, and beginners would have had to learn to negotiate the dangerous areas. Some of the art appears to have required the artist to stand for long periods on rocky outcrops, perched precariously at dizzying heights. In some cases we cannot fathom how the artist ever reached the place chosen to be worked. In other cases the artist was forced to lie in a cramped position on the cold, damp cave floor. It seems that the artists sometimes sought out the most inaccessible spaces, almost as if it were a challenge to find ever more forbidding surfaces to work.

There were more than physical challenges. Artists had to sustain strong mental concentration for the time required to complete what were, in some instances, huge, mural-size paintings or large, complex carvings. A remarkable level of self-discipline and a capacity for intellectual focus is evident. Creativity, expressed in art making, could often be hard work physically, but it was always mentally demanding.

CREATIVE HUMOR

Ha-ha and ah-ha are related.

—DEL CLOSE

A firm relationship appears to link creativity with wit and humor. We see this linguistically in the similarity between the natural expletives *ah-ha* and *ha-ha.* Scholars of humor (itself a humorous idea) agree that incongruity is the essence of humor. Schopenhauer wrote: "The cause of laughter in every case is simply the sudden perception of the incongruity between a concept and the real object."[14] It may not always result in a laugh, but there must be a collision of two ideas that results in a conceptual shift. Henri Bergson, in his analysis of humor *Le rire,* wrote about this collision, which he called "reciprocal interference": "A situation is always funny when it belongs at the same time to two absolutely independent series of events and can be interpreted at the same time in two different ways."[15] Arthur Koestler called the same phenomenon "double association."[16] My infant granddaughter, Madeleine, must have realized this before she could speak when, with a devilish look for my reaction, she placed the nipple of her bottle in her ear. In earlier chapters we saw examples of visual double association; the result is visual wit or visual puns. We might call our reaction to many of the optical illusions we looked at "double takes," or the perception of double entendres. We saw this duality of interpretation as we switched back and forth from figure to ground, concave to convex, and rightside-up to inverted, and as we looked at spatially ambiguous, "cohabiting" figures. We experienced double takes when things that seemed mimetically real were proved to be false. Our minds looked at objects in their original form and then in their new incarnations as found objects or as the results of closure or projection. Exaggeration is the basis of caricature and cartooning, a notorious source of humor. In this case, the humor is based on a mental comparison

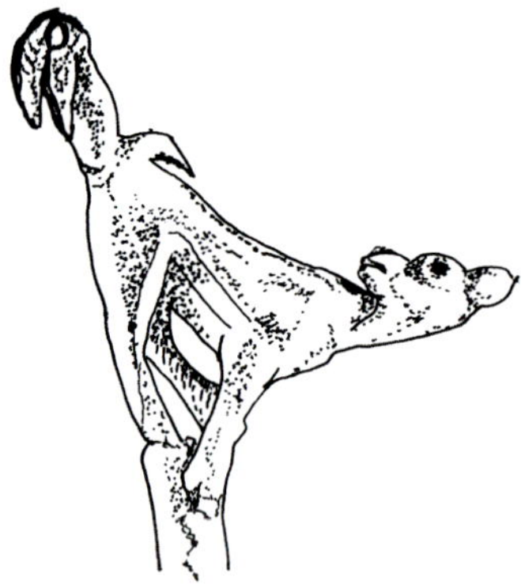

Figure 7.1. The "bird-turd" spear thrower from Mas d'Azil.

between the original and its exaggeration and on the fact that the original can still be recognized in the new version, despite the artist's editorial comment.

We cannot be certain that our reactions to the Ice Age drawings that appear to us as caricatures are the same as those of the artists who drew them. We cannot be sure that they elicited the same sense of irony, but we do know that caricature has a long history. Our reactions range from surprise to amusement, from a titter to a burst of laughter. It is hard not to think that the artist was being witty in one carving from Mas d'Azil. The sculpture forms the end of a spear thrower. A fawn, with head turned backward, is regarding its tail. Feces emerge from under the tail, and a bird is perched on them, no doubt assessing their dietary potential. Archaeologists refer to the subject matter as "bird-turd" (fig. 7.1). Ten similar pieces have been found despite the inevitable destruction of artifacts over so vast a time. This suggests that there were many such examples and the subject was popular. We can assume that its wit appealed to Ice Age people for the same reason it appeals to us now. And it may be relevant to mention that humor based on scatology is one of the first and most enduring sources of infant, child, and even adult humor.

THE MIND'S EYE

To be an artist is not a matter of making paintings or objects at all. What we are really dealing with is the state of our consciousness and the shape of our perception.

—ROBERT IRWIN

Gatherers and hunters survived by their skills of perception. We know, through their art, that these earliest artists scrutinized the world intently. We saw earlier how precise their observation was in the engraving of the antlered reindeer head on the baton from Lortet. That head was a detail from the larger scene engraved on the baton. Made from a piece of antler, it is a tour de force in which the artist envisaged an entire scene consisting of two reindeer crossing a stream with salmon swimming between their legs. The artist engraved the scene on the cylindrical tine in such a way as to cause no distortion or overlap. Because it was impossible for the artist to have viewed the whole engraving at one time, it was first imaged in the mind's eye and then adapted to the long, thin antler (fig. 7.2).

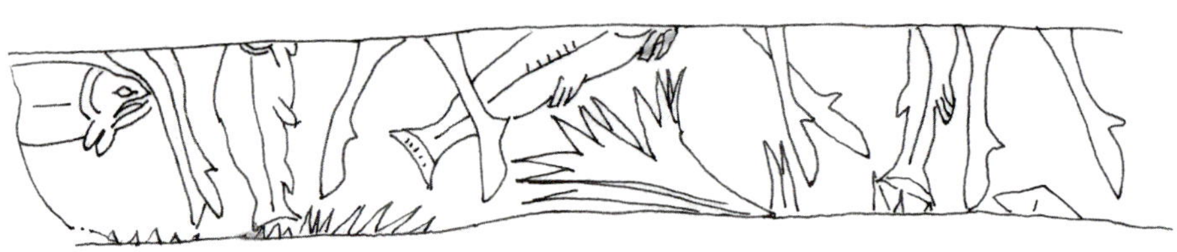

Figure 7.2. One view of a scene on a reindeer antler baton. Engraving goes completely around the antler. Each end is broken.

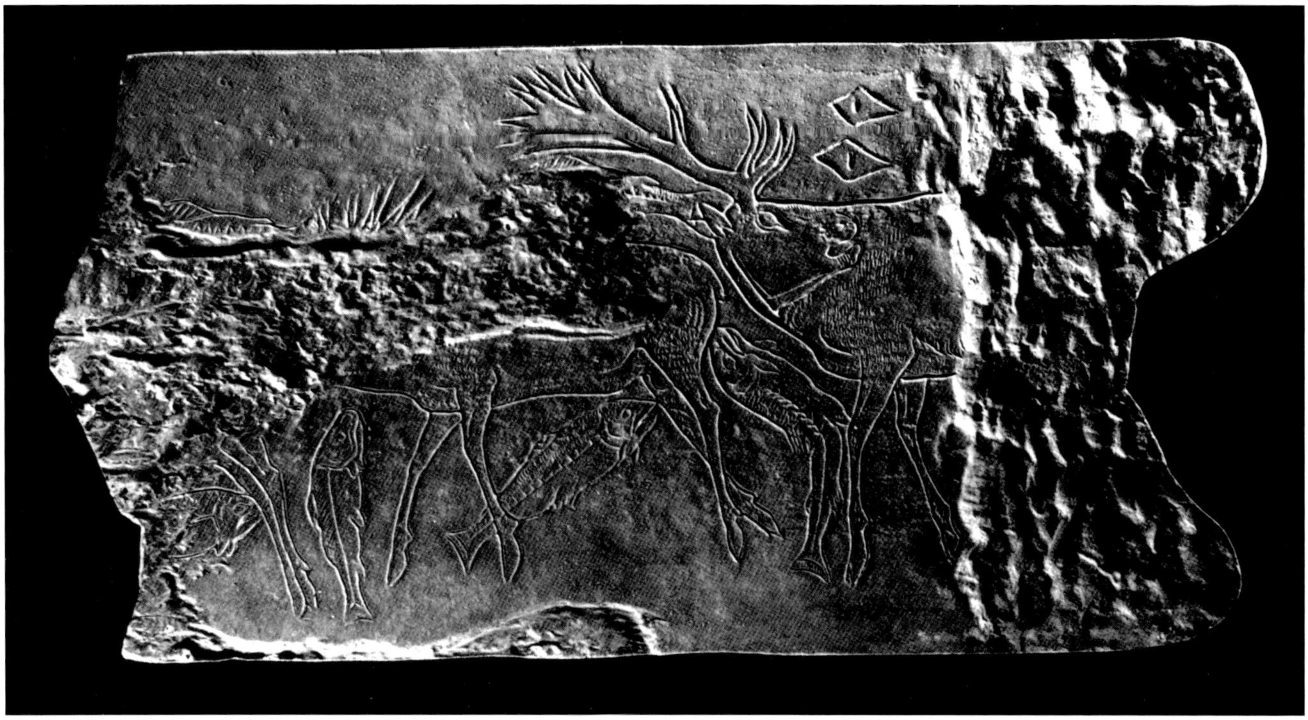

After the piece was found in modern times, it was rolled out onto a plasterlike substance to make a negative in which the engraved lines were raised rather than incised. This cast was imprinted on another substance, reproducing the original intaglio, shown here (fig. 7.3). The scene that emerged is aesthetically astounding in its accurate use of perspective, its visual realism, and its complex composition. The artist observed the texture of the coats of the deer and even the detail of the part of the eye where the tear duct is located. We are shown, in one instance, a salmon's skeleton in a kind of x-ray view, and in another, the scales on its skin (fig. 7.4). Ice Age artists had the inventiveness to seek graphic solutions that would replicate their perception. The English painter Francis Bacon wrote: "Real imagination is technical imagination. . . . it is the search for the technique to trap the object at a given moment."[17] These first known artists applied their intelligence and imaginations to a search for techniques.

Figure 7.3. The Lortet antler baton. Photograph of one of the rollouts of the scene on the antler. The reindeer in front is very eroded, so that only the rump and legs are clear. Photo: L. Hamon. © MAN de Saint-Germain-en-Laye.

Figure 7.4. Salmon, detail from the Lortet antler.

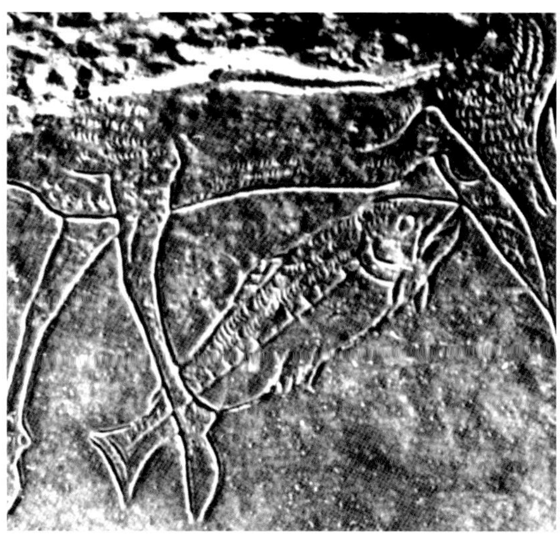

We have seen that Ice Age artists found all the techniques I have discussed in this book: outline, contour line, cross-contour line, parallel hatching, cross hatching, cameo and intaglio marking, smudging, shading, overlapping, stenciling and imprinting. They also discovered foreshortening, use of friezes and use of plane and void perspective. In sculpture they did carving in relief and in the round, champlevé carving, piercing for beads and pendants, modeling in clay and even, in at least one area, kiln firing of clay figures. Ice Age artists made early forays into what would later be called Pointillism, Cubism, and Surrealism. These inventions were not unique to Ice Age artists and did not end with them. When, in subsequent periods, artists wanted once again to depict the reality they saw, they would reinvent the same techniques. I use the term *reinvent* because Ice Age art was hidden and unknown until the nineteenth century. An understanding of Ice Age art-making techniques was only gradually revealed in the twentieth century. These techniques are now staples in the tradition of art-making up to the present.

The artists derived their images from what they were seeing or had seen. There are two different ways of recording reality. Artists who draw directly from life make a record at the moment of perception. The electromagnetic stimuli reaching the senses are translated into a graphic surrogate almost simultaneously with the act of visual perception. Alternatively, artists may work from memory. The deep caves were difficult of access and far removed from the animals that were depicted. It would have been difficult, if not impossible, to bring animals into the caves as models. One might think that the high-relief clay sculpture of the two bison at Tuc d'Audoubert required the information provided by models. But the thought of bringing animal models into this cave is ludicrous. Moreover, as hunters, these people knew the animals literally inside-out. After all, they cut them up or saw them cut up shortly after the kill.

Much of what these artists saw was evanescent, but some images were selected to be stored in the temporal lobes of their brains. Neuroscientists tell us that internally generated images are continually being evoked and compared with new ones. The neurologist Adam Zeman described this process vividly: "New experience always percolates through old, leaving a hint of its flavor as it passes."[18] Remembered images are often powerful, for they activate the cortex in a similar way and with almost the same intensity as the original perception itself. These images can be recalled as if they were projected onto an inner screen that we call the mind's eye. But the screen metaphor is actually misleading, because the images are composed of neuronal combinations which the Ice Age artists could summon, just as we do now.

Whether images derive from immediate perception or from past perception, they are not themselves pictures, even though they may give us the feeling of being pictures. They are "not facsimiles of the particular object, but rather results of the interactions between each of us and an object. . . . There is a set of correspondences between physical characteristics of the object and modes of reaction of the organism according to which a unique internally generated image is constructed."[19]

IMAGINATION

When we activate a memory, we excite areas in the visual cortex, and this in turn evokes the sensations we experienced when we first viewed the object. Recalling a visual memory, therefore, gives rise to an imagined visual experience, perhaps less strong than the original but having the feel of reality. Memory takes us back down the trajectory of perception to the initial sensation. It was this phenomenon that Adam Zeman referred to when he wrote, "Imagination is akin to recognition in reverse."[20]

. . . it is much better to draw only what you still see in your memory. This is a transformation in which imagination collaborates with memory.

—EDGAR DEGAS

Imagination has another meaning that refers to manipulation and transformation of remembered information to create new inventions or images. In her work with children, the psychologist Annette Karmiloff-Smith found that by about the age of 10, children achieve the mental flexibility that allows them to record what they remember seeing. What is more, at that age they are able to rearrange and invent imagery. When asked to draw a pretend animal or person, the children sometimes drew one with exaggerated appendages, or with multiple appendages, or with two heads, or images that were made up of a collage of body parts, some human and some animal.[21] These are the same inventions made by mature artists. And they are the same inventions we have seen beginning in Ice Age art.

We have seen the Ice Age imagination at work in dramatic form in the creation of incongruous hybrids such as part-human, part-animal figures and other fantasy creatures. We have looked at anamorphism and seen how Ice Age artists could take an image from memory and distort it systematically so that from another vantage point the image would appear normal. They possessed the ability to reduce the scale of large animals while retaining correct proportions. That is interesting but not remarkable, for all of us perform image reduction without much thought when we draw, for example, a house or a person on a small sheet of paper. What is surprising is that Ice Age artists were also able to maintain correct proportions in images while enormously enlarging them. In the Rotunda at Lascaux, the aurochs are impressively large—one is 5.5 meters long. This is a feat achieved during the Renaissance and in subsequent ages by using grids, and more recently by mechanical photographic projection.

In the ceiling of the Polychrome Chamber at Altamira, circled with large bison, a uniformity of approach suggests that one artist created the entire group. The artist used natural outcroppings of rock to create the forms of many of the bison, and fine cracks in the limestone as parts of their outlines. Most of the animals were first engraved, then redrawn with charcoal, and finally painted. This is counterintuitive: it would have been easier to draw animals of such large size using a brush or at least a charcoal crayon. The largest bison is about 1.7 meters long, and the deer measures over 2 m long. It would normally be hard for any artist to maintain proper proportions at this scale, especially using a small tool without the possibility of correction. An artist would tend to get lost in the details and lose the sense of the whole form. Yet these Ice Age artists did not.

The achievement was even more remarkable because the ceiling, now excavated to some distance from the floor, was just a few feet above the floor during the Ice Age. The artist could not have seen an entire figure at one time. Yet this artist was somehow able to depict whole animal forms using a fine burin. The feat suggests that the drawing, in some mysterious fashion, already existed in the artist's imagination and could be re-created on the ceiling. Looking again at the engraving on the Lortet baton (fig. 7.2), we can see how the artist transformed a mind's-eye image. To accurately place the scene on a cylindrical antler about 20.3 cm long, the artist had to carefully visualize the image. Then its scale had to be adjusted with fine precision, so that it fit exactly in the available, tightly curved area, filling the entire surface without leaving excess space or allowing the top and bottom of the image to touch. Adding to the challenge, the engraved line, made by a small burin that was difficult to hold, could not be changed. The artist had only one chance to get it right. This may be one of the criteria for art. A work of art may be thought of as an acrobatic feat on a high wire, and the greatest artistic achievements as leaps of daring executed without a safety net.

EMOTION AND CREATIVITY

If [the artist] feels accurately he will think accurately.

—PAUL CÉZANNE

Henri Matisse, who is generally considered to have been not an emotional painter but rather one who aspired to calm contemplation, nevertheless wrote something that delved more deeply into his inspiration: "I do not literally paint that table but I paint the emotion it arouses in me."[22] Escher, with whose observations I began this journey into the caves, continued to describe his visit to Lascaux: "The head of the bull appears on the rock wall. . . . it looks as if the damp nostrils tremble. Our brother depicts the bull with such intense emotion that the distance of 700 or 1,000 centuries that separates us from him shrinks to nothing."[23] He somehow got his chronology wrong; Lascaux is dated to about 17,000 years before the present—170 centuries, still an awesome distance. The feelings of the artists had been frozen in time and then came to life again for the viewer about 1,000 generations later.

Vision is tied to the brain's emotional centers. Sensory input arrives first to specialized visual areas and then to areas in which varied information is combined—for example, to the limbic region, where it may be selected to be stored in memory. The limbic system is also the center for emotion, and remembered images may have emotional content. The area of the brain most involved with emotion seems to be the one most involved with associative and imaginative reactions. For the moment it seems that the region dealing most directly with emotion overlaps the region most involved with human creativity.

Robert Motherwell, the American painter, was about to lose possession of his painting *Elegy to the Spanish Republic* as the result of a divorce settlement. Because it was such an important work in his opus he decided to make an exact copy. Motherwell pursued this project on sun-filled days at his seaside studio in Provincetown. By that time he was a well recognized artist, content both in his professional and personal life. Yet as he worked on the painting, a profound despair gripped him. So black were the moods that they propelled him to thoughts of suicide, all the more disturbing because he could not understand why he felt this way. It finally became clear to him. He was experiencing all over again the emotions he had felt when he originally painted the picture in the 1930s, in the bleak aftermath of the Spanish civil war. A painting composed of strong shapes in black and white carried its emotional content back to the man who had made it years before.[24]

How it is that drawn lines and painted surfaces can convey emotions is mysterious. When the American painter Mark Rothko painted, he chose fields of color that, when juxtaposed, were uniquely and inexplicably affecting. The English painter Francis Bacon remarked on this difference when he said, "It's a very close and difficult thing to know why some paint comes across directly on to the nervous system and other paint tells you the story in a long diatribe through the brain."[25] Anything we perceive at intense moments is more apt to be selected immediately for long-term memory. We remember where we were and what we were doing when President John F. Kennedy was assassinated, or when the airplanes struck the World Trade Center, even though we might not remember anything else about the day before or the day after. John Pfeiffer, in his book *The Creative Explosion,* speculated on the importance of drama and danger in caves for teaching important information to Ice Age initiates. Emotional content may be a requirement for art. The prehistorian Emmanuel Anati, who holds this view, refers to art as "psychograms," conveyors of emotion.[26] With this in mind, let us look once more at the antler from Lortet.

In the rollout of the scene (fig. 7.3, p. 191), the stag's nostrils are sensing the air. Its mouth is open, ready to give warning. Despite the small size of the image, the animal's eye is portrayed carefully, with attention given even to the lacrimal duct. The artist seems to have empathized with the emotion of the animal. In addition, the artist appears to have been sensitive to the sheer beauty of the scene. It may describe spring, when the salmon run. Close attention to the details of spring might have recalled the artist's feelings upon the return of warmer weather. These mingled emotions communicate to us in layers, so that we are able to experience both the fearfulness of the deer and the feelings of the artist simultaneously.

The finding of a new solution to a problem can, by itself, produce a sense of exhilaration. This can be true of the pictorial solutions an artist might find while working. An optimal creative experience, or, as the painter Robert Henri called it, the "state of high functioning," can come as a feeling that a floodgate has been opened and there is a surge of energy. The psychologist Mihaly Czikszentmihaly called this condition *flow.*[27] It is a state of high creativity. At times there may be a climactic moment of revelation. Some Ice Age art manages to convey to us the excitement and enlightenment experienced by an ancient artist as the accompaniment to a creative, art-related discovery. This is true of more recent art as well. Camille Corot wrote: "Be guided by feeling alone. . . . If you really have been touched you will convey to others the sincerity of your emotions."[28]

RECURSION

Art is vision becoming conscious of itself.

—ADAM ZEMAN, *Consciousness: A User's Guide*

One of the tests used to learn whether an animal or a child has self-awareness is to see whether or not it recognizes its own image in a mirror.[29] Children begin to recognize themselves in mirrors at between 18 and 24 months of age. It was thought that only our closest primate relatives—chimpanzees, bonobos, orangutans, and gorillas—have the capacity for self-recognition. It now seems that elephants and to some extent dolphins also possess this ability.[30] In some video footage in which Koko the gorilla is confronted by her image in a mirror and asked, "Who is that?" she points first to the image and then to herself, replying in sign language, "Me."

Recursion begins when another mirror is added, so that the viewer can see the image of himself looking at his own image. "When we become conscious of our own mental activity," wrote the neurologist Richard Restak, "the process is like the infinity of self-reflecting mirrors.[31] The term *recursion* derives from the verb "to return." In the self-reflecting mirrors we return to see our face over and over again, each time at one more remove from the original. In Escher's *Drawing Hands,* he recursively drew his own hand, which is drawing his hand, which is also drawing his hand. Some years after making this print, Escher saw an almost identical image in a book by the American cartoonist Saul Steinberg. Neither had seen the other's drawing; they had been concerned independently with the same conundrum, and both were intrigued by it.

It is one thing to recognize one's face in a mirror and another level of distancing or recursion to paint oneself looking at one's own face in a mirror. René Magritte painted himself wearing his signature bowler hat, looking at himself in a mirror. Then, never content with the obvious, he turned the image around and painted himself from the rear looking into a mirror, which, disconcertingly, reflects not the front but the back of his head. In another painting, again recursively looking at himself from the rear, he painted himself staring into a mirror. But the mirror is eerily empty. This is perverse because what the artist seeks is a clearer view of the self, whereas here he confronts only a blank mirror.

Art making can be a mirror. In it we can catch ourselves in the act of perceiving, remembering, imagining, or feeling. For example, we can train ourselves to focus on only one aspect of seeing as we draw: we can concentrate only on edges, we can look only at pixel-like information, we can focus our attention on enclosed shapes or on more generalized masses, we can look at the world primarily in terms of color, or we can concentrate on movement alone. We can be conscious of one kind of visual processing and then switch gears to focus on another type. One can almost hear a click as our concentration changes from one mode to another.

This shift of mind is even more self-conscious when we work with optical illusions and multistable figures, switching with deliberation from one type of perception to another. Unlike the engaged attitude in which we are poised to act at any minute, recursion allows the luxury of contemplation. We know that Ice Age artists were self-aware, because their art reveals that they were aware that they experienced optical illusions. We can know this because they sometimes played with these illusions and left evidence of this self-awareness in their art. Neurologists describe self-awareness as one of the most evolved brain functions. It has been described as the beginning of real thought and the beginning of imaginative reasoning. As far as we know we are the only organism in the universe that seeks to understand itself.

Art making may be a means of self examination. It is rooted in the brain but is not merely as abstract and solipsistic as that implies. Concepts become reified. Art making involves a dialogue, an interplay of the mind and hand of the artist with the diverse variety of materials available in our world, beginning with stone and bone, antler and clay, moving along to copper and bronze, and finally including all kinds of materials—gold and silver, blood and urine, junk and jewels, film and flesh. We must include this visceral aspect in our understanding of the sensuous appeal of art.

AFTERWORD

The brain, in its quest for knowledge about the visual world, discards, selects and, by comparing the selected information to its stored record, generates the visual image in the brain, a process remarkably similar to what an artist does.

—SEMIR ZEKI, *Inner Vision*

It is nothing new to say that the anatomically modern brain is the source of human creativity. In the early sixteenth century Michelangelo wrote, "A man paints with his brains and not his hands."[32] It is surprising, however, to learn from neuroscientists such as Semir Zeki that this brain works in much the same way that artists themselves work. Zeki is a specialist in vision and has been active in the field of neuroaesthetics. Not only has he stated that the brain works in a manner similar to that of the artist, but he has compared artists to scientists, writing that "artists are in some sense neurologists studying the brain with techniques that are unique to them."[33]

Looked at another way, the artist often pursues a process very like that used by the brain itself. The reality presented to our exploring eyes is selected and worked. Experience can be thought of as found material which may be fashioned into collages or assemblages. Some of it may be stored for future use or eventual transformation. Experience may be accompanied with a gush of chemicals that suffuse it with emotion. Or it may be contemplated in a purely aesthetic mode. There is further similarity. The point of both the brain's inquiry and the artist's quest is to forge meaning out of the neutral electrochemical stimuli with which the brain is assaulted. In a similar spirit, Robert Solso, another neuroscientist who is particularly interested in the arts, wrote: "When we create or experience art, in a very real sense we have the clearest view of the mind. We do not 'see' art, we see the mind."[34] Great art is, in this sense, translucent.

The immediate reaction of almost every viewer of Ice Age art is to ask what the art means. There can be no single answer to this question. Ice Age art was made over a vast geographical area, from the Atlantic Ocean to the Urals and from the Baltic Sea to the Mediterranean, for at least 20,000 years. And although the record is less clear, there is some evidence of art making in other parts of the world, such as Africa, beginning almost 30,000 years ago. Its specific purposes must have varied from place to place and from one time period to another in human history. Yet the ability and compulsion to make graphic and sculptural art appears to be a human characteristic. A certain number of people in every population have been drawn to express themselves by this means. Their art may be very different in appearance and meaning, but beneath the evident differences lie deep universals.

The human brain is the source of these universals. Humans bear, poised precariously on the tips of their spines, an enlarged brain, a relentless electrochemical machine serried with "cell assemblies." These networks of cells interact with one another, possibly by vibrating in synchrony. The neuroscientist Charles M. Gray is among those who believe that consciousness involves sets of oscillating neurons that vibrate in synchronous rhythm patterns moving at 25 to 100 cycles per second.[35] Cells incessantly hum with neural activity, confabulating in a ceaseless buzz of conversation, each neuron contacting up to 10,000 others at rates of up to 100 messages per second.[36] For some people this burden might be unbearable without a means of releasing expressive energy. Whether for societal or solipsistic reasons, art offers the possibility of creating something beyond the individual, something larger in scope than normal activity provides and more enduring than our individual lives. For some, art making may become a compulsion and a solace too great to resist. Whatever the individual impetus, art making appears to be an inevitable result of our breathtakingly interconnected brain.

Armed with this marvel of complex interconnection, Ice Age humankind unleashed creative powers that enabled them to make images that remain inventive and astonishing to us 1,000 generations later. With one hundred thousand million connections (10 with 14 zeros), our electrochemical brain has, in a sense, become incandescent. We can liken it to the flames in the lamps used to illuminate the dark and hidden caves. Bearing their lamps, restless humans explored underground passages and seemingly were compelled to leave behind engravings, drawings, paintings, and sculptures. Remote, dark spaces now teemed with virtual life. Ice Age people left these caves forever changed, in the same way we, their descendants, would eventually change the entire planet.

NOTES

INTRODUCTION

1. M. Escher, *Escher on Escher* (New York: Abrams, 1986), 11. At approximately the same time Maurits Escher viewed Lascaux, the American poet Robert Frost wrote a poem about some Ice Age pebbles found at the site of Mas d'Azil. In *A Missive Missile,* his gist was that these ancient artifacts could not speak to him at all:

Someone in ancient Mas d'Azil
Once took a little pebble wheel
And dotted it with red for me,
And sent it to me years and years—
A million years to be precise—
Across the barrier of ice:

Far as we aim our signs to reach,
Far as we often make them reach,
Across the soul-from-soul abyss,
There is an aeon-limit set
Beyond which they are doomed to miss.

Frost played with loaded dice. Unlike Escher, who examined figurative art, Frost looked at ancient markings that were entirely geometric, composed only of dots and lines. It would have been impossible for them to mean anything to a viewer who did not know the code. In addition, he was more than imprecise when he dated them at "a million years to be precise"—he was off by at least 990,000 years. Escher was off by a mere 50,000–80,000 years when he gave a date of 70,000 to 100,000 years for cave art at Lascaux.

2. Flutes made of animal bones have been found in caves at Neanderthal and *Homo sapiens sapiens* sites. In France they were made mostly of hollowed bird bones; in central Europe, of reindeer or bear bone. Remains of 30 crane bone flutes dating from about 9,000 years ago have been found in central China. Most of the flutes have three to seven holes. One with seven holes is still playable. See J. Pfeiffer, *The Creative Explosion* (New York: Harper and Row, 1982), 180–82.

3. Conversations with Philip Lieberman, author of, among many other books, *Eve Spoke: Human Language and Human Evolution* (Cambridge, MA: Harvard University Press, 1998).

4. Leroi-Gourhan and Annette Laming-Emperaire believed that the cave animals represented a male-female dualism. Leroi-Gourhan concluded that the bison represented a female force, and the horse, a masculine one. Laming-Emperaire concluded that the horse was feminine and the bison masculine. P. Ucko and A. Rosenfeld, *Palaeolithic Cave Art* (New York: McGraw-Hill, 1967), 145–46.

5. A group of scientists, historians, futurists, and artists was asked to propose a means of communicating to humans as much as 250,000 years in the future to warn of the "fiendishly toxic" plutonium buried at the Waste Isolation Pilot Project site in Carlsbad, New Mexico, which will be dangerous for that long. That is as far from us in the future as *Homo erectus,* maker of hand axes, is from us in the past. None of our symbols can be relied upon to convey meaning over such a time span. It was decided that only realistic pictures would be able to communicate. One of the suggestions was to depict human faces expressing horror and revulsion. This corresponds to my view that pictorial realism, even with our current sophistication, is the surest means of conveying information over vast stretches of time. Charles Piller, "Carlsbad's Information," *Los Angeles Times,* May 9, 2006.

6. The term *neuroaesthetics* was coined by the neuroscientist Semir Zeki.

7. G. Edelman, *Bright Air, Brilliant Fire: On the Matter of Mind* (New York: Basic Books, 1992), 176.

8. The art historians Rudolf Arnheim, in *Art and Visual Perception: A Psychology of the Creative Eye* (Berkeley: University of California Press, 1954), and Ernst Hans Gombrich, in *Art and Illusion* (London: Phaidon, 1960), used Gestalt psychology for this purpose beginning in the mid-twentieth century.

Gombrich later co-edited a book with the neuropsychologist Richard L. Gregory, *Illusion in Nature and Art* (New York: Scribner, 1973). Psychologists have written about the creative process. Among the most prominent books on the subject are Howard Gardner's *Art, Mind, and Brain* (New York: Basic Books, 1982) and Robert L. Solso's *The Psychology of Art and the Evolution of the Conscious Brain* (Cambridge, MA: MIT Press, 2003). Archaeologists such as Michel Lorblanchet and Mathilde Múzquiz-Pérez-Seoane have examined the creative process as well. Steven Mithen, in *The Prehistory of the Mind: The Cognitive Origins of Art, Religion, and Science* (London: Thames and Hudson, 1996), analyzed tool making to probe the early mind. A number of books have appeared in recent years by scientists who have applied developments in brain research to an understanding of the creative mind, although they do not deal with specific examples of art. Among them are V. S. Ramachandran's *The Emerging Mind* (London: Profile Books, 2003), his *A Brief Tour of Human Consciousness: From Imposter Poodles to Purple Numbers* (New York: Pi Press, 2004) and his and Sandra Blakeslee's *Phantoms in the Brain: Probing the Mysteries of the Human Mind* (New York: William Morrow, 1998). With the philosopher William Hirstein, Ramachandran wrote "The Science of Art" (*Journal of Consciousness Studies* 6, no. 6–7 [1999]: 15–51).

9. M. Lorblanchet, "From Man to Animal and Sign in Paleolithic Art," in *Animals into Art,* ed. H. Morphy (Boston: Unwin Hyman, 1989), 110–11.

10. F. Boas, *Race, Language, and Culture* (New York: Macmillan, 1940), 589.

11. B. Holm, *The Art and Times of Willie Seaweed, a Kwakiutl Master* (Seattle: University of Washington Press, 1983), 59.

12. E. H. Gombrich, *The Story of Art* (London: Phaidon, 1950), 5.

PART ONE. UNIVERSALS OF ART MAKING

The epigraph is from Ramachandran, *Brief Tour of Human Consciousness,* 4.

CHAPTER 1. ELEMENTS

Epigraphs in this chapter are from H. Matisse, *Jazz* (New York: George Braziller, 1983), xvi; M. Verstockt, *The Genesis of Form: From Chaos to Geometry* (London: Muller, Blond and White, 1987), 46; Arnheim, *Art and*

Visual Perception, 54; S. Fein, *First Drawings: Genesis of Visual Thinking* (Pleasant Hill, CA: Exelrod Press, 1993), 10; R. B. Hale, *Drawing Lessons from the Great Masters* (New York: Watson Guptill, 1964), 87; T. Lenain, *Monkey Painting* (London: Reaktion, 1997), 99. The epigraph attributed to P. Klee is an extremely common quote, invariably used without source. It is probably from his teaching at the Bauhaus School in Berlin. A similar idea, less pithily expressed, appears in his 1925 *Pedagogical Sketchbook* (New York: Praeger, 1967), 16.

1. For analysis of ideas regarding missing digits, see E. Hadingham, *Secrets of the Ice Age* (New York: Walker, 1979), 144–49.

2. M. Lorblanchet, "Palaeolithic Paint Job," *Discover* 14, no. 7 (1993): passim.

3. M. Berenguer, *Prehistoric Man and His Art: The Caves of Ribadesella* (London: Souvenir Press, 1973), 82.

4. M. Múzquiz-Pérez-Seoane, *Altamira* (New York: Abrams, 1999), 82–84.

5. A. Marshack, *The Roots of Civilization* (New York: McGraw-Hill, 1972), passim.

6. F. J. Dockstader, *Indian Art in North America* (New York: Graphic Society, 1961), 212.

7. Shitao, inscription on a landscape album, collection of the Nelson Atkins Museum, St. Louis, Missouri.

8. D. Baffier and V. Feruglio, "Premières observations sur deux nappes de ponctuations de la Grotte Chauvet," *International Newsletter of Rock Art* 21 (1998): 1–4.

9. Dong Quichang, inscription on "boneless landscape" painting titled *Landscape after Wang Meng,* 1615. Collection of the Nelson Atkins Museum, St. Louis, Missouri.

10. Hale, *Drawing Lessons,* 91.

11. Ibid., 87, 104.

12. D. Pelli, a professor of psychology and neural science at New York University, experimenting on the large face paintings of Chuck Close, found that whether one saw a series of marks or a unified image depended on the width of the mark relative to the viewing distance. Reported in *Science,* August 1999.

13. Quoted from an interview with Chuck Close by John Clay, http://www.artzar.com/content/close/page 1.html.

14. H. Morphy, "From Dull to Brilliant: The Aesthetics of Spiritual Power among the Yolngu," in *Anthropology, Art and Aesthetics,* eds. J. Coote and A. Sheldon, 182–208 (Oxford: Clarendon Press, 1992).

15. J. D. Lewis-Williams and T. A. Dowson, *Images of Power: Understanding Bushman Rock Art* (Johannesburg: Southern Book Publishers, 1989), passim.

16. S. Turpin and J. Zintgraff, *Pecos River Rock Art* (San Antonio, TX: Sandy McPherson, 1991) 34, 46, 58.

17. Conversation with Jim Zintgraff, 1999.

18. P. A. Helvenston and P. G. Bahn, *Waking the Trance Fixed* (Louisville, KY: Wasteland Press, 2005), 12–13.

19. H. Gardner, *Artful Scribbles: The Significance of Children's Drawings* (New York: Basic Books, 1980), 28–29.

20. Hadingham, *Secrets of the Ice Age,* 72.

21. C. Scarre, "Painting by Resonance," *Nature,* June 10, 1993, 382.

22. The Gestalt group of psychologists was founded in Berlin, primarily by Max Wertheimer. Most prominent in the twentieth century were Wertheimer, Kurt Koffka, and Wolfgang Köhler.

23. A. Marshack, "On the Dangers of Serpents in the Mind," *Current Archaeology* 26, no. 1 (1985): 106, 139–45.

24. H. Breuil, *Four Hundred Centuries of Cave Art* (New York: Hacker, 1979), 39.

25. P. G. Bahn, *Journey through the Ice Age* (Berkeley: University of California Press, 1997), 25, 32.

26. F. D'Errico, C. Henshilwood, and P. Nilssen, "An Engraved Bone Fragment from c. 70,000 Middle Stone Age Levels at Blombos Cave, South Africa," *Antiquity* 75, no. 288 (2001): 308–18. It is curious that crisscross markings like the ones on the Blombos pieces are occasionally found in early artifacts worldwide.

27. D. Gucwa and J. Ehmann, *To Whom It May Concern: An Investigation into the Art of Elephants* (New York: Norton, 1985), 3–4.

28. B. Holm, *Northwest Coast Indian Art: An Analysis of Form* (Seattle: University of Washington Press, 1965), 92–93.

29. H. Rosenberg, http://www.painterskeys.com/auth_search.asp?name=Harold%20.

30. I. Rock, "Perception," in *Scientific American Library* (New York: W. H. Freeman, 1984), 101.

31. K. Nicolaides, *The Natural Way to Draw* (Boston: Houghton Mifflin, 1941), 5.

32. P. Cézanne to A. Vollard, August 1936, quoted in D. Cooper and J. Richardson, *Claude Monet: An Exhibition of Paintings Arranged by Association with the Edinburgh Festival Society* (London, 1957), 41.

33. Gardner, *Artful Scribbles,* 59.

34. J. M. Kennedy, *A Psychology of Picture Perception* (San Francisco: Jossey Bass, 1974), 79–83.

35. R. L. Gregory, "How We Interpret Images," in *Images and Understanding* (Cambridge: Cambridge University Press, 1990), 310–13.

36. In 1959, the neurobiologists Torsten Wiesel and David Hubel did research on the visual cortex that led them to the discovery of the way visual processing works. They were awarded a Nobel Prize for this work in 1981.

37. D. D. Hoffman, *Visual Intelligence: How We Create What We See* (New York: Norton, 1998), 66–68.

38. My primary sources of information on the use of red ocher in the Paleolithic are Bahn, *Journey through the Ice Age;* L. S. Barham, "Systematic Pigment Use in the Middle Pleistocene of South-Central Africa," *Current Anthropology* 43, no. 1 (2002); C. Chippindale and P. S. C. Taçon, *Archaeology of Rock-Art* (Cambridge: Cambridge University Press, 1998); S. McBrearty and A. Brooks, "The Revolution that Wasn't," *Journal of Human Evolution* 39 (2000): 524–28; R. Rudgley, *The Lost Civilizations of the Stone Age* (New York: Free Press, 1999); D. Stubbs, *Prehistoric Art of Australia* (New York: Charles Scribner, 1974); G. L. Walsh, *Australia's Greatest Rock Art* (Bathurst: Brill-Brown, 1988); E. E. Wreschner, "Red Ochre and Human Evolution," *Current Anthropology* 21, no. 5 (1980): 631–44; and C. Couraud and A. Laming-Emperaire, "Les colorants," in *Lascaux inconnu,* eds. A. Leroi-Gourhan and J. Alain (Paris: Editions du Centre National de la Recherche Scientifique, 1979), 153–69.

39. B. Klima, "A Triple Burial from the Upper Paleolithic of Dolní Vestonice, Czechoslovakia," *Journal of Human Evolution* 16 (1988): 831–35.

40. N. Humphrey, *Seeing Red: A Study of Consciousness,* quoted by N. Angier in *Science Times,* February 6, 2002, D4.

41. The word for red in old Russian is the same as the word for beautiful.

42. Pipestone carvings exhibition catalog, Sioux Indian Museum and Craft Center, Rapid City, SD, 1997.

43. Quoted in T. Conway, *Painted Dreams* (Minocqua, WY: NorthWord, 1993), 44.

44. Louise Bourgeois, *New York Times,* December 25, 2001, E1–5.

45. O. Ballet et al., "Etude technique de poudres colorées de Lascaux," in Leroi-Gourhan and Alain, *Lascaux inconnu,* 170–74.

46. J. M. Masson and S. McCarthy, *When Elephants Weep: The Emotional Lives of Animals* (New York: Delacorte, 1995), 192–93.

47. Ibid., 193.

48. B. Tedlock, *The Beautiful and the Dangerous* (New York: Penguin, 1992), 232.

49. S. Zeki, *Inner Vision: An Exploration of Art and the Brain* (Oxford: Oxford University Press, 1999), 66.

50. Quoted in E. Protter, *Painters on Painting* (New York: Grosset and Dunlap, 1971), 182.

51. Quoted in O. Sacks, *An Anthropologist on Mars* (New York: Knopf, 1995), 293–94.

52. Ramachandran and Blakeslee, *Phantoms in the Brain,* 177.

53. Zeki, *Inner Vision,* 185–89.

54. O. Sacks, "A Neurologist's Notebook: To See and Not See," *New Yorker,* May 10, 1993, 65.

55. L. Weschler, "An Afrikaner Dante," *New Yorker,* November 8, 1993, 96–97.

56. S. Lackner, *Beckmann* (New York: Abrams, 1991), 50.

57. B. Bova, *The Beauty of Light* (New York: Wiley, 1988), 16.

58. Paul D. MacLean was the author of *the Triune Brain.* The three brains to which he referred were the neocortex, or neomammalian brain, the limbic, or paleomammalian, brain, and the reptilian brain, consisting of the brain stem and the cerebellum.

59. J. LeDoux, *The Emotional Brain: The Mysterious Underpinnings of Emotional Life* (New York: Simon and Schuster, 1996), passim.

CHAPTER 2. BASIC STRUCTURES

Epigraphs in this chapter are from I. Eibl-Eibesfeldt, *Beauty and the Brain: Biological Aspects of Aesthetics* (Basel: Birkhauser Verlag, 1988), 32; F. Boas, *Primitive Art* (New York: Dover, 1955), 6; D. Hofstadter, *Metamagical Themas: Questing for the Essence of Mind and Pattern* (New York: Basic Books, 1985); and E. H. Gombrich, *A Sense of Order* (Ithaca, NY: Cornell University Press, 1979), 9.

1. Gombrich, *Sense of Order,* 6–10.

2. A. Leroi-Gourhan, *The Dawn of European Art* (Cambridge: Cambridge University Press, 1982), 24–26.

3. M. C. Corballis and I. L. Beale, *The Psychology of Left and Right* (Hillsdale, NJ: Erlbaum, 1976), passim.

4. A.-C. Welté, "An Approach to the Theme of Confronted Animals in French Palaeolithic Art," in Morphy, *Animals into Art,* 215–37.

5. H. K. Crotty, "Formal Qualities of the Jornada Style of Pueblo IV Anasazi Rock Art," *American Indian Rock Art* 16 (1990): 151.

6. R. L. Anderson and K. L. Field, *Art in Small-Scale Societies* (Englewood Cliffs, NJ: Prentice Hall, 1992), 36ff.

7. Observation by C. Schuster, a researcher at the Museum of Natural History in New York City, in his notes, which after his death were edited by the archaeologist Edward Carpenter and published as *Social Symbolism in Ancient and Tribal Art* (New York: Rock Foundation, 1988), tome II (second of three boxed sets), vol. 1, 99–182.

8. Two-headed snakes occur occasionally in nature. One such king snake, with heads side by side, at the San Diego Zoo was named Dudley-Duplex. One of his heads tried to swallow the other, but the second head was rescued by zoo

staff. The endangered head took revenge by poisoning the aggressor head, thus ending the lives of both heads.

9. Greek legend proposed a mythical two-headed serpent called Amphisbaena that had a head at each end. It was spawned from the blood of Medusa when drops of blood from severed head(s) fell on the ground. But the image itself appears to be older and nearly universal.

10. M. J. Young, *Signs from the Ancestors* (Albuquerque: University of New Mexico Press, 1992), 97–98, 174.

11. B. Rensch, “Rekurrenzlust,” *Die Wirksamkeit Äesthetischer Faktoren bei Wirbeltieren Zeitschrift für Tierpsychologie* 15 (1958): 447–61.

12. T. J. Sejnowski, D. K. Kienker, and G. E. Hinton, “Learning Symmetry Groups with Hidden Units beyond the Perceptron,” Proceedings of the 22nd International Union of Pure and Applied Sciences (1985), *Physica* 22 D (Applied Physics) (1986): 75. Online journal distributed by the Nature Publishing Group.

13. I. Kant, *Kritik der Urteilskraft,* 3rd ed., part 5, paragraph 15, 1799.

14. Eibl-Eibesfeldt, *Beauty and the Brain,* 31, 178.

15. A. Zee, *Fearful Symmetry: The Search for Beauty in Modern Physics* (Princeton, NJ.: Princeton Science Library, 1999), 100, 280.

16. H. A. Einstein, *Einstein, A Centenary Volume* (Cambridge, MA: Harvard University Press, 1979), 172.

17. Ibid.

18. D. K. Washburn, *Symmetries of Culture* (Seattle: University of Washington Press, 1999), 553–54.

19. B. Zaslow, “Symmetry and Contemporary Hopi Art,” *Kiva: Journal of the Arizona Archaeological and Historical Society* 51, no. 4 (1986): 233, 245, 253.

20. D. K. Washburn, ed., *Living in Balance: The Universe of the Hopi, Zuñi, Navaho and Apache* (Philadelphia: University of Pennsylvania Museum, 2004), passim.

21. Ucko and Rosenfeld, *Palaeolithic Cave Art,* 154–55, fig. 72.

22. J. Clottes and J. Courtin, *The Cave beneath the Sea:*

Paleolithic Images at Cosquer (New York: Abrams, 1999), 101.

23. Quoted in B. S. Shapiro, *Edgar Degas: The Painter as Printmaker* (Boston: Museum of Fine Arts, 1984), 16.

24. C. W. Tyler, "Painters Centre One Eye in Portraits," *Nature* 392, no. 6679 (April 30, 1998): 877.

25. Escher, *Escher on Escher,* 122.

26. B. Rensch, "The Intelligence of Elephants," *Scientific American* 196, no. 2 (1957): 44–49.

27. The research by David Sulzer and Richard Lair is discussed in "A Band with a Lot More to Offer than Talented Trumpeters," *New York Times,* science section, December 16, 2000, 62.

28. L. F. Baptista and R. Keister, "Why Bird Song Is Sometimes Like Music," *Perspectives in Biology and Medicine* 48, no. 3 (2005): 426–43.

29. R. Payne, "Whale Songs: Musicality or Mantra," *Science*: 291, no. 5501 (2001), 52–54.

30. This comment by Bach is said to have been related by Friedrich Wilhelm Marpurg, who knew Bach. See H. David and A. Mendel, *The Bach Reader* (New York: W. W. Norton, 1966), 257.

31. Hofstadter, *Metamagical Themas,* 233, 259.

PART TWO. WINDOWS INTO THE MIND

The epigraph is from T. Roethke, "Prayer," in *The Modern Poets: An American-British Anthology,* eds. J. M. Brinnin and B. Read (New York: McGraw-Hill, 1963), 294.

1. *The Scientific American Book of the Brain* (New York: Scientific American Press, 2001); J. McCrone, *The Ape That Spoke: Language and the Evolution of the Human Mind* (New York: William Morrow, 1991), 50–54.

2. J. P. Frisby, *Seeing: Illusion, Brain and Mind* (Oxford: Oxford University Press, 1980), 35.

3. Quoted in J. Hadamard, *The Psychology of Invention in the Mathematical Field* (Princeton, NJ: Princeton University Press, 1949), 142.

4. G. Holton, *The Scientific Imagination* (Cambridge: Cambridge University Press, 1978), 142.

5. R. Fagen, *Animal Play Behavior* (Oxford: Oxford University Press, 1981), 470.

6. J. D. Watson, *The Double Helix* (New York: Signet New American Library, 1968), 116.

7. J. Glieck, *Chaos* (New York: Viking, 1987), 175.

8. B. Mandelbrot, talk presented at the Santa Fe Institute, Santa Fe, New Mexico, May 18, 2000.

9. J. N. Noble, "Sailing a Wheelchair to the End of Time," *New York Times,* March 24, 1998, B18.

10. G. Orwell, "Politics and the English Language," *Horizon* magazine (London, 1946), reprinted in *Shooting Elephants and Other Essays* (New York: Harcourt, Brace, 1950), 77–92.

11. J. J. Gibson, "The Information Available in Pictures," *Leonardo* 4: 27–35.

12. A. M. Leslie, personal communication; A. M. Leslie, "The Necessity of Illusion: Perception and Thought in Infancy," in *Thought without Language,* ed. L. Weiskrantz (Oxford: Clarendon Press, 1986), 185–210.

CHAPTER 3. ILLUSION

Epigraphs in this chapter are from R. L. Gregory, "The Confounded Eye," in *Illusion in Nature and Art,* eds. R. L. Gregory and E. H. Gombrich (New York: Scribner, 1973), 63; J. Halverson, "Art for Art's Sake in the Paleolithic," *Current Anthropology* 28, no. 1 (1987): 63–89; J. Teresi and D. Teresi, *The Three-Pound Universe* (New York: Macmillan, 1986), 47; E. H. Gombrich, http: www.quotationspage.com/quotes/E._H._Gombrich/; and Mark Twain, *A Connecticut Yankee in King Arthur's Court,* quoted in *Mark Twain Wit and Wisecracks* (White Plains, NY: Peter Pauper Press, 1961), 23.

1. R. White, "Beyond Art: Toward an Understanding of the Origins of Material Representation in Europe," *Annual Review of Anthropology* 21: 537–64.

2. Bahn, *Journey through the Ice Age,* 88.

3. R. White, "Visual Thinking in the Ice Age," *Scientific American,* July 1989, 95.

4. The clay appears to have been stiffened with the addition of bone. It is unknown whether this was necessary for making the clay workable, in the

same way grogg is used in clay today, whether it was a symbolic use of animal material, or whether it had some other purpose.

5. Pliny the Elder, *The Natural History,* vol. 9, book 35 (Cambridge, William Heinemann, 1961), 331. A similar anecdote was told about the eighteenth-century British animal painter George Stubbs. He painted the stallion Whistlejacket in so lifelike and animated a manner that it was said that Whistlejacket, on seeing the picture, bucked and kicked it.

6. Ibid., 309, 311.

7. J. White, *The Birth and Rebirth of Pictorial Space* (New York: Harper and Row, 1972), 241–42.

8. S. Eimerl, *The World of Giotto* (New York: Time-Life Books, 1967), 85.

9. Conversations with Ed Wapp, Sac and Fox American Indian flute virtuoso and teacher at the Institute of American Indian Art in Santa Fe, New Mexico, 1995.

10. Psychology and biology professors Meredith West and Andrew King, of Indiana University, wrote of the starling's musical ability in *American Scientist,* March–April 1990. Timothy Gentner, a neural physiologist, published experiments with starlings and music in May 2006 in *Nature*. He believes that starlings recognize song patterns that may resemble a beginning linguistic syntax.

11. Conversations with conductors Oliver Prezant and Bernard Rubinstein and with musicologist Mark Malkovitch, 1999–2000.

12. S. Whitfield and J. Elderfield, *Bonnard* (New York: Abrams, 1998), 34–35.

13. "Perhaps natural selection has wired up the visual areas in such a way that the reinforcement is actually stronger if it is obtained after 'work.'" Ramachandran and Blakeslee, *Phantoms in the Brain,* 288.

14. H. Matisse, *Retrospective Exhibition of Paintings, Drawings, and Sculpture* (Philadelphia: Philadelphia Museum of Art, 1938), 33–34.

15. I will not give a simplified definition of art here. The book builds to address the complex meaning of art in the concluding chapter.

16. Lorblanchet, "From Man to Animal," 115.

17. Clottes and Courtin, *Cave beneath the Sea,* 97.

18. Sze, *The Tao of Painting I,* 104, quoted in Gombrich, *Art and Illusion,* 208.

19. Quoted in Brassaï, *Picasso and Company* (Garden City, NY: Doubleday, 1966), 241.

20. R. G. Bednarik, "The Australopithecine Cobble from Makapansgat," *South African Archaeological Bulletin,* 1980, 53–58.

21. Eibl-Eibesfeldt, *Beauty and the Brain,* 177.

22. C. G. Gross, "Coding for Visual Categories in the Human Brain," *Nature Neuroscience* 3 (Sept. 2000): 855.

23. Ramachandran and Blakeslee, *Phantoms in the Brain,* 85–113.

24. Ibid.

25. A. Clark, "Action, Reason and the Grand Illusion," *Journal of Consciousness Studies* 9, no. 5–6 (2002): 194–201.

26. E. Tulving and D. Schecter, "Priming and Human Memory Systems," *Science* 247, no. 4940 (1990): 301–6.

27. Arnheim, *Art and Visual Perception,* 31.

28. J. A. Hobson, *The Chemistry of Conscious States* (Boston: Little Brown, 1994), 214.

29. F. Crick, *The Astonishing Hypothesis* (New York: Scribner, 1994), 57.

30. Pfeiffer, *Creative Explosion,* passim.

31. Conway, *Painted Dreams,* 93.

32. Young, *Signs from the Ancestors,* 98–99.

33. B. O. Alpert, "An Unusual Realistic Petroglyph in New Mexico" (manuscript).

34. Pliny, *Natural History,* 337–39.

35. S. Shimada, "Concerning the I-p' in Style of Painting," *Oriental Art,* new series 7, no. 2 (1961): 3–11.

36. Quoted in Gombrich, *Art and Illusion,* 188.

37. Leonardo da Vinci, *Treatise on Painting, Notebooks,* vol. 1 (New York: Dover, 1970), section 508, 254.

38. A. Cozens, *A New Method of Landscape* (London: Paddington Press, 1991), 5, 9.

39. Gombrich, *Art and Illusion,* 188.

40. L. B. Alberti, *De Statua,* quoted in English in Gombrich, *Art and Illusion,* 90.

41. Conversation in 1983 with Felipe Puente, chief guide of the Santander region (now Cantabria), who was Picasso's guide when he returned to Spain. As Puente described Picasso's visit, it was "clandestino."

42. Quoted in Brassaï, *Picasso and Company,* 70.

CHAPTER 4. ANALOGY

Epigraphs in this chapter are from R. Frost, quoted in W. F. Allman, *Apprentices of Wonder: Inside the Neural Network Revolution* (London: Bantam, 1989), 100; C. Raymo, *The Virgin and the Mousetrap* (New York: Viking, 1991), 178; B. Pascal, quoted in A. Ludovici, *Secret of Laughter* (New York: Viking, 1933), 27; A. Spiegelman, "Drawing Blood and the Art of Outrage," *Harper's,* June 2006, 45; and B. Harvey, quoted from an interview by Tracy Jones in the newspaper *Metro Pulse,* January 1993, 19–20.

1. J.-M.-G. Itard, *The Wild Boy of Aveyron* (Englewood Cliffs, NJ: Prentice Hall, 1962), 76–77.

2. F. H. Cushing, *The Mythic World of the Zuñi* (Albuquerque: University of New Mexican Press, 1988), 5.

3. J. K. Crellin, *A History of Healing* (New York: Marlowe, 1997), passim.

4. V. J. Vogel, *American Indian Medicine* (Norman: University of Oklahoma Press, 1970), 128, 294.

5. D. Morris, *The Biology of Art* (New York: Knopf, 1961), passim.

6. The source of the anecdote is Bernard D. Davis, Adele Lehman Professor of Physiology at Harvard Medical School, in a letter to the editor, *New York Times,* September 12, 1990.

7. M. Ruspoli, *The Cave of Lascaux: The Final Photograph* (New York: Abrams, 1986), 145.

8. A. Marshack, "The Meander as a System: The Analysis and Recognition of Iconographic Units in Upper Paleolithic Compositions," in *Form in Indigenous Art,* eds. P. J. Ucko and A. Rosenfeld, 286–317 (Canberra: Institute of Aboriginal Studies, 1977).

9. J. W. Fewkes, *Hopi Snake Ceremonies: An Eyewitness Account* (Albuquerque, NM: Avanyu Press, 2000), passim.

10. R. Eisler, *Sacred Pleasures* (San Francisco: HarperCollins, 1995), 5; D. Slifer, *The Serpent and the Sacred Fire* (Santa Fe: Museum of New Mexico Press, 2000), 80.

11. R. Bunzel, *Pueblo Potter: A Study of Creative Imagery in Primitive Art* (New York: Columbia University Press, 1929), 136.

12. B. O. Alpert, "Cupoles, Circles, and Mandalas," in a special edition of *Anthropologie* devoted to symbolism in Paleolithic art, published by the Moravske Muzeum, Brno, Czech Republic, 1996.

13. Young, *Signs from the Ancestors,* 67, 82.

14. Quoted in Verstockt, *Genesis of Form,* 63.

15. Marshack, *Roots of Civilization,* 33ff.

16. For a number of similar examples, see M. Gimbutas, *The Language of the Goddess* (New York: HarperCollins, 1991), 228–31.

17. Sackler Collection, Fogg Museum Collection, Harvard University, catalogue no. 59.

18. Quoted in D. Sieberling, "The Female View of Erotica," *New York Magazine* 7 (Feb. 11, 1974): 56.

19. Young, *Signs from the Ancestors,* 105–6.

20. A. Seowtewa, "Adding a Breath to Zuñi Life," *Native Peoples* (Flagstaff, AZ), Winter 1992, 10–16.

21. M. C. Corballis, *The Lopsided Ape: Evolution of the Generative Mind* (Oxford: Oxford University Press), 146.

22. R. A. Gardner and B. T. Van Cantfort, *Teaching Sign Language to Chimpanzees* (Albany: State University of New York Press, 1989), 81.

23. Ibid.

24. S. Savage-Rumbaugh and R. Levin, *Kanzi: The Ape at the Brink of the Human Mind* (London: Wiley, 1994), 278.

25. F. Patterson, "Conversations with a Gorilla," *National Geographic,* October 1978, 438–65.

26. Raymo, *The Virgin and the Mousetrap,* 177.

27. G. Lakoff and M. Johnson, *Metaphors We Live By* (Chicago: University of Chicago Press, 1980), 56, 185–86.

28. A. Gopnik and A. Meltzoff, *Words, Thoughts, and Theories* (Cambridge, MA: MIT Press, 1997), passim.

29. Ramachandran, *Brief Tour of Human Consciousness,* 73–74.

30. A. C. R. Damasio, *Descartes' Error: Emotion, Reason, and the Human Brain* (New York: Putnam, 1994), 26–27.

31. Conversation with Reggie Miller, an Australian Aboriginal man from Arnhem Land, 1995.

32. For a discussion and exhaustive examples of Kokopelli, see Slifer, *Serpent and Sacred Fire.*

33. M. Titiev, "The Story of Kokopele," *American Anthropologist* 41, no. 1 (1939): 41.

34. F. Kabotie, *Designs from the Ancient Mimbreños, with a Hopi Interpretation* (San Francisco: Grabhorn Press, 1949), fig. 24.

35. A. Sieveking, *Engraved Magdalenian Plaquettes,* BAR International Series 369 (Oxford: Oxford University Press, 1987), 3.

36. H. Seidelman and J. Turner, *The Inuit Imagination: Arctic Myth and Sculpture* (Vancouver, BC: Douglas and McIntyre, 1993), 42.

37. E. O. Christensen, *Primitive Art* (New York: Viking, 1995), 245, fig. 202.

38. Quoted by H. M. Sheets in a review of *Francis Bacon: A Retrospective,* by D. Farr, S. Yard, and M. Pappiatt, *New York Times,* January 1999.

39. Sargent's sketchbook no. 2, 1869, p. 1, shows three faces. This notebook was made while Sargent was 13. Sketchbooks in the collections of the Fogg Art Museum, Harvard University.

40. G. M. Mallery, *Picture-Writing of the American Indians,* vol. 2 (New York: Dover, 1972), 506.

41. Sargent, notebook of April 22, 1913. In sketchbooks made toward the end of his life, Sargent made two similar faces.

42. Ramachandran and Hirstein, "Science of Art," 18–21.

43. I. Rock, *An Introduction to Perception* (New York: Macmillan, 1975), 102.

44. Ibid.

45. P. Churchland, *The Engine Is the Seat of the Soul* (Cambridge, MA: MIT Press, 1995), 32–38.

46. H. Barlow, C. Blakemore, and M. Weston-Smith, *Images and Understanding* (Cambridge: Cambridge University Press, 1990), 60.

47. D. Pearson, E. Hanna, and K. Martinez, "Images and Understanding," *Memory and Cognition* 20, no. 4 (1992): 433–40.

48. Quoted in Whitfield and Elderfield, *Bonnard,* 170.

49. V. Van Gogh to Theo Van Gogh, 1885, quoted in Protter, *Painters on Painting,* 13–14.

50. Quoted in M. De Zayas, "Picasso Speaks," *The Arts* (New York) 3 (1923): 315–26.

51. Shakespeare, *As You Like It,* II, iii, 1.18.

52. Bahn, *Journey through the Ice Age,* 24, 32.

53. C. Archambeau pointed out this bison to me in 1996.

54. This piece is in the collection of the Instituto Nacional de Antropología e Historia, Mexico City.

55. D. Vialou, *L'art des cavernes* (Paris: Le Rocher, 1987), 36 (my translation).

56. T. A. Dowson, *Rock Engravings of Southern Africa* (Johannesburg: Witwatersrand University Press, 1992), 105.

57. B. Spencer and F. J. Gillen, *The Native Tribes of Central Australia* (Oosterhout, Netherlands: Anthropological Publications, 1999), 67–68.

58. Brassaï, *Conversations avec Picasso* (Paris: Gallimard, 1969), 76.

59. T. Jones, interview with B. Harvey, *Metro Pulse,* January 1989, 19–20.

60. M. Lorblanchet and J.-C. Marquet, "A Neanderthal Face? The Proto-figurine from La Roche-Cotard, Langlais, Indreat-Loire, France," *Antiquity* 77, no. 298 (2003): 661–70.

61. B. Netanyahu, ed., *The World History of the Jewish People at the Dawn of Civilization* (New Brunswick, NJ: Rutgers University Press, 1964), 80–83.

62. Quoted in "The Wizard of Eyes: Evolution Creates Novelty by Varying the Same Old Trick," *New York Times,* science section, November 2001.

CHAPTER 5. AMBIGUITY

Epigraphs in this chapter are from Gombrich, *Art and Illusion,* 314; M. Escher, quoted in Teuber, "Sources of Ambiguity," 92; Crick, *Astonishing Hypothesis,* 8; and B. Reid, *Form and Freedom: A Dialogue on Northwest Coast Indian Art* (Houston: Institute for the Arts, Rice University, 1995), 3.

1. L. Thomas, *The Lives of a Cell* (New York: Viking, 1974), 91–95.

2. For information on the Gestalt group see R. Sterling, *Cognitive Psychology,* 4th ed. (Belmont, CA: Wadsworth, 2006).

3. Quoted in B. Edwards, *Drawing on the Artist Within* (New York: Simon and Schuster, 1986), 117.

4. P. Shammi and D. T. Stuss, "Humor Appreciation: A Role of the Right Frontal Lobe," *Brain: A Journal of Neurology* 122, pt. 4 (April 1999): 657–66.

5. S. Giedion, *The Eternal Present: The Beginnings of Art* (New York: Pantheon, 1962), 20–21.

6. E. Rubin, "Figure and Ground," in *Readings in Perception,* eds. D. C. Beardslee and M. Wertheimer (Princeton, NJ: Van Nostrand, 1958), 194.

7. J. Clegg, "Aesthetics, Rock Art and Changing States of Consciousness," *Aesthetics and Rock Art,* eds. T. Heyd and J. Clegg (Burlington, VT: Ashgate, 2005), 162–63.

8. Teuber, "Sources of Ambiguity," 92.

9. Ibid.

10. Conversation with Shaun Edwards, 1995.

11. Rock, *Introduction to Perception,* 101.

12. Ibid., 265.

13. Ibid., 267.

14. Ibid., 291.

15. P. Bahn, personal communication, 1992.

16. Quoted in J. J. Brody, *Mimbres Painted Pottery,* 2nd ed. (Santa Fe, NM: School of American Research Press, 2005), 20.

17. Da Vinci, *Notebooks,* 41.

18. R. L. Gregory, *The Intelligent Eye* (New York: McGraw-Hill, 1970), 128–31.

19. S. R. Lehky and T. J. Sejnowski, "Network Model of Shape from Shading," *Nature* 333 (June 1988): 452–54.

20. R. Baillargeon, "How Do Infants Learn about the Physical World?" *Current Directions* 3 (1994): 133–40.

21. *Fliegende Blätter,* October 23, 1892, 147; see also Gombrich, *Image and Eye,* 55.

22. *Harper's Weekly,* November 19, 1892, 1114.

23. J. Jastrow, *Keeping Mentally Fit: A Guide to Everyday Psychology* (New York: Greenberg, 1928).

24. E. Carpenter, *Eskimo Realities* (New York: Holt, Rinehart and Winston, 1973), 106.

25. Holm, *Northwest Coast Indian Art,* 89.

CHAPTER 6. PARADOX

Epigraphs in this chapter are from R. M. Restak, *Brainscapes* (New York: Hyperion, 1995), 127; L. Mumford, quoted in J. A. Hobson, *The Dreaming Brain* (New York: Basic Books, 1988), 220; Sieveking, *Engraved Magdalenian Plaquettes,* 3; D. R. Olson and E. Bialystok, *Spatial Cognition: The Structure and Development of Mental Representations of Spatial Relationships* (Hillsdale, NJ: Erlbaum, 1983), 15; U. Boccioni, "Futurist Manifesto of April 1910," in R. Goldwater and M. Treves, *Artists on Art: From the Fourteenth to the Twentieth Century* (New York: Pantheon, 1945), 434–35; and P. Picasso, quoted in D. Ashton, *Picasso on Art* (New York: Viking Press, 1972), 61.

1. R. M. Restak, *The Brain* (New York: Bantam, 1984), 240–46; and Restak, *Brainscapes,* 101.

2. J. D. Lewis-Williams and T. A. Dowson, "The Signs of All Times: Entoptic Phenomena in Upper Paleolithic Art," *Current Anthropology* 29, no. 2 (1988): 211.

3. Vialou, *L'art des cavernes,* 112–15. Other viewers have seen different animal parts in this image.

4. N. W. Smith, *Analysis of Ice Age Art* (New York: Peter Lang, 1992), passim.

5. Pfeiffer, *Creative Explosion,* 114–18.

6. N. J. Conard, "Paleolithic Ivory Sculptures from Southwestern Germany and the Origins of Figurative Art," *Nature,* December 18, 2003, 830–32.

7. Mallery, *Picture-Writing,* 737.

8. H. J. Shafer, *Ancient Texans* (Houston, TX: Gulf Publishing, 1986), 150.

9. Lewis-Williams and Dowson, "Signs of All Times," 211.

10. A. Solomon, "Ethnography and Method in Southern African Rock-Art Research," in Chippindale and Taçon, *Archaeology of Rock-Art,* 277.

11. M. Donald, *Origins of the Modern Mind* (Cambridge, MA: Harvard University Press, 1999), 279.

12. Quoted in J. Hooper and D. Teresi, *Three-Pound Universe* (New York: Macmillan, 1986), 325.

13. Clottes and Courtin, *Cave beneath the Sea,* 20.

14. Mallery, *Picture-Writing,* passim.

15. Marquette's account is in R. G. Thwaites, *The Jesuit Relations and Allied Documents: Travels and Explorations of the Jesuit Missionaries in New France,* vol. 59 (Cleveland: Burrows Bros.), 102.

16. Quoted in Goldwater and Treves, *Artists on Art,* 70.

17. Magritte to Paul Nouge, November 1927, quoted in H. Torczyner, *Magritte: Ideas and Images* (New York: Abrams, 1966), 213.

18. Hobson, *Dreaming Brain,* 297.

19. Sieveking, *Engraved Magdalenian Plaquettes,* passim.

20. E. Piette, *L'art pendant l'age du renne* (Paris: Masson, 1907), 70.

21. E. Kedourie, ed., *The Jewish World, Revelation, Prophecy and History* (London: Thames and Hudson, 1975), 39.

22. S. Dalí, "Communication: Paranoiac Face," *Le Surréalism au Service de la Révolution* (Paris), no. 3 (December 1931): 40.

23. Ibid.

24. L. Etienne, *Palindromes bilingues* (Bannes: Edition de Fourneau, 1984), passim.

25. Hobson, *Chemistry of Conscious States,* 93.

26. E. Carpenter, *Eskimo Realities* (New York: Holt, Rinehart and Winston), 37.

27. B. Chatwin, *Songlines* (New York: Viking, 1987), passim.

28. Pliny, *Natural History,* 303.

29. Arnheim, *Art and Visual Perception,* 80–86.

30. C. Bouleau, *The Painter's Secret Geometry: Study of Composition in Art,* trans. J. Griffin (New York: Harcourt Brace and World, 1963), 31.

31. G. Rowley, *Principles of Chinese Painting* (Princeton, NJ: Princeton University Press, 1959), 61–63.

32. For a discussion of cave lighting, see B. Delluc and G. Delluc, "L'eclairage," in Leroi-Gourhan and Alain, *Lascaux inconnu,* 121–39.

33. N. Aujoulat, *Lascaux: Motion, Space and Time* (New York: Abrams, 2005), 215–26.

34. Ibid.

35. Pfeiffer, *Creative Explosion,* 142–43.

36. Traditional Renaissance one-point perspective requires that a stationary viewer use only one eye to arrive at a systematic recession within a perspectival space, which is then translated onto a real or virtual window glass. The glass is equivalent to the picture plane.

37. M. Eastham, "The Analysis of Scan Sequences Embedded in Palaeolithic Parietal Images," *Rock Art Research* 16, no. 1 (1999): 89–108.

38. D. Lewis-Williams, *Fragile Heritage* (Johannesburg: University of Witwatersrand Press, 1998), 95.

39. M. Livingstone, *Vision and Art:The Biology of Seeing* (New York: Abrams, 2002) 190–91.

40. The philosophers J. K. O'Regan and A. Noë argue that seeing is not the creation of an image as in seeing a picture but rather a process of exploration of the visual world. Noë was having his portrait drawn by an artist friend and was struck by the artist's frenzied looking activity, "an uninterrupted pattern of looking back and forth between me and the canvas." This experience led to his theory that our visual experience results from the process of exploration of the visual world ("Is the Visual World a Grand Illusion?" *Journal of Consciousness Studies* 9, no. 5–6 [2002]: 7 n. 9). Actually this is a technique long used by artists particularily since the Renaissance. Alternately, for most of history over most of the world, artists have drawn from inner sources. My six-year-old

grandson told his mother, "God's best gift to us is that we have pictures in our head." In general, when he draws, he appears to draw from these inner pictures, which can be extremely detailed and which contain a large amount of information. Extremely intense, long-lived, and elaborate imagery is called eidetic. Although sometimes confused with photographic memory, it is something different. About 8 percent of children have this ability, and most of them lose it by age 11.

My grandson appeared to draw only from such inner images until a few months short of seven. He asked to be given a starfish with the intent of drawing from it. In the end, however, he ignored the actual artifact and went back to his inner picture. A few days later he was visiting a relative and had nothing of interest to do. He requested paper and attempted to copy a complicated image from a coloring book. This was the first time I saw him employ the "frenzied" back-and-forth approach mentioned by Noë. Apparently he was able to switch from one mode to the other, although at most times he still preferred the inner image. In general artists are able to switch from one mode of perception to another. When examining reality, they can choose to concentrate on line, mass, contrast, or color. But usually this is a decision made to deviate from our normal response-directed vision.

41. Vialou, *L'art des cavernes,* 46 (my translation).

42. Ramachandran, *A Brief Tour of Human Consciousness,* 48.

43. Ashton, *Picasso on Art,* 61.

44. D. Hockney, quoted by curator in appended commentary in his landscape show at the Boston Museum of Fine Arts, 1998.

CHAPTER 7. THE CREATIVE BRAIN

Epigraphs in this chapter are from Zeki, *Inner Vision,* 21; P. Picasso, quoted in Ashton, *Picasso on Art,* 61; D. Close, http//www.improvcomedy.org/hall/close.html; R. Irwin, brochure for 1998 exhibition at Dia Center for the Arts; E. Degas, quoted in P. G. Jeanniot, *Souvenirs sur Degas* (Paris: Revue Universelle, 1993); P. Cézanne, quoted from an interview in C. Brinton, *The Modern Spirit in Contemporary Painting* (New York: John Lane, 1916); and A. Zeman, *Consciousness: A User's Guide* (New Haven, CT: Yale University

Press, 2002), 191. Del Close, a comedian with Second City, is most notorious for having left his skull to the theater for use in *Hamlet,* with the proviso that he be listed in the playbill as Yorik.

1. Personal conversation with the Comte de Bégouën, 1996.

2. J. Huizinga, *Homo Ludens: A Study of the Play Element in Culture* (Boston: Beacon Press, 1950), passim.

3. B. O. Alpert, "Des preuves de sens ludique dans l'art du Pleistocene Supérieur," *L'Anthropologie* (Museé de l'Homme, Paris) 96 (1992): 219–44. The nineteenth-century psychologist Karl Groos associated animal play with art making. Such linkage has long been anathema to art historians, who felt that play associated with art lacked gravitas and trivialized the art. As a backlash, the linkage of art with play has until recently been considered frivolous. Play is now a subject of serious study. I am not reviving Groos's theories of play here but rather considering the fundamental human cognitive state called *ludic.* The English language lacks a word that might better distinguish it from *play,* and so I have translated the word as "playful."

4. F. Gilot, *Matisse and Picasso: A Friendship in Art* (New York: Doubleday, 1990), 151.

5. Quoted in H. B. Chipp, *Theories of Modern Art* (Berkeley: University of California Press, 1958), 189.

6. Escher, *Escher on Escher,* 21.

7. Quoted in N. J. Hadamard, *Psychology of Invention in the Mathematical Field* (Princeton, N. J. : Princeton University Press, 1945), 142.

8. R. P. Feynman, *Surely You're Joking, Mr. Feynman: Adventures of a Curious Character* (New York: Norton, 1984), 173–75.

9. Ibid.

10. J. A. Byers and M. Bekoff, *Animal Play* (Cambridge: Cambridge University Press, 1998), passim.

11. Fagen, *Animal Play Behavior,* 470.

12. Restak, in *The Brain,* 136, quotes P. MacLean (*The Triune Brain*), who found that after destruction of part of the limbic system, young mammals cease to play.

13. Spencer and Gillen, *Native Tribes of Central Australia,* 617. The term *play-work* applied only to art that was not on sacred sites.

14. Quoted in J. Morreal, "Humor and Emotion," *American Philosophic Quarterly* 20 (1983): 297–365, n. 15.

15. H. Bergson, *Le rire* (Baltimore, MD: John Hopkins University Press, 1986), 27.

16. A. Koestler, *The Act of Creation: A Study of the Conscious and Unconscious in Science and Art* (New York: Macmillan, 1967), 2.

17. Quoted in Chipp, *Theories of Modern Art,* 620.

18. Zeman, *Consciousness,* 181.

19. A. Damasio, *The Feeling of What Happens: Body and Emotion in the Making of Consciousness* (New York: Harcourt Brace, 1999), 321.

20. Zeman, *Consciousness,* 183.

21. A. Karmiloff-Smith, "Constraints on Representational Change: Evidence from Children's Drawing," *Cognition* 34 (1990): 57–83.

22. H. Matisse, quoted by journalist and artist Clara T. MacChesney in an interview for the *New York Times.* A quote was taken from this interview by J. D. Flam, ed., *Matisse on Art* (London: Phaidon, 1973), 51.

23. Escher, *Escher on Escher,* 11.

24. R. Motherwell, speech made to graduating class at the Rhode Island School of Design, 1980.

25. Quoted in Chipp, *Theories of Modern Art,* 5.

26. E. Anati, *Les origines de l'art et la formation de l'esprit humain* (Paris: Albin Michel, 1989), 176, passim.

27. M. Czikszentmihaly, *Flow* (New York: HarperCollins, 1991), passim.

28. Quoted in Goldwater and Treves, *Artists on Art,* 241; see also J. Stolnitz, *Corot in Italy* (Boston: MIT Press, 1960), 158.

29. J. I. Hubbard, *The Biological Basis of Mental Health* (Boston: Addison Wesley, 1975), 86–87, 167.

30. Self-awareness appears to be centered in the superior frontal gyrus. The mirror test provides the most objective proof of the existence of self-awareness. Research described in the October 30, 2006, issue of *Proceedings of the*

National Academy of Sciences shows that elephants can also pass such a test. According to the primatologist Franz de Waal and other scientists, indications of self-awareness seem also to exist in other forms in animals that do not pass the mirror test.

31. Restak, *Brainscapes,* 130.

32. Quoted in Goldwater and Treves, *Artists on Art,* 70.

33. Zeki, *Inner Vision,* 10.

34. R. Solso, "A Cognitive Neuroscience of Art," *Journal of Consciousness Studies* 7, no. 8–9 (2000): 123.

35. *Science News* 153, no. 8 (1998): 129.

36. Hobson, *Chemistry of Conscious States,* 28.

SUGGESTED READING

BOOKS ABOUT ICE AGE ART

Anati, Emmanuel . *Les origines de l'art et la formation de l'esprit humain*. Paris: Albin Michel, 1989.

Bahn, Paul and Vertut, Jean, *Journey through the Ice Age*. Berkeley: University of California Press, 1998.

Breuil, Henri, *Four Hundred Centuries of Cave Art*. New York: Hacker, 1979.

Delporte, Henri, *L'Image des Animaux Dans l'Art Préhistorique*. Paris: Picard, 1990

Hadingham, Evan, *Secrets of the Ice Age*. New York: Walker, 1979.

Leroi-Gourhan, André, *Treasures of Prehistoric Art*. New York: Abrams, 1966.

Lorblanchet, Michel. *La Naissance de l"Art: Genèse de l'Art Préhistorique*. Paris: France, 1999.

Marshack, Alexander, *The Roots of Civilization* (2nd ed.). New York: Moyer Bell 1991.

Pfeiffer, John E. , *The Creative Explosion: An Inquiry into the Origins of Art and Religion*. New York, Harper & Row, 1982.

Piette, Edouard, *l'Art Pendant l"Age du Renne*. Paris: Masson, 1907.

Sieveking, Ann, *The Cave Artist*. London: Thames & Hudson, 1979.

Ucko, Peter and Rosenfeld, Andrea, *Palaeolithic Cave Art*. New York: McGraw-Hill, 1967.

Vialou, Denis, *L'art des cavernes*. Paris: Le Rocher, 1987.

White, Randall, *Prehistoric Art: The Symbolic Journey of humankind*. New York, Abrams, 2003.

BOOKS ABOUT SPECIFIC AREAS OF ICE AGE ART

Aujoulat, Norbert, *Lascaux: Motion, Space and Time*. New York: Abrams, 2005.

Bégouën, Henri and Breuil, Henri, *Les Cavernes du Volp: Trois Frères- Tuc d'Audoubert*. Paris: Arts et Métiers Graphiques. 1958.

Chauvet, Jean Marie and Clottes, Jean et al. *La grotte Chauvet: l"Art des Origines*. Paris: Seuil, 2001.

Clottes.Jean and Courtin, Jean, *The Cave beneath the Sea: Paleolithic Images at Cosquer*. New York, Abrams. 1994.

Clottes, Jean, *Les Cavernes de Niaux: Art Préhistorique en Ariège*. Paris: Seuil, 1995.

Múzquiz-Pérez-Seoane, Matilde, *Altamira*. New York: Abrams, 1999.

Pales, Léon and Tasson de Saint-Pereuse, M., *Les Gravures de la Marche*. Mémoire no. 7 Vol. 1. Bordeaux: Institut de Préhistoire de l'Université de Bordeaux, 1969.

Piette, Edouard, *L'Art Pendant l'Age du Renne*. Paris: Masson, 1907.

Ruspoli, Mario,*The Cave of Lascaux: The Final Photographs*. New York: Abrams, 1986.

Sieveking, Ann, *Engraved Magdalenian Plaquettes*. BAR International Series 369, Oxford: Oxford University Press, 1987.

BOOKS ABOUT ART AND PERCEPTION

Arnheim, Rudolph, *Art and Visual Perception: A Psychology of the Creative Eye*. Berkeley: University of California Press, 1954.

Gombrich, Ernst Hans, *Art and Illusion*. London: Phaidon, 1960

R. L. Gregory, "How We Interpret Images," in *Images and Understanding*. Cambridge: Cambridge University Press, 1990.

Mithen, Steven. *The Prehistory of the Mind:The Cognitive Orignis of Art, Religion and Science.* New York, Thames & Hudson, 1996..

Ramachandran, Vilayanur S. *A Brief Tour of Human Consciousness: From Imposter Poodles to Purple Numbers.* New York: Pi Press, 2004

Ramachandran, Vilayanur S. and Blakeslee, Sandra, *Phantoms in the Brain: Probing the Mysteries of the Human Mind.* New York: William Morrow, 1998.

Rock, I, *An Introduction to Perception.* New York: Macmillan, 1975

Solso, Robert L. *The Psychology of Art and the Evolution of the Conscious Brain.* Cambridge, MA: MIT Press, 2003.

Zeman, Adam. *Consciousness: A User's Guide.* New Haven, CT: Yale University Press, 2002.

Zeki, Semir. *Inner Vision: An Exploration of Art and the Brain.* Oxford: Oxford University Press, 1999.

ILLUSTRATION CREDITS

Drawings by author unless otherwise noted.

1.1 Photograph by J. Vertut, courtesy Centre National de Préhistoire., Ministère de la Culture et de la Communication.

1.2 Drawing by H. Breuil, from A. del Rio, H. Breuil, and L. Sierra, *Les cavernes de la région cantabrique (Espagna)* (Monaco: A. Chéne, 1911), fig. 20.

1.3 Drawing after a photograph by J. Chauvet, in J. Clottes, *Dawn of Art: The Chauvet Cave* (New York: Abrams, 1996), fig. 8

1.4 Drawing after H. Breuil, *Four Hundred Centuries of Cave Art* (New York: Hacker, 1979), fig. 259.

1.5 Drawimg after a photograph by M. D. Davis.

1.6 The Metropolitan Museum of Art, purchase, Joseph Pulitzer Bequest, 1955 (55.21.1). Reproduced by permission of The Metropolitan Museum of Art, New York City.

1.7 Drawing by H. Breuil, reproduced from Breuil, *Four Hundred Centuries of Cave Art,* fig. 22.

1.8 Drawing by H. Breuil after a photograph by A. Lémozi, from Breuil, *Four Hundred Centuries of Cave Art,* fig. 307.

1.9 Drawing after a photograph by Chris Henshilwood.

1.10 Drawing after a photograph by J. Clottes, in J. Clottes, *Cavernes de Niaux* (Paris: Abrams, 1997), fig. 173.

1.11 Drawing after a tracing by E. H. Pacheco, 1919, in the collection of the Museo Nacional de Ciencias Naturales, Madrid.

1.12 Drawing after G. M. Mallery, *Picture-Writing of the American Indians,* vol. 1 (New York: Dover, 1972), fig. 523.

1.13 Drawing by H. Breuil from a photograph by M. E. Boyle, reproduced from Breuil, *Four Hundred Centuries of Cave Art,* fig. 339.

1.14 Drawing by H. Breuil, *Four Hundred Centuries of Cave Art,* figs. 374 and 375.

1.15 Drawing after a 1918 tracing by H. Obermaier and Conde de la Vega del Sella, in the collection of the Museo Nacional de Ciencias Naturales, Madrid.

1.16 Tracing by H. Breuil from H. Bégoüen, *Les cavernes du Volp* (Paris: Arts et Métiers Graphiques, 1958), figs. 65 and 136.

1.17 Drawing after a tracing by L. Pales, who simplified and interpreted the intricately tangled lines of the plaque, in L. Pales and Tasson de Saint-Pereuse, *Les gravures de la Marche,* vol. 1 (Bordeaux: Institut de Préhistoire de l'Université de Bordeaux, 1969).

1.18 Drawing inspired by a figure devised by the psychologist J. M. Kennedy,

1.19 Tracing by H. Breuil from del Rio, Breuil, and Sierra, *Les cavernes de la région cantabrique,* fig. 10.

2.1 Photograph by M. Bégouën, reproduced from del Rio, Breuil, and Sierra, *Les cavernes de la région cantabrique.*

2.2 Drawing after photograph and artifact in the collection of the University Museum of Archaeology and Ethnology, Cambridge, England.

2.3 Drawing after a photograph by A. Turk. The tool is in the Musée National de Préhistoire, Les Eyzies.

2.4 Drawing by H. Breuil, from G. H. Luquet, *The Art and Religion of Fossil Man* (New Haven, CT: Yale University Press, 1930), fig. 43.

2.5 Drawing after a photograph in G. Bosinski, *Der Löwenmensch: Tier und Mensch in der Kunst der Eiszeit* (Sigmaringen: J. Thorbecke, 1994). Object is in the Museum für Archäologie des Eiszeit, Neuwied, Germany.

2.6 Drawing after a photograph by M. Ruspoli in his book *The Cave of Lascaux: The Final Photographs* (New York: Abrams, 1987), 59.

2.7 Tracing by H. Breuil, from del Rio, Breuil, and Sierra, *Les cavernes de la région cantabrique,* fig. 154.

2.8 Drawing from a photograph by B. D. Alpert.

2.9 Photograph by L. Yost..

2.10 Drawing by G. M. Mallery, reproduced from Mallery, *Picture-Writing of the American Indians,* vol. 2 (New York: Dover, 1972), fig. 1177.

2.11 Drawing after a drawing by E. Piette, in E. Piette, *L'art pendant l'age du renne.* (Paris: Masson, 1907). Piece is now in St. Germain-en-Laye.

2.12 Drawing after a photograph and sketch by J. Gaussen, in J. Gaussen, *La grotte ornée de Gabillou* (Bordeaux: l'Institut de Préhistoire de l'Université de Bordeaux, 1964), pl. 11.

2.13 Drawing by H. Breuil, reproduced from del Rio, Breuil, and Sierra, *Les cavernes de la région cantabrique,* fig. 154.

2.14 Drawing from a reproduction in M. Gimbutas, *The Goddesses and Gods of Old Europe* (Berkeley: University of California Press, 1974), fig. 90.

2.15 Drawing after Mallery, *Picture-Writing of the American Indians,* vol. 1, fig. 135.

2.16 Photograph by J. Kerr, reproduced by permission of the Maxwell Museum of Anthropology, University of New Mexico, Albuquerque.

2.17 Drawing after photograph by B. D. Alpert.

2.18 Photograph by the author.

2.19 Photograph by Ekkehart Malotki from *Stone Chisel and Yucca Brush: Colorado Plateau Rock Art*, Kiva Publishing, Walnut CA., 2002

2.20 © British Museum. Reproduced with permission.

2.21 Drawing after tracings by H. Breuil and A. Glory.

2.22 Drawing on site.

3.1 Photograph by J. Vertut

3.2 Photograph courtesy of R. White.

3.3 Drawing of head of the Commarque horse made by author on site.

3.4 Drawing by E. Piette from Piette, *L'art pendant l'age du renne*

3.5 Drawing after a photograph by F. Windels, in Breuil, *Four Hundred Centuries of Cave Art,* fig. 304.

3.6 Drawings after Leroi-Gourhan

3.7 Drawing after Chart 30 in A. Leroi-Gourhan, *Treasures of Prehistoric Art* (New York: Abrams, 1987), 512

3.8 Image © The Metropolitan Museum of Art, New York City, NY.

3.9 Photo by P.A. Saura Ramos. Museo de Altamira, Spain.

3.10 Author's sketches made on site.

3.11 Drawing after H. Breuil

3.12 Photograph courtesy of J. Clottes.

3.13 Photograph by the author.

3.14 Photograph by B. D. Alpert.

4.1 Drawing by A. Glory from A. Leroi-Gourhan and J. Alain, eds., *Lascaux inconnu* (Paris: Editions du Centre National de la Recherche Scientifique, 1979), pl. 27.

4.2 Drawing after a tracing by H. Breuil and R. de St. Périer from A. Marshack, *The Roots of Civilization* (New York: McGraw-Hill, 1972), fig. 60.

4.3 Drawing after a photograph by A. Frolov, in E. Anati, *Origini dell'arte e della concettualità* (Milan: Jaca, 1989), 174.

4.4 Drawing permission of Dennis Slifer.

4.5 Drawing after a photograph by A. Marshack, in Marshack, *Roots of Civilization,* fig. 200.

4.6 Drawing after a photograph by W. Duff, in R. L. Carlson, ed., *Indian Art Traditions of the Northwest Coast* (Seattle: University of Washington Press, 1983), 55.

Piece in the collection of the Museum of the American Indian, Smithsonian Institution.

4.7 Drawing after image in M. Gimbutas, *The Language of the Goddess* (New York: HarperCollins, 1991), fig. 46.

4.8. After a photograph by H. Delporte, in H. Delporte, *L'image de la femme dans l'art préhistorique* (Paris: Picard, 1979).

4.9 Drawing after photo by A. Marshack reproduced in Gimbutas, *Language of the Goddess,* fig. 357.

4.10 Drawing from A. M. Sackler Collection, Freer Gallery, Washington, D.C.

4.11 Other, less well preserved female figures and one male figure form part of the frieze, now in the Musée d'Aquitaine, Bordeaux, France. Photo Erich Lessing./Art Resource, New York.

4.12 Photograph by B. D. Alpert.

4.13 Drawing after photograph by D. Slifer.

4.14. Drawing after a photograph by E. Hadingham, in E. Hadingham, *Secrets of the Ice Age: The World of the Cave* Artists.

4.15 Drawing after a photograph by B. D. Alpert.

4.16 Photograph by S. A. LeBlanc by permission of S. A. LeBlanc and the owner of the vessel.

4.17 Photograph by C. Emmer / Art Resource, New York.

4.18 Drawing after an image in A. I. Martynov, *The Ancient Art of Northern Asia* (Chicago: University of Chicago Press, 1991), fig. 143.

4.19 Drawing after a photograph in the collection of the Hermitage Museum, St. Petersburg, Russia.

4.20 Drawing by H. Breuil from *Four Hundred Centuries of Cave Art,* figs. 188 and 189.

4.21 Drawing after a photograph by B. D. Alpert.

4.22 Drawing after a photograph in the collection of the Peabody Museum of Archaeology and Ethnology, Harvard University.

4.23 Drawing after a photograph by B. D. Alpert.

4.24 Drawings after H. Breuil, A. Leroi-Gourhan and L. Pales.

4.25 Drawings (a) by Bernini, (b) based on petroglyph at Marsoulas and (c) based on petroglyph at Labastide.

4.26 Drawing based on photograph from Associated Press.

4.27 Drawings after a photograph in C. Grant, *Rock Art of the American Indian* (New York: Crowell, 1967) 131.

4.28 Drawing after sketch in Sargent's Sketchbook no. 2, p. 1, 1869 collection of the Fogg Art, Museum, Harvard University

4.29 Drawing by G. M. Mallery, *Picture-Writing of the American Indians,* vol. 2, fig. 713.

4.30 Photograph by P.A. Saura Ramos © Museo de Altamira.

4.31 Drawing after artifact in the museum at Mas d'Azil.

4.32 Drawing made on site at exhibition of Northwest Coast art.

4.33 Courtesy of the Instituto Nacional de Antropologia e Historia, Mexico City.

4.34 Photograph by B. D. Alpert by permission of J. Minter.

4.35 Drawing after a photograph available on the Internet.

4.36 Photographs by Holly Hughes. Reproduced by permission of the Capitol Art Collection, State Capitol building, Santa Fe, New Mexico.

5.1 Drawing after photographs and drawings by S. Giedion, in, *The Eternal Present: The Beginnings of Art* (New York: Pantheon, 1962), 520, 521. Artifact in museum at Les Eyzies.

5.2 Drawing after the figure devised by E. Rubin.

5.3 Photograph by S. A. LeBlanc, with permission of LeBlanc and the owner of the pot.

5.4 Drawing made at site.

5.5 Drawing from pot in the collection of the School for Advanced Research, Santa Fe, NM.

Photograph by S. A. LeBlanc, by permission of LeBlanc and the owner of the vessel, Thomas W. Weisel.

5.7 Reproduced from R. H. Mathews, *The Aboriginal Rock Pictures of Australia* (Brisbane: Transactions and Proceedings of the Royal Geological Society of Australasia, 10, 1895), 67–70.

5.8. Drawing after a section of the Picasso etching 347 series, no. 8, 1968.

Drawing after a section of Maurits Escher's work *Study of Regular Division of the Plane with Birds,*1938 from J. L. Locher, ed., *The World of M. C. Escher* (New York, Abrams, 1988), fig. 101.

5.10. Reversible images in *Slave Market with The Disappearing Bust of Voltaire.* ©2008 Salvador Dali / Artists Right Society (ARS) N.Y.

5.11 Drawing of section of Animal *Magnetism* by permission of William Steig.

5.12 Linoprint in collection of the author.

5.13 Figure devised by the Swiss crystallographer L. A. Necker in 1832 to demonstrate multistable perception.

5.14 Photograph by P.A. Saura Ramos © Museo de Altamira

5.15 Drawing made at the site.

5.16 Drawing after a photograph by J. Clottes.

5.17 Drawing after a photograph by A. Solomon.

5.18 Photo Credit: Erich Lessing/Art Resource, NY.

5.19 Photograph © 2005 The M. C. Escher Company–Holland. All rights reserved. Original in the Rosenwald Collection of the National Gallery.

5.20 Drawing after a tracing by L. Pales, based on his interpretation of the intricately tangled lines, in Pales and Saint-Pereuse, *Les gravures de la Marche.*

5.21 Drawing by H. Breuil, reproduced from H.Bégouën, *Les cavernes du Volp,* figs. 110 and 111.

5.22 Drawing after a photograph in Breuil, *Four Hundred Centuries of Cave Art,* fig. 52.

5.23 Drawing after a photograph by M. Pillot.

5.24 Drawing after a photograph by P. Lieberman.

5.25 Drawing on site.

5.26 Drawing after study for the above mentioned painting. formerly in the collection of A. F. Petit Gallery, Paris.

5.27 Drawing after a tracing by Breuil, *Four Hundred Centuries of Cave Art.*

figs. 283–85.

5.28 Drawing on site.

5.29 Drawing after a image in Leroi-Gourhan and Alain, *Lascaux inconnu,* fig. 316.

5.30 Reproduced by permission of the Maxwell Museum of Anthropology, University of New Mexico, Albuquerque.

5.31 Duck-rabbit from *Fliegende Blätter,* October 23, 1892, 147.

5.32 Courtesy of Frederick Schultz, Daedalus Gallery, New York, and the owner J. R. Myers.

5.33 Burke Museum of Natural History and Culture, catalogue no. 1.2E634. Photograph by Barry McWayne, courtesy of the Anchorage Museum of History and Art.

5.34 Collection of the Menil Foundation, Houston, Texas. Photograph by Hickey and Robertson, reproduced by permission of E. Carpenter.

5.35 Photo Credit: Erich Lessing/Art Resource, NY

5.36 Drawing of section of painting in the private collection of a bank in Basel, Switzerland.

5.37 Drawing after original, in the collection of the Victoria and Albert Museum.

5.38 Drawing after original in the collection of the Metropolitan Museum of Art, New York City, NY.

5.39 Reproduced by permission of the *Atlanta Journal* and the *Atlanta Constitution.*

5.40 The Museum of Modern Art, New York, Mrs. Simon Guggenheim Fund. Reproduced by permission of The Museum of Modern Art, New York.

5.41 Reproduced by permission of *New Yorker* magazine.

5.42 Courtesy of the Clifford Odets Estates, collection of H. K. Harrisburg and Michael Rosenfeld Gallery, New York.

5.43 Reproduced by permission of Nicholas McCarthy.

5.44 Reprise of illustration 5.20

5.45 René Magritte, The Rape © 2008 Salvador Dali foundation/Artists Right Society (ARS) New York.

5.46 Reproduced by permission of the Statens Konstmuseer, Nationmuseum/ Moderna Museet, Sweden.

6.1 Photograph by F. Windels, from Breuil, *Four Hundred Centuries of Cave Art,* fig. 114.

6.2 Drawing by H. Breuil, from H. Breuil and E. Cartailhac, *La caverne d'Altamira à Santillane près Santander* (Monaco: A. Chéne, 1912).

6.3 Drawn at site.

6.4 Drawing after Martynov, *Ancient Art of Northern Asia,* fig. 38.

6.5 Reproduced from T. Özgüç, *Les Hittites* (Ankara: Museum of Anatolian Civilization, undated), 53.

6.6 Photograph by S. Mancini.

6.7 Photograph by S. Mancini.

6.8 Drawing by G. M. Mallery from *Picture-Writing of the American Indians*, vol. 1, fig. 135.

6.9 Drawing by H. Breuil from Bégouën, *Les cavernes du Volp*, pl. 20.

6.10 Drawing by H. Breuil from Bégouën, *Les cavernes du Volp*, fig. 58.

6.11 Drawing by H. Breuil from Bégouën, *Les cavernes du Volp*, fig. 63.

6.12 Drawing after E. Piette's tracing from *L'art pendant l'age du renne*, 34.

6.13 Photograph by T. Stephan. Collection of the Ulmer Museum, Germany.

6.14 Drawing after figure.Collection of Anadolou Medeniyetleri Müzesi (Museum of Anatolian Civilizations), Ankara, Turkey.

6.15 Drawing after photo by D.Bakker, *Ancient Art of the American Woodland Indian*, Plate 76.

6.16 Drawing after photograph by J. Zintgraff.

6.17 © D. Lee

6.18 Drawing after a tracing by E. Piette from, *L'art pendant l'age du renne*, 72.

6.19 Drawing by H. Breuil from Bégouën, *Les cavernes du Volp*, pl. 9.

6.20 Drawing after photograph by F. Staud.

6.21 Photograph by B. D. Alpert.

6.22 Drawing after photograph by B. D. Alpert.

6.23 Drawing after photograph by J. Vertut of bas reliefs at Musée D'Aquitaine, Bordeaux, France.

6.24 Photo credit: Scala/Art Resource, N.Y.

6.25 Drawing after photo by Delvert

6.26 Drawing after tracing by E. Piette in *L'art pendant l'age du renne*.

6.27 Drawing after rendition in A. Marshack, *Roots of Civilization*, fig. 135D.

6.28 Drawing after M. Gimbutas, *Language of the Goddess*, fig. 253.

6.29 Drawing after photo courtesy E. Carpenter

6.30 Photograph by the author.

6.31 Drawing after photograph by D. Slifer.

6.32. Photograph courtesy of Taylor A. Dale Antiquities.

6.33 Drawing after a tracing of petroglyph by D. Vialou.

6.34 Drawing after a reproduction in E. Kedourie, ed., *The Jewish World, Revelation, Prophecy and History* (London: Thames and Hudson, 1975), 33.

6.35 Drawing after section of Chagall's *Homage to Gogol.*

6.36 Published as an example of what Dali called "paranoia" in the periodical *Surrealisme au service de la révolution* in 1931.

6.37 Reissued from an edition of 1894 (New York: Dover, 1964), 47.

6.38 Photo J. Chauvet ©Courtesy of J. Clottes

6.39 Photo J. Vertut, courtesy Centre National de Préhistoire..

6.40 Drawing after Leroi-Gourhan, *Treasures of Prehistoric Art,* fig. 201.

6.41 Drawing based on tracing by L. Pales, in *Les gravures de la Marche,* vol. 11, *Les humains,* (Paris: Editions Ophyrs, 1976), observations 155–62.

6.42 Drawing after a photograph by M. Bégouën from Ruspoli, *Lascaux: The Final Photographs,* 63.

6.43 Drawing after a photograph by J. Chauvet, in Clottes, *Dawn of Art,* fig. 86.

6.44 Photo Loic Hamon. Detail of Lortet antler © MAN de Saint-Germain-en-Laye

6.45 Drawing from two different positions at the site.

6.46 Drawing after H. Breuil, *Four Hundred Centuries of Cave Art* , 54.

6.47 Photograph courtesy D. Slifer.

6.48 Drawing by H. Breuil from del Rio, Breuil, and Sierra, *Les cavernes de la région cantabrique,* fig. 208.

6.49 Photograph courtesy of B. Draper.

6.50 Drawing by H. Breuil, from Bégouën, *Les cavernes du Volp,* fig. 75.

6.51 Photograph by Yan, courtesy CNP-MCC.

6.52 Drawing after photograph by author.

6.53 Drawing of section of a sketch from Picasso's notebook of 1946.

7.1 Drawing from piece in collection of the Musée du Mas d'Azil.

7.2 Drawing of Lortet antler by E. Piette from *L'art pendant l'age du renne.*

7.3 Roll out of the Lortet antler. Photo Loic Hamon © MAN de Saint-Germain-en-Laye.

7.4 Detail of 7.3.

INDEX

(Sites listed only by department are in France)

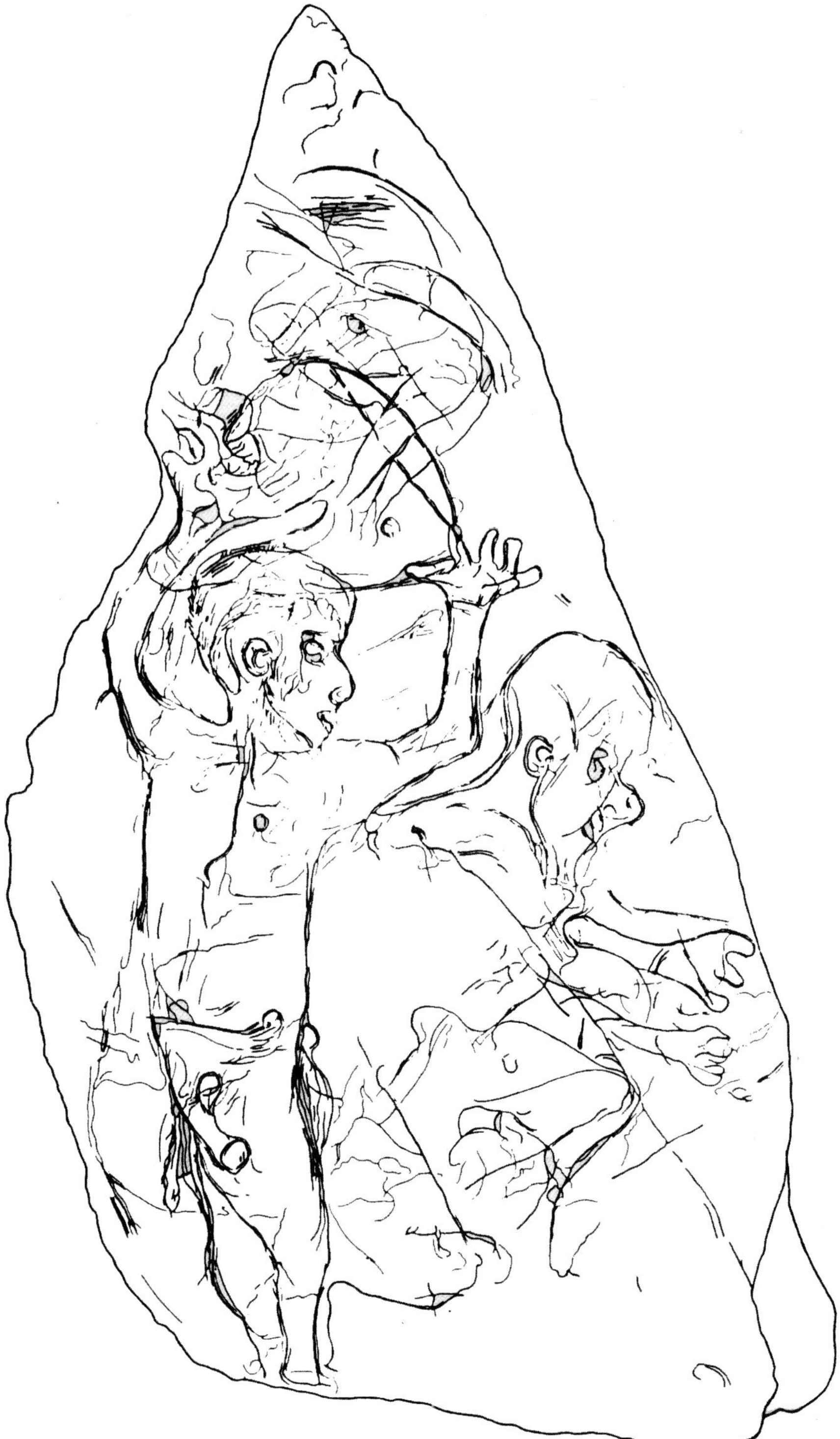

L. Pales.